D1591639

MRI OF THE SHOULDER

Second Edition

MRI OF THE SHOULDER

Second Edition

Michael B. Zlatkin, MD, FRCP (C)

National Musculoskeletal Imaging
Sunrise, Florida

Voluntary Professor of Radiology
University of Miami School of Medicine
Miami, Florida

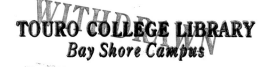
LIPPINCOTT WILLIAMS & WILKINS
A **Wolters Kluwer** Company
Philadelphia • Baltimore • New York • London
Buenos Aires • Hong Kong • Sydney • Tokyo

Acquisitions Editor: Beth Barry
Developmental Editor: Delois Patterson
Supervising Editor: Mary Ann McLaughlin
Manufacturing Manager: Ben Rivera
Cover Designer: Kevin Kall
Compositor: Michael Bass & Associates
Printer: Walsworth Publishing

© 2003 by LIPPINCOTT WILLIAMS & WILKINS
530 Walnut Street
Philadelphia, PA 19106 USA
LWW.com

Printed in the USA

Library of Congress Cataloging-in-Publication Data
  Zlatkin, Michael B.
    MRI of the shoulder / Michael B. Zlatkin.—2nd ed.
      p. ; cm.
    Includes bibliographical references and index.
    ISBN 0-7817-1590-3
    1. Shoulder—Magnetic resonance imaging. I. Title.
    [DNLM: 1. Shoulder—injuries. 2. Magnetic Resonance Imaging. 3. Shoulder—
  radiography. WE 810 Z82m 2002]
  RC939.Z53 2002
  617.5'7207548—dc21

                                                              2002030193
                                                              CIP

                                              10 9 8 7 6 5 4 3 2 1

*For my special and beautiful wife, Marilyn, and
my wonderful children, Nancy, Robert, Alyssa and Chad.
They supported me throughout the writing of this book
and waited patiently while I worked.*

*To my cherished mother, Gert.
Through thick and thin, always behind me.*

*The second edition of this book is dedicated to the memory of my late father, Rafael
(Ralph) Zlatkin. My beloved father died unexpectedly during the course of my working
on this book. He was a man who was born into very harsh conditions in a small
town in rural Poland. At the young age of sixteen, he was separated from his family
and taken to Hitler's concentration camps, including the infamous Auschwitz. He
survived, miraculously, and came to North America to start a new life. He was a
man with little formal education, but he was one of the most knowledgeable men I
have known in my life. He loved learning, and had the most inquisitive mind. He
taught me the value of education and through his efforts gave me the opportunity to
pursue my medical studies, without financial burden. He taught me the value of
hard work, dedication to one's craft, and persistence towards the completion of a
task. Through his example he also taught me the value of honesty and integrity.
I have been fortunate in my career to have many excellent teachers and mentors,
some of whom are the best in our craft, and for that I am grateful. But my father
was my best and most enduring teacher and mentor in life, and I miss him and
will continue to miss him greatly, every day.*

CONTENTS

CONTRIBUTING AUTHORS

Javier Beltran, MD   Professor of Clinical Radiology, Department of Radiology, Maimonides Medical Center, New York University School of Medicine, Brooklyn, New York

Jenny Bencardino, MD   Department of Radiology, Long Island Jewish Medical Center, Albert Einstein College of Medicine, New Hyde Park, New York

Michael A. Blake, MRCPI, BSC(Hons), FFR(RCSI), FRCR   Instructor in Radiology, Department of Radiology, Division of Abdominal Imaging and Intervention, Massachusetts General Hospital, Boston, Massachusetts

Brian D. Cameron, MD   Stevens Orthopedic Group, Edmonds, Washington

Robert Edelman, MD   Professor of Radiology, Director of Magnetic Resonance Imaging, Department of Radiology, Beth Israel Deaconess Medical Center, Boston, Massachusetts

Mary G. Hochman, MD   Chief of Musculoskeletal Radiology, Instructor of Radiology, Department of Radiology, Beth Israel Deaconess Medical Center, Boston, Massachusetts

Cary J. Hoffman, MD   National Musculoskeletal Imaging, Sunrise, Florida

Joseph P. Iannotti, MD, PhD   Chairman, Department of Orthopedic Surgery, The Cleveland Clinic Foundation, Cleveland, Ohio

Scott A. Mirowitz, MD   Associate Professor of Radiology, Chief of Radiology, Barnes-Jewish Hospital North, Co-Director of Body MRI, Mallinckrodt Institute of Radiology, Washington University School of Medicine, St. Louis, Missouri

David A. Molyneaux, DE   Vice President, MRI Devices Corporation, Gainesville, Florida

Steven Needell, MD   Boca Raton Community Radiology Group (BCRG), Boca Raton, Florida

William E. Palmer, MD   Director Musculoskeletal Imaging, Department of Radiology, Massachusetts General Hospital, Harvard Medical School, Boston, Massachusetts

Thomas E. Schubert, BS Engineering Mechanics   President/CEO, MRI Devices Corporation, Waukesha, Wisconsin

Marianne Shih, MD   Washington University School of Medicine, St. Louis, Missouri

Michael B. Zlatkin, MD, FRCP (C)   National Musculoskeletal Imaging, Sunrise, Florida; Voluntary Professor of Radiology, University of Miami School of Medicine, Miami, Florida

PREFACE

Much has changed in medicine, radiology and MR imaging since the publication of the first edition of this text. Specifically with regard to MRI of the shoulder, this imaging procedure is now without question the most important and widely utilized diagnostic study in evaluating patients with painful shoulders. Over this period of more than ten years, there has been a plethora of new information on the clinical, pathophysiologic, and imaging aspects of derangements of this joint. Whereas in the first edition it was my task to gather the work of myself, my colleagues, and a few others into what was considered then a comprehensive review of knowledge, in this edition the task of gathering all the relevant information for inclusion in the text was far more daunting. It is impossible in light of this to be all inclusive.

Another factor that made my job of compiling this second edition very difficult is the changed circumstance facing many of us in medicine today. Whereas we are blessed with so much new information and much easier access to such through the Internet, the time available in both academic and especially, as in my case, in clinical practice to carry out these endeavors is increasingly limited. Thus the work to complete this text took far longer and was much more challenging than I had anticipated when I agreed to revise it.

The second edition of this text bears little resemblance to the first as it had to be largely rewritten to keep pace with all of the changes. The basic outline of the text, its goals and its intended audience, however, remain similar. There are chapters devoted to the basics of MR imaging, which I hope the reader (whether new to MRI or well versed in the topic) will find useful as a general introduction and review, compiled by my good friend and colleague Robert Edelman and his associates. We have added a chapter on techniques and pitfalls in shoulder MRI, compiled by Scott Mirowitz, who is a recognized authority in this area of musculoskeletal MRI. MR imaging of joints is also dependent on having the appropriate local coils, and Tom Schubert and his colleagues at MRI Devices Corporation. have compiled a useful chapter on the principles of local coils and how they apply specifically to the small joints. Although the topic of MRI arthrography is dealt with in the context of the other chapters in the text, I have greatly admired the work that Bill Palmer has done in this important area. His chapter on this topic helps to summarize many of the key concepts—at times with a different perspective than I have provided—but I am sure the reader will benefit from the sometimes differing points of view.

My collaboration with Joe Iannotti during my years at the University of Pennsylvania was the foundation of the concepts in the first edition of this book. Although we have gone along separate paths over the ensuing years, I was fortunate to have him and his colleagues update the clinical chapter in this text to provide the orthopaedic surgeon's perspective on the evaluation of the patient with shoulder pain and the usefulness of MRI in this endeavor.

The remaining chapters deal with the important topics of anatomy, rotator cuff disease and shoulder instability. In the anatomy chapter I was aided by my partner Cary Hoffman, who helped bring a fresh perspective to some of the basic concepts of general shoulder anatomy as well as that seen with MRI. We also spent considerable time and effort describing and illustrating the variational anatomy that is so important in understanding shoulder MR imaging. The excellent illustrations done by Salvador Beltran should be of significant benefit in that regard. My former fellow Steven Needell, with his meticulous labeling of images, provided a comprehensive atlas of both conventional and MRI arthrographic anatomy. The chapters on rotator cuff disease and shoulder instability should help put into perspective many of the newer concepts we have learned through close collaboration with our orthopaedic colleagues. These chapters should aid us in translating the MRI appearance of many of the processes that our colleagues have come to understand through their increasing skill and continued study with the shoulder arthroscope. There is a separate chapter in the current text on the difficult topic of the postoperative shoulder, which we have gained increased experience in managing over the last number of years. Finally, Doctors Javier Beltran and Jenny Bencardino had the difficult task of reviewing the multitude of other processes that affect the shoulder, including biceps tendon disorders, and their wide array of material in these areas should help to elucidate these diverse topics.

We have come a long way in our understanding of MR imaging of the shoulder since the publication of the first edition of this text. Nonetheless there is still much that we don't understand, much that we are not clever enough yet to discern, and some that we will see only with further improvements in technique and technology, and with continued sharing of information and expertise with our orthopaedic colleagues. I hope that this text will provide the background and knowledge for many to continue in this challenging area of orthopaedic MRI.

Michael B. Zlatkin, M.D., F.R.C.P. (C)

PREFACE TO THE FIRST EDITION

The work leading up to this book really began in 1986. As an orthopedic radiology fellow at the University of California, San Diego, I chose a research project, the goal of which was to try to better understand the cross-sectional anatomy of the shoulder capsular mechanism, as it appeared on computerized tomography (CT) arthrography. It was during the early stages of this project that I began to realize the complex, yet fascinating nature of this joint. In Southern California at that time magnetic resonance imaging (MRI) of the knee was beginning to have a strong impact on diagnoses, and I thought this new technique could be applied to the shoulder. We began by imaging cadaver specimens. These were quite successful, and some of the images done at that time are included in this book. But cadaver shoulder specimens can be placed anywhere and in any position in the magnet and they do not move, unlike six-feet-tall football players. When we added software to our General Electric machine to allow off-center and oblique imaging, we found ourselves imaging the neck instead of the shoulder. I was fortunate to meet Murray Reicher from Mercy Hospital who had many of these problems solved on his Technicare scanner. As is his gift, he had already convinced half the orthopedic surgeons in San Diego County of the tremendous potential of this technique. While working with him and Leland Kellerhouse we began to understand the appearance of both the normal and injured shoulder. Which this experience in hand I began a close association at the University of Pennsylvania with Joseph Iannotti. The results of my collaboration with him are the foundation of the concepts expressed in this book.

After an initial slow start, MR of the shoulder has become, in many centers, the second most common joint imaged in the musculoskeletal system. It potentially has even greater clinical benefit because, as opposed to the knee where arthroscopy is well understood and widely applied, shoulder arthroscopy is still in its early stages. Shoulder MR is the procedure of choice for imaging the rotator cuff and has nearly completely replaced arthrography for this application. It is extremely useful in imaging patients with shoulder instability, and in many institutions has replaced CT arthrography for this clinical problem. Other areas of application include imaging of biceps tendon disorders, avascular necro-

sis, synovial processes, other posttraumatic disorders, and the staging and evaluation of musculoskeletal neoplasms.

This book translates and summarizes what is currently known about MR of the shoulder, from my own work and experience and from that of others. It emphasizes the areas of greatest clinical application—imaging of rotator cuff disease and shoulder instability—but also includes discussions of many of the other disease processes that make up the spectrum of shoulder joint pathology. It is an effort to make more comprehensible what has so far been a difficult area for radiologists, orthopedic surgeons, and others charged with interpreting the images of this joint. My intent is not only to illustrate and describe the MR patterns, but also to try to understand and explain the anatomy and pathophysiology of the relevant disease states. In Chapter 2 the normal and variational general and MR anatomy of the shoulder is reviewed. Chapters 4, 5, and 6 contain comprehensive discussions of the relevant pathophysiology prior to describing the spectrum of MR imaging findings in detail. It is also necessary for the radiologist and clinician to have some understanding of the basic principles of MR in a global sense, as well as grasping how they apply to imaging of this joint. Chapter 1 provides these details in a simple and clear manner. I believe that the depth of this discussion is not too complex for the beginner, nor too elementary for the sophisticated reader. It is also important for the radiologist to have a knowledge of the clinical presentations and decision-making processes involved in dealing with the patient with shoulder pain. Chapter 3 deals with these problems. It provides a clear explanation of these principles for the imager and is a useful review for the clinician.

I have attempted to be comprehensive in the illustrations of both the anatomy and pathology. Too often one hears the complaint when lecturing or presenting scientific papers that the best and most obvious images are shown and the difficult cases are what is left to deal with in practice. Although it is not possible to present all the variations, I have tried to illustrate the widest spectrum of cases possible within the confines of what I had available and what could be reasonably included in a book of this size.

There is still much that we do not understand about MRI of the shoulder including many of the technical aspects, as well as a complete understanding of the normal and pathologic appearances. This is, nonetheless, an area of MRI with great potential. The information is there for us to behold, we only have to be bright enough to find it and comprehend it. It is only through careful study of the anatomy and pathology of this joint, combined with our knowledge of the principles of MR imaging, that we will be able to make sense of what we see in the display on our scanners and the images that result.

Michael B. Zlatkin, M.D.

ACKNOWLEDGEMENTS

A work of this nature is not possible without the aid of many individuals. I am always grateful to the many technologists I have worked with over the years who have continued to provide me with images of excellent quality despite the increasing demands on all of us to go faster and increase our imaging throughput. I have been fortunate in my career to have earned the support and trust of many orthopaedic surgeons, who continue to provide me with a vast array of clinical material to include in the illustrations in this text, and continue to teach me important clinical concepts.

I am very grateful to my medical photographer, Joey Accordino for his excellent work and his dedication to his craft. He took images from all sources including old slides, cut film, digital formats and translated them into a standard format of high quality and resolution that kept me from worrying about this aspect of the book's production. Salvador Beltran MD is responsible for the high quality of the majority of the new illustrations in this text.

I am also thankful for the patience and support shown to me by my publisher. I made many promises and missed too many deadlines, but they stuck with me through it all, and never had a harsh word, or put undue pressure on me, and allowed me to work at my own pace. In particular I would like to single out Beth Barry in that regard, who was constantly and consistently there to support and encourage me throughout this long and sometimes arduous process.

BASIC PRINCIPLES OF MRI INCLUDING FAST IMAGING

MICHAEL A. BLAKE
MARY G. HOCHMAN
ROBERT EDELMAN

Magnetic resonance imaging (MRI) is a powerful technique for the diagnosis of shoulder pathology. Understanding the principles of MRI is critical in optimally exploiting its unique ability to provide multiplanar, high tissue contrast, high-resolution imaging. Interpretation relies on a combination of sound anatomical and pathological knowledge and an appreciation of the factors determining signal appearance (1–7).

All sequences, both conventional and advanced, are based on the same underlying principles. This chapter seeks to describe these fundamental principles on which effective, high-quality MR shoulder imaging depends. We have attempted to highlight specific ways in which understanding of MR essentials can be applied to be helpful in daily clinical practice.

OVERVIEW OF THE MRI PROCESS

The production of an MRI image may be summarized as follows: First, randomly oriented tissue nuclei are aligned by a magnetic field producing a longitudinal magnetization. Next, radiofrequency pulses tilt all or a portion of the equilibrium magnetization into the transverse plane, and as the nuclei relax (recover equilibrium), radiofrequency signals are generated and can be measured (read out) at selected times. Different tissue nuclei recover at different rates based on T1 and T2 (or T2*) relaxation times, thereby producing tissue contrast (Table 1.1).

Finally, spatial encoding of the nuclei is allowed by altering the magnetic field in an orderly pattern (field gradients).

PRODUCING A MAGNETIC RESONANCE SIGNAL

Most clinical MR imaging is based on proton behavior, although techniques for imaging of sodium and other nuclei

also exist. The human body is composed predominantly of water (approximately 70%) with a total nearing 5×10^{27} hydrogen nuclei. The hydrogen nucleus consists of a single proton and by virtue of its spinning charge can be considered analogous to a tiny bar magnet with a magnetic moment (Fig. 1.1). In the absence of an external magnetic field, these

TABLE 1.1 APPEARANCES OF TISSUES ON MR IMAGES

Tissue	T1-weighted Image	T2-weighted Image
Fat[a]	Very bright	Intermediate to dark
Cysts		
Water	Very dark	Very bright
Proteinaceous	Intermediate to bright	Very bright
Bone marrow		
Yellow[a]	Very bright	Intermediate to dark
Red[b]	Intermediate	Dark
Cortical bone	Very dark	Very dark
Cartilage		
Fibrocartilage	Very dark	Very dark
Hyaline[c]	Intermediate	Intermediate
Osteophyte		
Marrow	Bright	Intermediate to dark
Calcified	Dark	Dark
Tendons	Dark	Dark
Ligaments	Dark	Dark
Muscle	Dark	Dark
Gadolinium enhancement		
Low concentration	Very bright	Bright
High concentration	Intermediate to dark	Very dark

[a]Bright on fast spin echo T2-weighted images.
[b]Dark on out-of-phase image.
[c]Bright on proton density–weighted image.

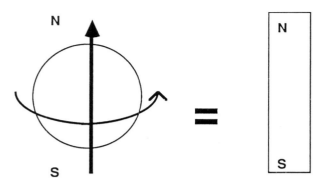

FIGURE 1.1. The spinning nucleus behaves magnetically as if it were a tiny bar magnet with the orientation of the magnet along the axis of the nucleus.

tiny magnetic moments are distributed randomly. When subjected to an external field, they tend to align either parallel (lower energy level) or antiparallel (higher energy level) to the applied field direction. The thermal energy of the system determines the relative concentrations; at room temperature, there are nearly equal populations. Of every million nuclei placed in a 1.5 Tesla magnetic field, at 25°C, only approximately five will be preferentially aligned with the magnetic field. The remaining protons effectively cancel out, leaving a small net magnetization vector (with magnitude and direction) usually referred to as M (Fig. 1.2).

M may be considered to have two components: longitudinal magnetization parallel to the Bo field and transverse magnetization perpendicular to this axis (Fig. 1.3). M is stable in a constant magnetic field (Bo) and is called the *equilibrium longitudinal magnetization*. It can be disturbed by applying a second magnetic field, B1, produced by a radiofrequency field with a specific frequency called the *Larmor frequency*. This Larmor frequency can be calculated from the equation

$$\omega L = \gamma Bo$$

where ωL = Larmor frequency; γ = the gyromagnetic ratio; Bo = static magnetic field.

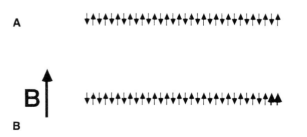

FIGURE 1.2. A: A group of spins in the absence of an applied magnetic field; there is a net cancellation of all magnetization. **B:** When the spins are placed in a magnetic field, there is a difference in the steady state populations between those parallel and antiparallel to the magnetic field. This results in the creation of a net magnetization, *M*.

The applied B1 field at the Larmor frequency causes the spins to precess in concert around the axis of the B1 field. The net effect is to rotate the longitudinal magnetization into detectable transverse magnetization. The angle of precession or flip angle is determined by the energy of the radiofrequency pulse. Following the application of the excitatory pulse, both the transverse and longitudinal components return to the equilibrium state. The motion induced by recovery may be described as a conelike gyration that collapses onto

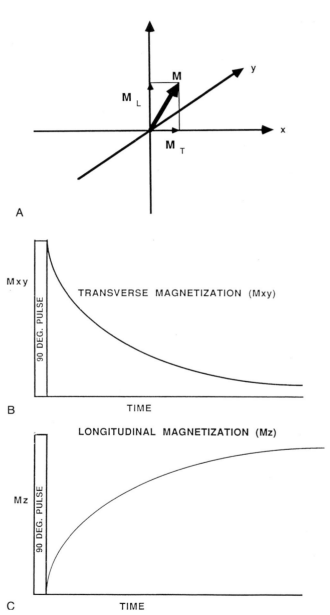

FIGURE 1.3. A: The magnetization vector can be split into transverse and longitudinal components. **B:** The transverse magnetization (M_{xy}) decays to zero with a time constant of T2. **C:** The longitudinal magnetization returns to its equilibrium value with time constant T1.

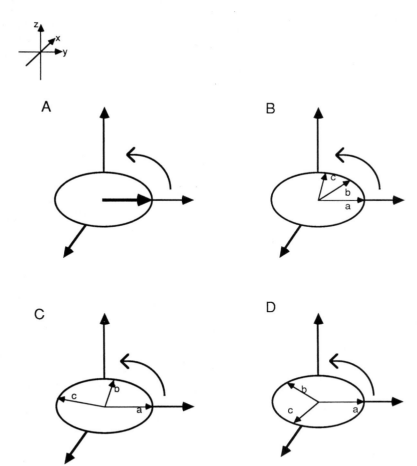

FIGURE 1.4. The effect of field inhomogeneity on the transverse magnetization. The different components of the transverse magnetization (*a, b, c*) experience slightly different magnetic fields and precess at different rates. As time progresses, the components of the transverse magnetization diverge until the vector sum becomes zero.

the longitudinal axis, followed by a slower one-dimensional return in longitudinal magnetization to the equilibrium value. The gyrational portion, known as *Larmor precession,* is characterized by a relaxation time T2*. The one-dimensional recovery of longitudinal magnetization is characterized by the recovery time T1. The precessing transverse magnetization is capable of electrical signal induction and is the sole contributor to the measurable MR signal intensity.

The principal mechanism by which MR signal decays is loss of phase coherence among the individual contributors to the signal. Protons exposed to differing magnetic field strength will gyrate at different frequencies and thus lose phase coherence (Fig. 1.4). The more inhomogeneous the magnetic field, the faster the decay and the shorter the T2* value.

The relaxation mechanisms are important to the understanding of tissue contrast. The process of recovery of magnetization to its equilibrium value is mediated by the tissue environment and thus provides the basis for different tissue contrast in MRI. The longitudinal or T1 magnetization recovers by giving off its absorbed energy to its surrounding lattice. Transverse magnetization decays to zero by giving off energy as in T1 relaxation and also by losing phase coherence due to nonrefocusable spin–spin field inhomogeneity (T2).

The random variations caused by individual proton interactions determine the value of T2 and reflect predominantly the microscopic mobility of water molecules. If the refocusable static field inhomogeneities are also considered, as in gradient echo sequences, the time constant is T2*. T2* will always therefore be shorter than its corresponding T2 value, because T2* is influenced by all types of transverse dephasing processes.

SPATIAL ENCODING OF THE MR SIGNAL

As the tissue protons are perturbed and then realign with the main magnetic field, they produce characteristic radiofrequency signals. This phenomenon is the basis for nuclear magnetic spectroscopy. To produce images however, this information must be capable of being localized. This is achieved by spatially encoding the magnetic spins (Fig. 1.5). The most common way of achieving spatial encoding is to employ two-dimensional Fourier transform (2DFT) imaging. By applying incremental changes across the magnetic field, three orthogonal axes are imposed on the system as follows:

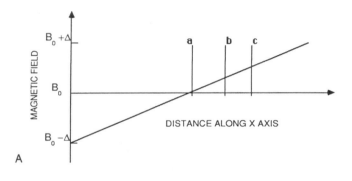

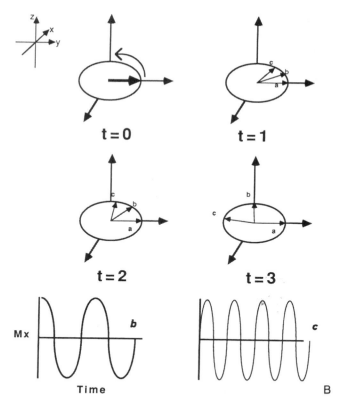

FIGURE 1.5. **A:** The linear gradient applied along the *x*-axis makes the Bo field a function of position along that axis. Spins a, b, and c are positioned at different locations and therefore experience increasing Bo fields. **B:** The rates of precession of these three spins are therefore different, as demonstrated by their angular position as a function of time. The signal from each spin is thus sinusoidal, each with a different frequency.

1. *Slice selection:* One gradient is applied at the same time as the RF pulse to selectively excite the spins in a specific slice.
2. *Frequency encoding:* A second gradient encodes location along one in plane dimension based on the frequency of the MR signal.
3. *Phase encoding:* A third gradient encodes along the other in plane dimension based on the phase differences of the MR signal.

These three gradients define three orthogonal planes and they may be aligned arbitrarily to produce any desired oblique projection.

Three-dimensional Imaging

Three-dimensional (3D) methods phase-encode spatial information along the slice selection (*z*) direction as well as the *y* direction, and they also employ a 3D FT algorithm reconstruction. 3D-gradient echo imaging provides thin sections, facilitating detection of small cartilage defects and allowing for reformatting in any plane. Fast-spoiled contrast-enhanced 3D gradient echo sequences have been successfully combined with image postprocessing to render virtual arthroscopic views (8). Fast imaging techniques allow 3D acquisition in a time tolerable to the patient; permit dynamic imaging of exogenous contrast agents to better characterize

tissue microvasculature, perfusion, and permeability; and allow for advances in kinematic joint imaging (9).

IMAGE RECONSTRUCTION

The raw data generated by most sequences is separated into phase and frequency components by a mathematical procedure called *Fourier transformation*. To generate an anatomic image, the raw data must be inverse Fourier transformed. The Fourier codomain of the image space is referred to as the *k-space*. k- and image spaces have an identical matrix size and contain equivalent imaging information in terms of spatial resolution and contrast. An exact one-to-one relationship does not exist, however, as the signal contains information from the entire image. The k-space data points are ordered according to the phase and frequency conferred on them by the spatial encoding process. The data points nearest the center of k-space contain the strongest signal elements because they are the least dephased by spatial encoding gradients. In contrast, data points at the periphery of k-space, though weaker, are responsible for reproducing the finer details in the image.

Fourier-transformed MRI pulse sequences are said to scan on a k-line by k-line basis. In conventional pulse sequences, the trajectory moves upward in an orderly pattern

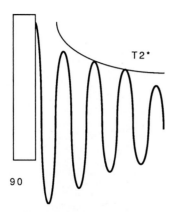

FIGURE 1.6. The NMR signal after a 90° pulse is called *free induction decay* (FID). It consists of a sinusoidal voltage decaying with a time constant T2*.

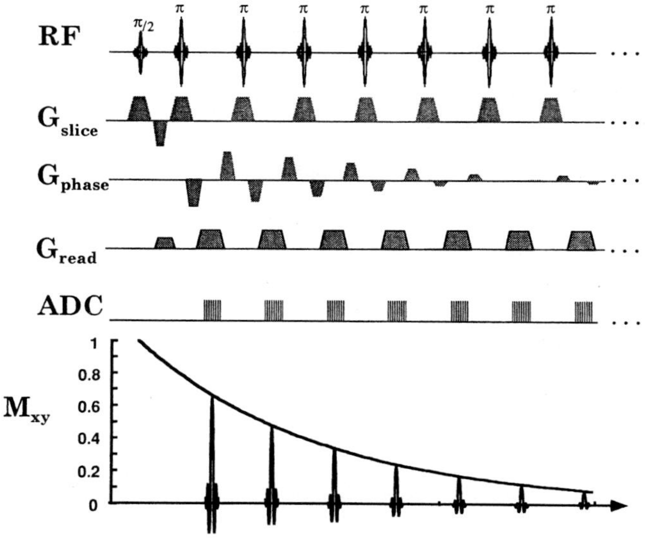

until all k-lines are acquired. We will see later how many of the new faster pulse sequences make use of more efficient and rapid ways of traversing k-space.

PULSE SEQUENCES

By varying the type, length, and relative timing of the radio-frequency (RF) pulses and gradients, one can generate images that emphasize different kinds of contrast among different tissues. The term *pulse sequence* refers to the sequence, type, and duration of the RF pulses applied and their relationships to the gradients imposed. The RF pulse sequence determines the type of MR signal generated. The simplest pulse sequence (fast field echo or gradient echo) consists of a single RF pulse per TR cycle that generates an FID signal that decays rapidly (T2* time constant) (Figs. 1.6, 1.7). The spin echo sequence uses two pulses, a 90° excitation pulse

FIGURE 1.8. Turbo spin echo diagram showing T2 decay that occurs from one echo to the next. (From Edelman RR, Hasselink JR, Zlatkin, MD, eds. *Clinical magnetic resonance imaging,* 2d ed. Philadelphia: WB Saunders, 1996, with permission.)

followed by a 180°- refocusing pulse, to generate signals that are compensated for static magnetic field inhomogeneities (Figs. 1.8, 1.9). Gradient echo and spin echo are the parent sequences from which the majority of other pulse sequences are derived.

Due to the simple contrast behavior of spin echo pulse sequences and the relative insensitivity to image artifacts, spin echo methods are still routinely used in clinical practice. Gradient echo methods have proved invaluable for specific applications such as fast imaging and for high-resolution 3D joint applications. The critical drawback of the conventional spin echo sequences is image acquisition time, which

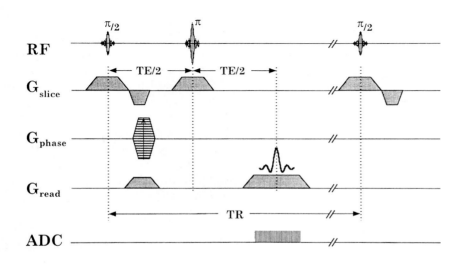

FIGURE 1.7. Spin echo pulse sequence diagram. After a π/2 excitation pulse, a π refocusing pulse is applied at TE/2 that causes a spin echo to occur at TE. (From Edelman RR, Hasselink JR, Zlatkin, MD, eds. *Clinical magnetic resonance imaging,* 2d ed. Philadelphia: WB Saunders, 1996, with permission.)

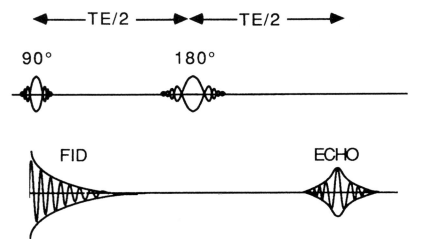

FIGURE 1.9. Simplified diagram of spin echo sequence. After a 90° excitation pulse, a 180° refocusing pulse is applied at TE/2 that causes a spin echo to occur at TE. (From Edelman RR, Hasselink JR, Zlatkin, MD, eds. *Clinical magnetic resonance imaging,* 2d ed. Philadelphia: WB Saunders, 1996, with permission.)

typically varies from a few minutes to 10 minutes or longer. With long scan times, throughput is hampered, and the likelihood of patient motion increases. For conventional sequences, the image acquisition time can be calculated from the following equation:

$$\text{Acquisition time} = TR \times NPE \times NSA$$

where TR = repetition time; NPE = number of phase-encoding steps; NSA= number of signal averages.

Fast imaging employs various methods to produce a faster filling of k-space and thus a reduction in acquisition time. Decreasing any of the contributors to acquisition time can incur other penalties, however. For instance, collecting fewer phase-encoding steps degrades spatial resolution, using fewer signal averages reduces the signal-to-noise ratio, and short TR times have a penalty in terms of contrast resolution. Multislice 2D scanning makes use of the relatively long inactive period in conventional spin echo sequences required for T1 relaxation between each echo to interrogate other unexcited slices, but the overall scan duration is still long.

In hybrid pulse sequences, multiple k-lines are acquired following each RF excitation. Each signal is individually phase encoded and read out, and the series of echoes is called the *echo train* (Fig. 1.8). Important parameters describing these sequences include the number of k-lines acquired during each readout (the echo train length [ETL]), the time interval between consecutive spin echo signals (the echo spacing [ES]), and the effective echo time (TE$_{eff}$), which determines the degree of T2 weighting and refers to the time of acquisition of the zero phase encoding k-line with reference to the RF excitation. There is a major time savings as the overall acquisition time is reduced according to the new equation:

$$\text{Acquisition time} = TR \times NPE \times NSA/ETL$$

Another strategy that can be employed is to acquire only some of the k-space lines and use these to predict the remainder of the lines by a process known as *symmetrical con-*

jugate synthesis. This is the basis of half Fourier acquisition single shot turbo spin echo (HASTE) imaging.

PULSE SEQUENCES
Gradient Echo

Gradient echo methods have proved invaluable for specific applications such as fast imaging and for high-resolution 3D joint applications. Gradient echo imaging of the rotator cuff has also been used with reports indicating accuracy rates for full-thickness tears that are equivalent to fast spin echo imaging (9,10). Kinematic imaging can be performed using a gradient echo sequence that is repeated as the patient moves the upper extremity from maximal internal to maximal external rotation. The technique has been proposed as a noninvasive method of assessing the anterior labrum and joint capsule (11).

Fast Spin Echo

Fast or *turbo spin echo sequences* are adaptations of the rapid acquisition with relaxation enhancement (RARE) technique. The hybrid RARE readout involves acquiring multiple spin echo signals with different phase encodings. Fast or turbo spin echos (FSE/TSE) acquire MR images in a fraction of the time it takes with conventional spin echo imaging while maintaining contrast and overall quality. In FSE/TSE, multiple refocusing 180° pulses follow each 90° pulse (Fig. 1.10). Time savings are proportional to the number of 180° pulses (echo train length), and the increased efficiency can be used to improve resolution or the signal-to-noise ratio. The accuracy of fast spin echo imaging has been shown to be equivalent to that of conventional spin echo sequences at a considerable savings in time (12).

Some significant differences between conventional and fast spin echo sequences must be emphasized. Fat appears

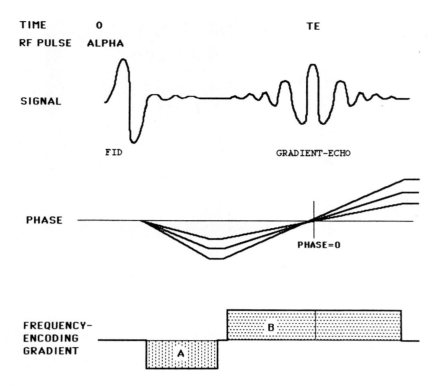

TIME   **0**   **TE**

RF PULSE   **ALPHA**

SIGNAL

FID   GRADIENT-ECHO

PHASE

PHASE=0

FREQUENCY-
ENCODING
GRADIENT

A   B

FIGURE 1.10. Simplified diagram of gradient echo sequence. Dephasing gradient pulse A produces a negative phase shift, while the rephasing gradient B produces a compensatory positive phase shift. At time TE, the phase shifts are precisely canceled. (From Edelman RR, Hasselink JR, Zlatkin, MD, eds. *Clinical magnetic resonance imaging,* 2d ed. Philadelphia: WB Saunders, 1996, with permission.)

brighter on FSE/TSE than on conventional spin echo, which can interfere with the ability to detect soft-tissue edema. Use of a longer echo time or superimposed fat saturation can help minimize this problem. Reduced susceptibility is a feature of FSE/TSE sequences as the serial refocusing pulses reduce dephasing and maintain signal (13). There is subtle intrinsic blurring in the FSE/TSE sequences compared to conventional spin echo imaging that can be minimized by using a short ETL, short ES, and appropriate rendering of the phase-encoding steps.

Echoplanar Imaging

Echoplanar imaging (EPI), based on the gradient echo technique, also mirrors RARE imaging in that a train of echoes is generated by multiple gradient reversals. In fact, the entire k-space can be filled in one excitation with this technique (14). The initial excitation may be embodied within a spin echo sequence or a gradient echo radiofrequency pulse, and very rapid gradient refocusing capability is required. Gradient echo spin echo hybrid (GraSE) combines gradient reversals and refocusing 180° pulses so that the images carry both gradient and spin echo information. Enhanced susceptibility increases meniscal tear conspicuity without the usual gradient echo bone distortion due to the compensatory spin echo effect.

The major drawback of EPI is the distortion by magnetic susceptibility and chemical shift artifact. The efficacy of echo planar sequences is unclear for current shoulder imag-

ing, though their subsecond imaging time permits very high temporal resolution; thus, they might eventually play a role in kinematic musculoskeletal applications.

Additional Techniques

Fat Saturation

High signal from fat on fast spin echo sequences may obscure bright signal from pathology (e.g., subacute hemorrhage on a T1-weighted image or soft-tissue edema on a T2-weighted image). Fat saturation is helpful in diagnosing marrow abnormalities, reduces chemical shift and motion artifacts, provides better distinction between fat and water on T2-weighted sequences, and improves the dynamic range for display of tissue signal. Fat-saturated T1-weighted images are also frequently used for assessing cartilage thickness and for imaging after gadolinium administration (e.g., to perform MR arthrography or to detect tumor enhancement).

A variety of methods attempt to suppress the signal from fat, including spectral, inversion recovery, out-of-phase imaging, and asymmetrical-echo Dixon techniques.

1. *Spectral:* The local chemical environment subtly modifies a proton's resonance frequency so that the frequency difference between a proton in a water molecule and one on a CH_2 group in fat is about 3.5 ppm. The signal intensity of fat can be selectively suppressed by applying an RF pulse at the Larmor frequency of fat protons and then dephasing

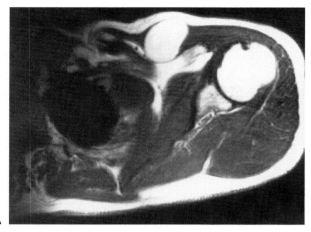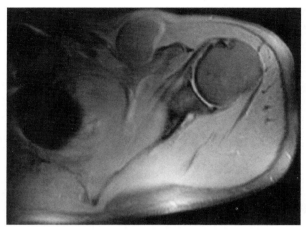

A   B

FIGURE 1.11. T1 weighted axial image **(A)** demonstrates a supraclavicular mass of high signal intensity with uniform reduction of signal on chemically selective fat suppression **(B)** in keeping with a lipoma (note chemical shift artifact).

them with a strong spoiler gradient before slice selection (Fig. 1.11). The addition of spectral fat suppression aids in differentiating fluid from the peribursal fat normally present around the rotator cuff tendons (15). The main limitations of this type of fat suppression are static magnetic field inhomogeneities (a problem when imaging away from the isocenter, as required for shoulder imaging, or when metal prostheses are present nearby). Effective spectral fat saturation requires a uniform strong magnetic field and therefore is not available at lower field strengths.

2. *Inversion recovery: Short tau inversion recovery* (STIR) imaging refers to a pulse sequence in which a preparatory 180° inversion pulse rotates the spins from the +z to the −z axis. The inversion time (TI) from the 180° pulse to the excitatory 90° pulse allows protons to reequilibrate partly. This occurs at different rates according to T1, and dramatic contrast differences can be achieved (Fig. 1.12). Fast spin echo has allowed a resurgence of IR methods that were previously considered too time-consuming for clinical practice. STIR imaging now plays a key role in detecting subtle bone and soft-tissue edema (Fig. 1.13). It is especially useful when low field strength or field heterogeneity makes spectral fat suppression suboptimal. The suppression is, however, non-

FIGURE 1.12. T1 recovery curves. After inversion, spins recover longitudinal magnetization at a rate dependent on their T1. Short T1 components such as fat reach the null point quickly, whereas long T1 components such as water recover slowly. The T1 appropriate to null a specific component thus varies with its T1 and the TR of the sequence. Assuming the TR is much greater than T1, spins with a T1 of 300 ms are nulled when T1 is 200 ms, and spins with T1 of 1,000 ms are nulled when T1 is 700 ms, as illustrated. (From Edelman RR, Hasselink JR, Zlatkin, MD, eds. *Clinical magnetic resonance imaging*, 2d ed. Philadelphia: WB Saunders, 1996, with permission.)

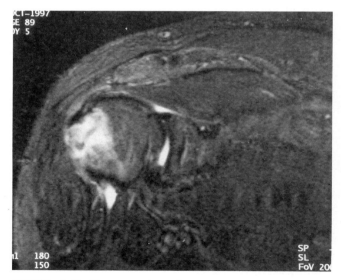

FIGURE 1.13. Short tau inversion recovery coronal oblique image demonstrating linear low signal with surrounding globular high signal in the greater tuberosity representing a fracture and associated marrow contusion.

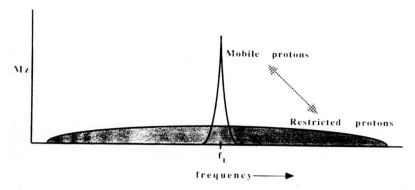

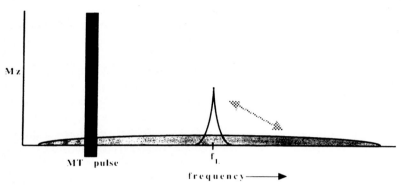

FIGURE 1.14. Principle of magnetization transfer (MT). The mobile protons have a relatively long T2 and resonate over a narrow range of frequencies. This pool of protons continually exchanges magnetization with a pool of protons having restricted motion, short T2, and a wide range of resonance frequencies. Application of an off resonance MT pulse saturates the restricted pool. The mobile pool also becomes saturated because of the exchange of magnetization between the two pools, and resulting MT contrast can help increase the conspicuity of subtle lesions. (From Edelman RR, Hasselink JR, Zlatkin, MD, eds. *Clinical magnetic resonance imaging,* 2d ed. Philadelphia: WB Saunders, 1996, with permission.)

specific, so that many substances with short T1 can be suppressed; these can include hemorrhage and gadolinium.

3. *Out-of-phase imaging:* The different resonant frequencies of fat and water may be exploited in out-of-phase imaging. As the echo time increases, fat and water protons cyclically either support or cancel their respective signals. Out-of-phase imaging is particularly useful where there are relatively similar amounts of fat and water, such as in the bone marrow.

4. *Dixon techniques:* This sequence depends on using a spin echo technique in which the 180° pulse is moved slightly, which results in phase differences between fat and water. With the three-point Dixon method, separate fat and water images can be reliably created. Image acquisition time, however, is increased threefold from a spectrally fat-suppressed acquisition.

Magnetization Transfer

Not all protons are MR visible owing to their physicochemical environment. Protons bound up in large macromolecular complexes can have an extremely short T2 with resulting poor detectability. Once excited, however, they can transfer their saturation to mobile (visible) protons (Fig. 1.14). Magnetization transfer suppresses signals predominantly from tissues containing abundant macromolecules, such as muscle. It has much less effect on fluid, blood, and fat. Magnetization transfer signal saturation has been advocated to aid

rotator cuff diagnosis as it may aid in identification of a persistent signal on T2-weighted imaging, which is an important discriminating feature between a rotator cuff tear and tendinosis/tendinitis.

Contrast Agents

Paramagnetic gadolinium contrast agents shorten T1 and result in signal enhancement on T1-weighted pulse sequences. After intravascular injection, most gadolinium chelates are distributed in the blood pool and the extracellular fluid space compartments of the body with half-lives between 1 and 2 hours. The gadolinium chelates at very high concentrations shorten T2 so much as to produce negative contrast enhancement even on T1-weighted pulse sequences. This explains the necessity to dilute gadolinium by a factor of at least 100 when injecting intraarticularly to outline joint structures (Fig. 1.15). Intravenous gadolinium chelate can result in intraarticular contrast enhancement due to diffusion from the synovium into the joint fluid; this effect is significantly increased if the patient exercises the joint for 10 to 15 minutes after injection (16).

Magnetic Resonance Angiography

Magnetic resonance angiography (MRA) allows noninvasive evaluation of the upper extremity vessels. Time-of-flight and phase contrast techniques have been available for over a

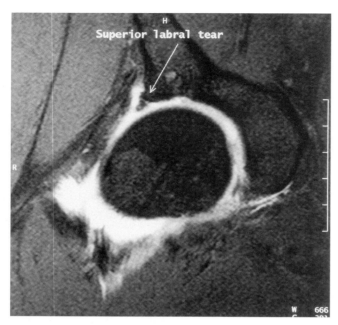

FIGURE 1.15. Post intraarticular injection of dilute gadolinium fat-suppressed T1-weighted image with high signal contrast outlining a superior labral tear.

decade. Time-of-flight techniques are based on the principle that blood flowing into an image section has higher magnetization than the partially saturated stationary tissue within the section. An alternative method, phase contrast MRA, relies on phase changes from motion to depict flowing blood. More recently, gadolinium-enhanced first-pass 3D MRA has become the MR method of choice for demonstration of the upper extremity arterial system. Correct timing of the contrast bolus allows capturing of the arterial phase. For venous demonstration, direct MR venography has been shown to be effective with infusion of dilute (1:20) gadolinium into a peripheral vein on the side of interest (17).

MR Spectroscopy

Magnetic resonance spectroscopy (MRS) uses the MR signal to give high-resolution information on the distribution of frequencies induced by chemical differences. With the advent of whole-body magnets of high field strength and homogeneity, early clinical studies focused on the phosphorus nucleus (18,19). Levels of phosphate-containing metabolites may be estimated using phosphorus MR imaging. A significant problem of phosphorus MRS, however, is its low sensitivity and resolution power. In recent years, there has been more interest in proton spectroscopy, particularly after it was demonstrated that it was possible to obtain high-resolution spectra from small well-defined regions in reasonably short scan times (20).

Many studies have demonstrated that musculoskeletal MRS applications can play a significant role in assessing both healthy and diseased muscle metabolism and function (21–26). Highly resolved spectra of normal muscle show the well-known resonances of lipids (methyl, methylene, olefinic, and other fatty acid resonances), creatine/phosphocreatine, choline/carnitine, taurine, and histidine with good intra-individual reproducibility. Pathological conditions such as myopathy, myositis, or irradiation damage increase the spectral lipid content, and after muscle irradiation, the localized 1H NMR spectrum may show a loss of the choline and creatine signals (21). Some metabolic myopathies, including McArdle's syndrome, are associated with failure to develop acidosis during exercise. For most pathological conditions, however, the metabolic findings of reduced phosphocreatine/phosphoinositol and greater acidosis during exercise with impaired recovery of phosphocreatine/phosphoinositol and pH are very similar (22).

Proton MRS has been shown to be a useful adjunct in the diagnosis and therapeutic monitoring of conditions such as adult-onset metabolic myopathy of carnitine palmitoyl transferase II (CPT II) deficiency. In their investigation of muscle CPT II deficiency, Videen et al. used proton MRS to reveal shortening of the T2 relaxation time, consistent with increased acetylation of the carnitine pool. Clinical symptoms resolved completely, and normal muscle MRS and T2 relaxation were recovered by appropriate dietary treatment (23).

MRS has also increased our understanding of muscle exercise and fatigue. Tartaglia et al. have assessed the effect of physical deconditioning on skeletal muscle's oxidative metabolism as evaluated by phosphorus-31 magnetic resonance spectroscopy (^{31}P MRS). Significant differences between the deconditioned and conditioned group were found, indicating that physical activity level should be taken into account when assessing patients' oxidative metabolism with (31)P MRS (24). Recording 1H MR spectra of human muscles during fatiguing exercise has further demonstrated that the spectral contributions of creatine/phosphocreatine (Cr/PCr) are also subject to change as a function of exercise (25). The inherent metabolic information of MRS will complement and reshape MR diagnosis in the 21st century and may perhaps partly replace orthodox histopathology. MRS certainly promises future insights into musculoskeletal biochemistry, and clinical applications continue to be developed (26).

MR Diffusion and Perfusion

The Brownian motion of water and the slow movement of blood can be measured by MR using diffusion and perfusion techniques, respectively. The most widely used perfusion technique for the evaluation of cerebral ischemia utilizes a bolus injection of a magnetic susceptibility agent that induces $T2^*$ shortening so that signal intensity is modified as it passes through the capillary bed. When a bolus-tracking technique is used and rapid imaging is performed, a transient signal loss is observed as the agent passes through the tissue. These changes in T2* signal intensity can be used to construct concentration time curves and hemodynamic maps (27).

Diffusion-weighted imaging maps water proton contrast that reflects translation of water over short distances in the microvascular water environment. A pair of gradient pulses is placed symmetrically on either side of the 180° refocusing pulse in a spin echo sequence (28). The diffusion image obtained shows signal intensity differences that are due to differences in water diffusion. By altering the time and amplitude of the pair of gradient pulses (the B value), images with variable sensitivity to diffusion can be obtained. Using multiple measurements, a diffusion coefficient, also known as the *apparent diffusion coefficient* (ADC), can be calculated (29). Both perfusion and diffusion research show great promise in the biological evaluation of the dynamics of the extracellular, interstitial, and intracellular tissue spaces (30).

Double Echo in the Steady State (DESS)

DESS represents a steady-state imaging sequence, which simultaneously allows in a single acquisition the formation of two MR echoes with clearly different contrasts. The contrast of the first echo is FISP-like, whereas the second is strongly T2 weighted; these two echoes are combined in the DESS image. Using steady-state techniques, the contrast of the images is principally controlled by varying the repetition time and the flip angle. 3D-DESS is particularly useful in imaging cartilage, and a study by Ruehm et al. concluded that the sequence is accurate in detecting patellar cartilage abnormalities. Compared with a sagittal turbo spin echo sequence, the axial 3D-DESS sequence was superior in diagnosing cartilage softening but not surface lesions (31).

IMAGE PROPERTIES

1. *Signal-to-noise ratio (SNR):* Image clarity is optimized by increasing the amount of data (signal) and decreasing the amount of noise. Noise consists of random or systematic errors. It is desirable to increase the overall SNR of an image, but there are important trade-offs among SNR, spatial resolution, and acquisition time.

Multiple factors contribute to an image's SNR, including the pulse sequence, the magnetic field strength, the local coils, the slice thickness, the field of view, the matrix dimensions, and the number of signal averages (NSA).

2. *Spatial resolution:* Spatial resolution is determined by the size of the volume elements that make up the image. The actual in-plane resolution depends on the size of the picture elements (pixels) that comprise the image. Spatial resolution is thus inversely related to voxel size; therefore, increased resolution results from reducing the slice thickness or any of the in-plane voxel dimensions. One can decrease these dimensions by reducing the field of view while maintaining the matrix size or by increasing the matrix size while maintaining the field of view. In general, however, spatial resolution is increased at the expense of signal to noise.

3. *Contrast-to-noise ratio:* Contrast-to-noise ratio is the difference in signal intensities between two tissues divided by the standard deviation of the background noise. Intrinsic image contrast, although manipulated by both repetition time and echo time, is primarily dictated by tissue type. Complex macromolecules recover longitudinal and lose transverse magnetization rapidly because of rapid energy transfer capabilities, while tissues with unpaired protons not influenced by macromolecules recover longitudinal and lose transverse magnetization more slowly.

T2* Weighting

Spin echo sequences can be designed by virtue of their TR and TE variables in such a way that the images contain predominantly T1- or T2-weighted information or a balance of both. The TR value weights the MR signal of a tissue according to its T1, with short T1 generating the highest signal. The TE value weights the MR signal intensity according to a tissue's T2, as tissue with short T2 values will have less signal after long TE than longer T2 tissues. With gradient echo imaging, T2 weighting is replaced by T2* weighting as the static inhomogeneities are not refocused, as previously discussed. Since the TR is very short in gradient echo imaging, often transverse magnetization is left at the end of the TR period that builds up, which is called *steady-state free precession*. This occurs preferentially for tissues with long T2*, and the resultant image has a mix of T1 and T2* with relatively flat contrast. The high intrinsic contrast of orthopedic MR, however, permits use of this sequence for musculoskeletal imaging, particularly as it relates to contrast between articular cartilage and adjacent fibrocartilage, as in the glenoid labrum. Spoiled gradient echo sequences with true T1 weighting are ones in which the transverse magnetization remaining after each pulse is eliminated, thus preventing steady-state free precession buildup.

FACTORS AFFECTING THE MR SIGNAL: IMAGE CONTRAST
Pulse Sequences

We have seen already the importance of pulse sequence design to the type of MR signal generated and the resulting image contrast. Other important factors include those discussed in the following sections.

Spin Density

Spin density is the number of MR visible spins per unit volume and varies between tissues by only a few percentage

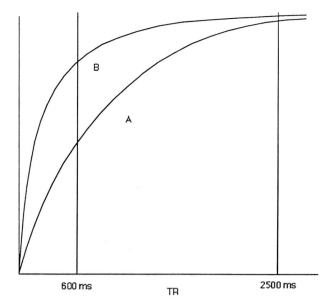

FIGURE 1.16. T1-weighted contrast. The signal intensity of two different tissues, A and B (A having the longer T1) are shown as a function of the TR. The T1 contrast at 600 ms is clearly greater than that at 2,500 ms.

points. T1 and T2 relaxation times characterize the longitudinal and transverse relaxations and can vary among tissues by a factor of 10. The number of protons in a given volume contributes to image signal. Images that have minimal T1 and T2 weighting have contrast based predominantly on visible proton density. Not all protons are MR visible because of their physicochemical environment. Protons bound up in large macromolecular complexes can have an extremely short T2 with resulting poor detectability. Areas of profound magnetic field inhomogeneity cause extremely short T2*, and protons in truly solid materials such as cortical bone and dense calcifications have extremely short T2 and long T1 values.

T1 Relaxation

The T1 or spin lattice relaxation constant relates to the period required to recover 63% of the equilibrium value after a 90° pulse excitation (Fig. 1.16). Most shoulder protocols include T1 or proton density sequences to assess anatomical detail.

T2 RELAXATION

Following RF excitation, the coherent precessing protons in the transverse plane produce the detectable MR signal. The amount of transverse magnetization that remains to form the spin echo at the TE time will depend on the T2 value of the tissue (Fig. 1.17). T2-weighted sequences demonstrate fluid and are the cornerstone of MR rotator cuff evaluation (Fig. 1.18). The mean T2 relaxation time of muscle is maximal immediately after exercise and then gradually decreases

to the preexercise level. Increases in skeletal muscle T2 relaxation time have been used to map whole muscle activity during exercise. Some studies further suggest that intramuscular variations in T2 after exercise can be used to map activity on a pixel-by-pixel basis by defining an active T2 threshold, though this methodology is yet to be proven (32). Yoshioka et al. have shown that differences in the T2 relaxation time of the soleus between the time immediately after exercise and at rest are smaller after successful intervention of arterial occlusive disease. T2 relaxation time may thus be a useful quantitative parameter in peripheral arterial occlusive disease as well as in other muscle studies (33).

Flow

Flow can produce either an increase or decrease in signal intensity, and the appearance of flowing blood depends strongly on the imaging sequence employed. A decrease may be due to flow-related dephasing or if the spins move between the 90° and 180° pulses and are not completely refocused. An increase on T1-weighted scans may be due to inflow of unsaturated new spins.

Magnetic Susceptibility

Magnetic susceptibility represents a material's tendency to distort a magnetic field. Paramagnetic materials like gadolinium have some electrons that tend to line up with the magnetic field, producing an additive effect. Supermagnetic substances like hemosiderin more strongly attract magnetic

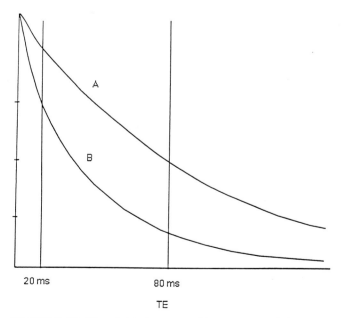

FIGURE 1.17. T2-weighted contrast. The response of the signal intensity of the two tissues, A and B (A having a longer T2) are shown. The percentage contrast is greater at a TE of 80 ms than that at a TE of 20 ms.

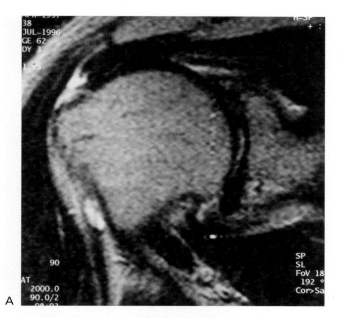

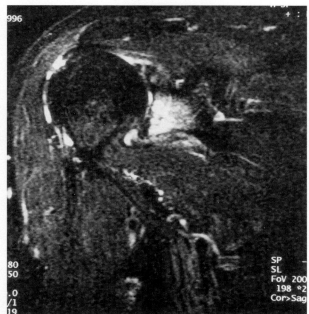

FIGURE 1.18. T2-weighted **(A)** and short tau inversion recovery (STIR) **(B)** coronal oblique images showing high signal traversing the supraspinatus tendon representing a full-thickness tear.

lines of force. Ferromagnetic substances (e.g., iron alloys) remain permanently magnetized after being removed from a magnetic field.

ARTIFACTS

Artifacts refer to image features that do not correspond to real anatomical structures. Recognizing artifacts and understanding their causes and remedies are critical for effective musculoskeletal imaging.

Motion Artifact

Motion artifact may be caused by physiological movements such as respiration and vascular pulsation as well as voluntary patient motion. Motion may be addressed directly by reducing imaging time and also by engaging in effective patient coaching and positioning at setup. If the forearm rests against the chest wall, respiratory motion will be transmitted to the shoulder with significant degradation of the resulting images. Careful positioning of the arm away from the chest and abdomen will minimize these artifacts. The phase-encoding artifact from axillary vessels can be eliminated by avoiding superior-inferior phase encoding. Motion artifact may also be minimized indirectly through averaging by increasing the NSA, reducing ghosts by fat saturation and presaturation pulses or correcting erroneous phases by ordered phase encoding.

Aliasing

Aliasing or *"wrap-around" artifact* refers to the artifact that occurs when a region not in the field of view appears within the image on the opposite side. This can occur in both the phase- and frequency-encoding directions but is more problematic in the phase-encoding direction. On modern equipment, aliasing in the frequency-encoding direction is avoided by using digital filters, which eliminate signals with frequencies outside the desired range, and in the phase-encoding direction by oversampling and the use of small local coils.

Chemical Shift

The local chemical environment subtly modifies a proton's resonance frequency. The difference between a proton in a water molecule and one on a CH2 group in fat is only about 3.5 ppm. This results in misregistration of fat signals compared to water (chemical shift artifact) (Fig. 1.19). The artifact is most severe with low bandwidth readout on a high-field magnet. As FSE sequences typically use a high bandwidth readout, chemical shift artifact is reduced.

Susceptibility Artifacts

Susceptibility artifacts are particularly important in postsurgical imaging as metallic hardware distorts the magnetic field and leads to signal loss due to geometric deformation and spatial misregistration. Artifacts are strongest at interfaces of two materials with different magnetic susceptibilities, such as at bone marrow/calcified bone and soft-tissue metal interfaces. Titanium causes the least amount of magnetic susceptibility artifact of the common metals left in place after orthopedic intervention; ferromagnetic metals are the worst offenders. The refocusing 180° pulse inherent in spin echo sequences (Fig. 1.20) (34) substantially alleviates susceptibility artifacts.

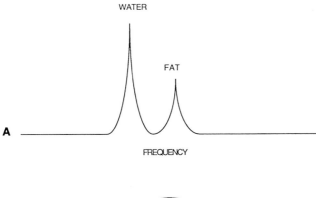

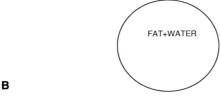

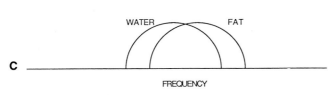

FIGURE 1.19. Chemical shift. **A:** The difference in precession frequencies between water and fat protons creates two peaks in the frequency spectrum of most tissues. If a tissue contains fat and water **(B)**, there will be a spatial misregistration of the fat relative to the water signal along the frequency encoding direction **(C)**.

Truncation Artifact

Abrupt changes in signal intensity at an interface can produce a "ring-down" artifact consisting of bright and dark bands whose intensity decreases with distance from the interface. The truncation of data in the conversion of a complex analogue signal to a finite set leads to these artifacts. The artifact can be reduced by increasing the spatial resolution of the image or by decreasing the contrast at the interface (e.g., by using fat suppression).

Magic Angle

At approximately 55° to the main magnetic field, dipole–dipole interactions between tendon molecules disappear so that tendon signal increases particularly on images acquired at echo times less than 30 ms; this is called the *magic angle phenomenon* (Fig. 1.21). Altering tendon obliquity or seeing the high signal vanish on longer TE images help in the recognition of this artifact, which can also occur in the glenoid labrum.

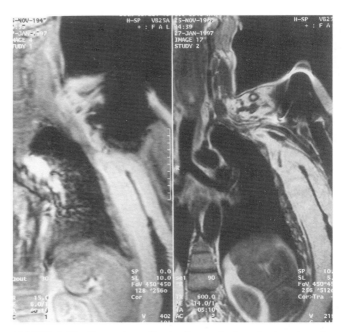

FIGURE 1.20. Coronal gradient echo and spin echo images of a patient with a left humeral metallic prosthesis producing magnetic susceptibility distortion, which is significantly reduced on the conventional spin echo image.

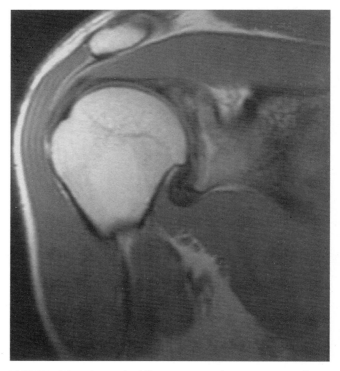

FIGURE 1.21. Coronal oblique proton density image of the shoulder demonstrating increased signal intensity in the rotator cuff, which disappeared on longer TE, T2-weighted scanning. Appearances could represent magic angle phenomenon or tendon degeneration. Repeating the scan with the tendon in a different orientation could help distinguish between these two possibilities.

HARDWARE CONSIDERATIONS

Magnetic Field

The choice of magnetic field strength involves trade-offs in terms of cost, image quality, and interventional MR capability. Dedicated open systems including an upright system have been developed. Low-cost dedicated extremity scanners and compact permanent magnets will also help shape the future role of MR shoulder imaging (35). Low-field magnets are less expensive, but image quality suffers from reduced SNR, and spectral fat suppression is problematic (Fig. 1.22). Scan times are usually longer since multiple NSAs are needed. An advantage of some low-field systems is their open design, reducing claustrophobia and allowing kinematic studies.

High field magnets most commonly have a superconductive coil design; open low-field magnet designs include permanent and resistive types. Open high-field magnet designs are also now available using superconductive technology.

Gradients

Gradient coils produce spatial-encoding magnetic fields. As described earlier, streams of electrical pulses are transmitted during the scan from the pulse sequence controller to the RF and gradient coils. Advances in gradient performance have comprised the most important progress, allowing for the recent dramatic improvements in fast, high-resolution MR imaging and shorter TR and TE times, as well as smaller field of views.

Radiofrequency Coils

Radiofrequency coils are specialized antennae that can convert electric current to and from electromagnetic radiowaves. A local coil is essential to ensure an adequate signal-to-noise ratio with thin-slice, high-resolution imaging. Many types of shoulder coils are available. Quadrature coils offer good signal-to-noise ratios when contoured to fit around the shoulder curvature. Still better SNR is obtained by use of multicoil arrays. These are local coils that are magnetically decoupled from each other and send their signals to separate receivers; thus, the signal from them is additive, but the noise is not. These important advances in coil design and their implications will be addressed more fully in the next chapter.

CONCLUSION

This chapter has attempted to introduce the basic concepts and principles of MRI, with emphasis on those concepts that are most applicable to musculoskeletal imaging and to shoulder MRI in particular. We hope it will enhance your understanding and appreciation of the succeeding chapters and be of benefit to you in your clinical MRI practice.

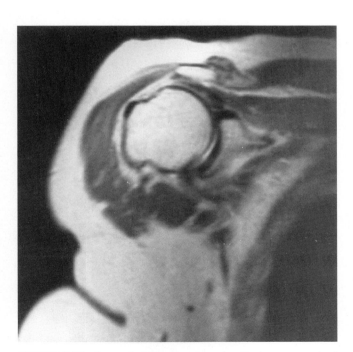

FIGURE 1.22. Coronal oblique proton density image acquired on a 0.2 T low-field magnet demonstrating high signal traversing the supraspinatus tendon representing a full-thickness tear.

REFERENCES

1. Edelman RR, Hasselink JR, Zlatkin, MB, eds. *Clinical magnetic resonance imaging,* 2d ed. Philadelphia: WB Saunders, 1996.
2. SJ Eustace. *Magnetic resonance imaging of orthopedic trauma.* Philadelphia: Lippincott Williams and Wilkins, 1999.
3. Stark DD, Bradley WG, eds. *Magnetic resonance imaging,* 3d ed. St. Louis: Mosby, 1999.
4. Higgins CB, Hricak H, Helms CA, eds. *Magnetic resonance imaging of the body,* 3d ed. Philadelphia: Lippincott-Raven, 1997.
5. Hashemi RH, Bradley WG. *MRI: the basics.* Baltimore: Williams and Wilkins, 1997.
6. Mitchell DG. *MRI principles.* Philadelphia: WB Saunders, 1997.
7. Rafii R. Update on the shoulder. *Magn Reson Imaging Clin N Am* 1997;5(4):661–897.
8. Weishaupt D, Wildermuth S, Schmid M, et al. Virtual MR arthroscopy: new insights into joint morphology. *J Magn Reson Imaging* 1999;9(6):757–760.
9. Sahin-Akyar G, Miller TT, Staron RB, et al. Gradient echo versus fat suppressed fast spin echo MR imaging of rotator cuff tears. *Am J Roentgenol* 1998;171:223–227.
10. Parsa M, Tuite M, Norris M, et al. MR imaging of rotator cuff tendon tears: comparison of T2*-weighted gradient-echo and conventional dual echo sequences. *Am J Roentgenol* 1997;168:1518–1524.
11. Sans N, Richardi G, Railhac J, et al. Kinematic MR imaging of the shoulder: normal patterns. *Am J Roentgenol* 1996;167:1517–1522.

12. Carrino JA, McCauley TR, Katz LD, et al. Rotator cuff: evaluation with fast spin echo versus conventional spin echo MR imaging. *Radiology* 1997;202:533–539.
13. Constable RT, Anderson AW, Zhong J, et al. Factors influencing contrast in fast spin–echo MR imaging. *Magn Reson Imaging* 1992;10:497–511.
14. Edelman RR, Wielopolski P, Schmitt F. Echo-planar MR imaging. *Radiology* 1994;192:600–612.
15. Quinn SF, Sheley RC, Demlow TA, et al. Rotator cuff tendon tears: evaluation with fat suppressed MR imaging with arthroscopic correlation in 100 patients. *Radiology* 1995;195:497–501.
16. Vahlensieck M, Peterfy CG. Wischwr T, et al. Indirect MR arthrography: optimization and clinical applications. *Radiology* 1996;200:249–254.
17. Li W, David V, Kaplan R. et al. Three-dimensional low dose gadolinium-enhanced peripheral MR venography. *J Magn Reson Imaging* 1998;8(3):630–633.
18. Radda GK. The use of NMR spectroscopy for the understanding of disease. *Science* 1986;233:640–645.
19. Luyten PR, Groen JP Vermeulen JQ, et al. Experimental approaches to image localized human 31P NMR spectroscopy. *Magn Reson Med* 1989;11:1–21.
20. Frahm J, Bruhn H, Gyngell ML, et al. Localized high resolution proton NMR spectroscopy using simulated echoes: initial applications to human brain in vivo. *Magn Reson Med* 1989;9:79–93.
21. Bongers H, Schick F, Skalej M, et al. Localized in vivo 1H spectroscopy of human skeletal muscle: normal and pathologic findings. *Magn Reson Imaging* 1992;10(6):957–964.
22. Kent-Braun JA, Miller RG, Weiner MW. Magnetic resonance spectroscopy studies of human muscle. *Radiol Clin N Am* 1994; 32(Mar,2):313–335.
23. Videen JS, Haseler LJ, Karpinski NC, et al. Noninvasive evaluation of adult onset myopathy from carnitine palmitoyl transferase II deficiency using proton magnetic resonance spectroscopy. *J Rheumatol* 1999;26(Aug,8):1757–1763.
24. Tartaglia MC, Chen JT, Caramanos Z, et al. Muscle phosphorus magnetic resonance spectroscopy oxidative indices correlate with physical activity. *Muscle Nerve* 2000;23(Feb,2):175–181.
25. Kreis R, Jung B, Slotboom J, et al. Effect of exercise on the creatine resonances in 1H MR spectra of human skeletal muscle. *J Magn Reson* 1999;137(Apr,2):350–357.
26. Moller HE, Vermathen P, Rummeny E, et al. In vivo 31P NMR spectroscopy of human musculoskeletal tumors as a measure of response to chemotherapy. *NMR Biomed* 1996;9(Dec,8):347–358.
27. Rosen RR, Belliveau JW, Vevea JM, et al. Perfusion imaging with NMR contrast agents. *Magn Reson Med* 1990;14(2):249–265.
28. Moseley ME, Wendland MF, Kucharczyk J. Magnetic resonance imaging of diffusion and perfusion. *Top Magn Reson Imaging* 1991;3(3):50–67.
29. Le Bihan D, Breton E, Lallemand D, et al. Separation of diffusion and perfusion in intravoxel incoherent motion MR imaging. *Radiology* 1988;168(2):497–505.
30. Baur A, Stabler A, Bruning R, et al. Diffusion-weighted MRI. *Radiology* 1998;207(2):349–356.
31. Ruehm S, Zanetti M, Romero J, Hodler J. MRI of patellar articular cartilage: evaluation of an optimized gradient echo sequence (3D-DESS). *J Magn Reson Imaging* 1998;8(Nov–Dec,6):1246–1251.
32. Prior BM, Foley JM, Jayaraman RC, Meyer RA. Pixel T2 distribution in functional magnetic resonance images of muscle. *J Appl Physiol* 1999;87(Dec,6):2107–2114.
33. Yoshioka H, Anno I, Kuramoto K, Matsumoto K, Jikuya T, Itai Y. Acute effects of exercise on muscle MRI in peripheral arterial occlusive disease. *Magn Reson Imaging* 1995;13(5):651–659.
34. Eustace S, Jara H, Goldberg R, et al: A comparison of conventional spin echo and turbo spin echo imaging of soft tissues adjacent to orthopedic hardware. *Am J Roentgenol* 1998;170(2): 455–458.
35. Peterfy CG, Roberts T, Genant K. Dedicated extremity MR imaging: an emerging technology. *Radiol Clin N Am* 1997;35:1–20.

LOCAL COILS

THOMAS E. SCHUBERT
DAVID A. MOLYNEAUX

A *local coil* is a radio frequency receiver coil (RF coil) placed in the locality of the area to be imaged. Such a coil may surround the tissue to be imaged (commonly known as a *volume* or *whole volume coil*), or it may be placed on the surface of the patient (commonly known as a *surface coil*). Variants of these concepts may partially surround the tissue of interest. These variants are known as *partial volume coils*.

Local RF coils are critical to MR imaging of the joints as they provide greater diagnostic capability through an increase in signal-to-noise ratio (SNR). Because noise is inherent in the tissue being imaged, it is important that an RF coil adequately covers the area of interest but as little unwanted tissue as possible.

In general, larger coils have lower SNR. The aim is to have as small a coil as is feasible to adequately cover the area of interest.

VOLUME COILS

Some of the fundamental work on volume coils was published by Hoult and Richards (1) in 1976, followed by Gadian (2) and Hayes (3). These publications discussed the basic concepts behind RF coil design (probes) and defined these concepts as having supreme importance in the performance of the MR systems. Solenoid, saddle, and loop coils were discussed in detail. A long solenoid is the best approximation to the ideal current distribution required for a uniform axial field within the interior of the solenoid. The solenoid coil was developed for applications where the sample would be inside of the coil, such as head, body, and extremity applications.

LOOP COILS

Some anatomical areas, such as the shoulders, do not lend themselves to cylindrical coil designs. Thus, surface coils consisting of simple loops were developed and optimized (4,5,6). A loop coil can be considered to be a single-turn so-lenoid coil. Hoult (4) determined that simple loops of wire wound in a plane can produce a transverse field, although highly nonlinear as a function of distance away from the surface of the coil. As the signal falls off from the surface of the coil, so does the obtainable SNR. The useful field of view of the coil is defined by its diameter.

Smaller loop coils have higher signal-to-noise performance, albeit less depth of penetration into the tissue of interest.

Although early work was with circular coils, further developments occurred (4,5) offering alternative geometries to the loop such as butterfly coils and rectangular coils. Figure 2.1 illustrates a loop coil, along with its associated magnetic flux vector. Figure 2.2 shows a butterfly coil, with its associated magnetic flux vector.

COIL PLACEMENT

All coils have a placement limitation based on their geometry. For a coil to work optimally, B1, the RF coil magnetic field, must lie in a plane perpendicular to the main magnetic field of the MR magnet, known as B0.

For example, for optimal reception, a loop coil should only be placed such that its B1 field lies in a plane that is orthogonal to the B0 field of the MR magnet. If the loop coil is placed such that its B1 axis is parallel or coincident with the B0 field of the magnet, there will be minimal radio frequency voltage induced in the coil and hence minimal RF signal received by the MR system.

Closed MR magnets have a B0 field that is horizontal and oriented down the axis of the body coil. Open MR magnets typically have a B0 field that is vertical.

Early methods of imaging the shoulder used general-purpose "loop" coils. Typically, these coils consisted of a one-turn solenoid. Enterprising practitioners would often use tape to fasten the coil in place over the humeral head. As along as the coil's B1 field lay approximately in a plane that was orthogonal to the B0 axis of the magnet, the results were reasonably good. Signal intensity would fall off quickly with distance from the plane of the loop.

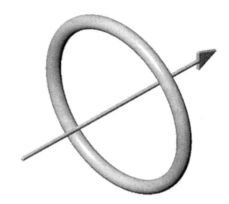

FIGURE 2.1. Loop coil. For optimal performance, the loop coil must be oriented such that the B1 field of the coil (arrow) lies in a plane that is orthogonal to the B0 field of the magnet.

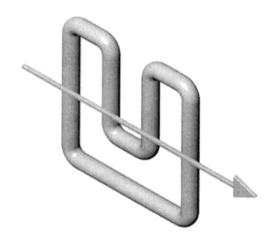

FIGURE 2.2. Butterfly coil. For optimal performance, the butterfly coil must be oriented such that the B1 field of the coil (arrow) lies in a plane that is orthogonal to the B0 field of the magnet.

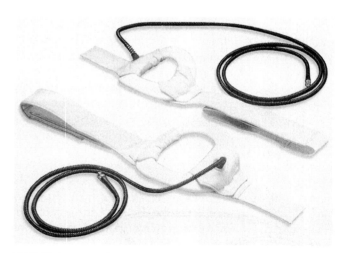

FIGURE 2.3. Set of large and small loop coils. (From IGC Medical Advances Inc., with permission.)

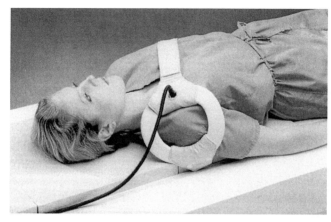

FIGURE 2.4. Linear one-turn solenoid loop coil (From IGC Medical Advances, Inc., with permission.)

As this technique gained acceptance, coil manufacturers began making single-turn solenoid "loop" coils with a larger hole in the middle. This allowed the humeral head to protrude into the middle of the loop, the area of highest signal intensity. The loops themselves were sometimes warped to better fit over the patient anatomy. Some were available in two sizes, to optimize SNR and tissue coverage on larger and smaller shoulders (Fig. 2.3). Better techniques of fastening the coil in place evolved. Figure 2.4 shows a loop coil positioned over the humeral head and held in place with a strap. This coil design is still in wide spread use today, and results can be difficult to improve upon when the MRI system is limited to a single channel. Coils with one element, such as the butterfly and loop coil, are known as *linear coils*.

THE HELMHOLTZ COIL

Helmholtz coils, often called *Helmholtz pairs*, consist of two parallel loops with the anatomy of interest sandwiched between them. The loops are connected electrically in parallel and produce a single-channel output to the MR system. This configuration has the benefit of reducing the falloff in signal intensity with distance from the coil and generally improving the uniformity of the resulting image. Typically, one coil element is positioned under the posterior aspect of the shoulder joint, while the other coil element is positioned above the anterior aspect of the joint (Fig. 2.5).

This approach also has some limitations. As the separation of the anterior loop and posterior loop changes due to patient size, the coil frequency also changes. The result is that signal-to-noise performance degrades as the separation changes. Some, but not all, MRI systems were designed to permit either automatic or manual tuning of coils, which could restore the Helmholtz coil to optimal performance

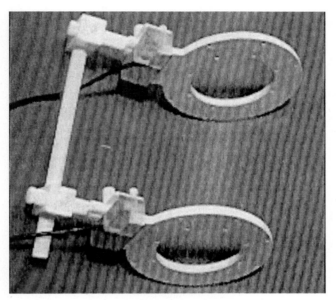

FIGURE 2.5. Helmholtz coil. Two general-purpose 5-in. coils, with connecting device.

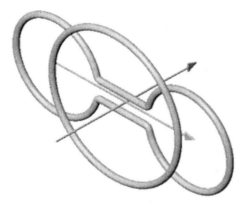

FIGURE 2.6. Planar quadrature coil consisting of a butterfly and a loop. The butterfly coil has a B1 field that is transverse to the B1 field of the loop coil. The signals from the coils are fed into a 90 degree combiner and produce a single-channel output.

levels. Manual or automatic coil tuning required additional time and was not always reliable.

As with all coils, proper positioning is very important. Various coil-positioning aids, similar to chemistry laboratory ring stands, were developed either by MRI manufacturers or MRI practitioners who had seized upon this technique. As quadrature and array coils became available, the use of Helmholtz coils was largely abandoned as a technique for shoulder imaging.

QUADRATURE OR CIRCULARLY POLARIZED COILS

RF coil design for shoulder imaging progressed from linear designs to quadrature designs. Quadrature refers to a coil with two orthogonal elements. The two elements are fed into a quadrature combiner, which shifts the phase of the two signals by 90 degrees and then adds the signals from the coils in an analog fashion, yielding a single-channel output to the MRI system. A perfect quadrature coil can realize a square root of two (41%) improvement in SNR in the center of the coil over a single-loop coil. Quadrature design coils are also known as *circularly polarized*, or CP, coils. As the name infers, CP coils have a polarity. If they are placed backward with respect to the B0 field of the MR magnet, the signals from the two elements will subtract from each other, rather than add, resulting in poor image quality.

The earliest work was by Hyde (5) in 1987 describing a quadrature detection system containing two surface coils. One of the two coils was a device called a *counterrotating coil*, which was basically a two-turn coplanar surface coil with the

turns wound in series to create a mode with a transverse field perpendicular to the plane of the coil. The second coil with two loops connected in parallel placed side by side and in the same plane as the first coil created a second mode with a B1 field parallel to the plane of the coil. Hence, quadrature detection at the origin was achieved. Isolation between the two coils was achieved by geometric decoupling, which occurs when the magnetic flux of one coil is not detected by the other coil due to canceling electromotive forces. This design was subsequently patented in U.S. patent 4,721,913 (6). Figure 2.6 illustrates the first quadrature planar surface coil.

Further enhancements in coil systems were published and patented by Mehdizadeh (7,8). This coil was a simple structure with a loop and a butterfly coil providing two orthogonal modes that were also geometrically isolated. It had the advantage of using rectangular rather than circular coils like Hyde (5), and it provided a true planar construction

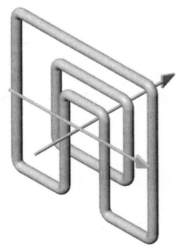

FIGURE 2.7. Planar quadrature coil. Variation of a butterfly and loop combined in quadrature.

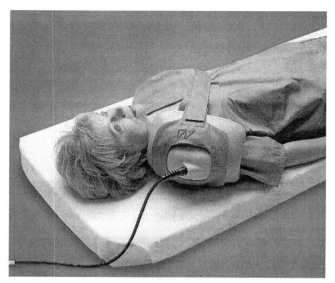

FIGURE 2.8. Quadrature shoulder coil. The coil may be positioned on the patient while the patient is sitting up. (From IGC Medical Advances, Inc., with permission.)

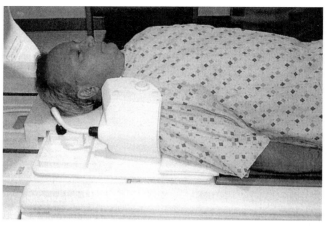

FIGURE 2.10. Vertical field shoulder coil positioned on patient. (From MRI Devices Corporation, with permission.)

both signal-to-noise and image uniformity, and they gained widespread acceptance among MRI practitioners. Figures 2.8 and 2.9 show coil designs using quadrature technology.

FLEXIBLE QUADRATURE COILS

Some MRI system manufacturers introduced general-purpose quadrature coils that were flexible. Such a coil yields true quadrature performance only when it is in a predetermined shape (Fig. 2.10). That is, when it is in a curvature of a given diameter. If the shape of the coil deviates from the optimal shape, performance can degrade sharply. When using a flexible quadrature coil, proper positioning and fixation of the coil is critical. These coils are widely available today. Some have a positioning aid, similar to the laboratory ring stand.

PHASED ARRAY COILS FOR SHOULDER IMAGING

At this point in the evolution of RF coil design, it was clear that any increases in both SNR and field of view would require a new technology to be developed. Roemer (9) developed a device called the *"NMR, Nuclear Magnetic Resonance," phased array*, a method for simultaneously acquiring and subsequently combining data from a multiplicity of closely positioned linear coils.

Closely spaced coils could be positioned so that the mutual inductance was minimal and a one-dimensional array could be formed to extend the useful field of view while providing the signal-to-noise performance of a smaller coil. Each coil's output was sent to its own preamplifier and analog-to-digital converter and then digitally combined into a large field of view and high SNR image.

By the mid-1990s, nearly all of the major MRI system manufacturers introduced systems with multiple receiver

methodology by allowing both coils to be etched on a substrate and packaged in a flat configuration. One output is phase shifted by 90 degrees and combined with the other output to give an improvement in signal-to-noise ratio as a result of the quadrature detection effect described previously. Figure 2.7 illustrates the planar version of a quadrature coil.

The theoretical SNR improvement was difficult to obtain, since in horizontal field magnets, human anatomy does not allow the placement of two orthogonal loops around the shoulder joint and still have the B1 axis of each coil element lie in a plane orthogonal to the B0 axis of the magnet. Planar quadrature coils were developed that wrapped around the shoulder. The quadrature improvement was maximal in only one place within the coil and was less everywhere else. Nevertheless, quadrature coils yielded an improvement in

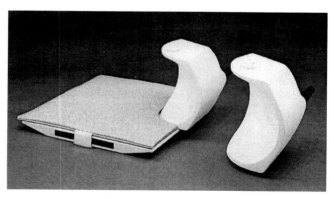

FIGURE 2.9. Large and small quadrature shoulder coils. Lockdown coil designs help prevent patient motion and ensure proper orientation of the coil with respect to the B0 field of the magnet. (From MRI Devices Corp., with permission.)

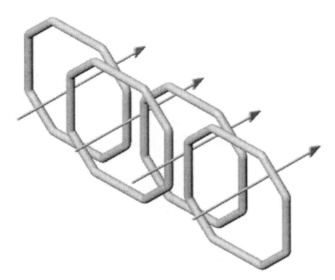

FIGURE 2.11. A four-channel array coil consisting of four linear coils arranged in a strip for an extended field of view. The arrows represent the B1 field of each coil in the array.

channels. These systems allowed receiving RF signals from an array of coils, usually as many as four. This ability to use multiple receiver channels is known variously as the multi-coil option, array option, or phased array.

The term *phased array*, borrowed from RADAR technology, is in common use. It is a misnomer, since the reception of RF signals from the coil elements is not phased. They are all receiving signal simultaneously.

The availability of multiple receiver channels in the MRI system allowed the creation of more sophisticated coils. Array coils have progressed beyond linear arrays into more sophisticated configurations. These configurations now use several array elements to image the same tissue, from different angles. Thus, the region of sensitivity of each array element encompasses a segment of the tissue of interest. By reducing the size of each element, a high SNR may be realized.

For array coil elements to work optimally, they must not "see" each other in an electrical sense. A property, known as *mutual inductance*, between array coil elements must be minimized. Minimizing the mutual inductance improves the electrical isolation of the elements of the coil array. If the individual elements of an array of coils are poorly isolated from each other, they behave as though they were one large coil, rather than four smaller coils (Fig. 2.11). The result is that the benefit of the coil array is lost, and the signal-to-noise performance approximates the performance of a single coil as large as the four array elements combined.

Array elements in close proximity to each other will detune each other. In other words, they will be poorly isolated from each other, and the benefits of the array will be lost or greatly diminished. A common technique to isolate array elements from each other involves overlapping them a precise amount. The solution for a four-coil array is vastly more complex than the example given earlier. The first element of the array must be isolated from the second, third, and fourth. The second element of the array must be isolated from the first, third, and fourth, and so on.

MRI system manufacturers are presently introducing systems and upgrades with the capability to use six or eight array channels. Future shoulder coil designs will make use of these additional channels.

REFERENCES

1. Hoult D. Laboratory frame NMR experiments. *J Magn Reson* 1976;24.
2. Gadian D. *Nuclear magnetic resonance and its application to living systems.* Oxford: Clarendon Press, 1982.
3. Hayes C, Edelstein W. *Radio frequency coils.* GE Medical Systems Publication, Milwaukee: 1985.
4. Edelstein W, Hayes C, Mueller O. Radio frequency coil for NMR. U.S. Patent # 4,680,548, 1987.
5. Hyde J, Jesmanowicz A. Quadrature detection surface coil. *Magn Reson Med* 1987;179–184.
6. Hyde J, Jesmanowicz A. Quadrature detection surface coil. U.S. Patent # 4,721,913, 1988.
7. Mehdizadeh M, Molyneaux D, Morich M. Quadrature planar surface coil. In: *Proceedings of SMRM.* 1988:271.
8. Mehdizadeh M, Molyneaux D, Morich M. Quadrature surface coils for magnetic resonance. U.S. Patent # 4,918,388, 1990.
9. Roemer P, Edelstein W. The NMR phased array coil. *Magn Reson Med* 1990;16:192–225.

Local Coils **25**

MRI OF THE SHOULDER: IMAGING TECHNIQUES AND DIAGNOSTIC PITFALLS

SCOTT A. MIROWITZ
MARIANNE SHIH

IMAGING TECHNIQUES

MR imaging of the shoulder has gained widespread utility in the evaluation of shoulder disorders since it offers excellent depiction of both soft tissue and osseous structures. Recent advances in MR imaging have contributed to shorter scanning times and higher-quality images. An understanding of imaging techniques, normal variants, technical artifacts, and diagnostic pitfalls will improve diagnostic accuracy on shoulder MRI studies.

Patient Positioning

Proper patient positioning is important to consider at the outset of the examination. The patient should be supine with the head directed toward the scanner bore. To avoid transmission of respiratory motion, the patient's arms should rest to the side of the body and should not be placed on the abdomen. The preferred positioning of the patient's arm is neutral to slightly externally rotated. Use of supports under the elbows can assist in maintaining this position. In external rotation, the posterior labrum is well visualized (1,2). Internal rotation of the arm should be avoided. Internal rotation causes laxity of the anterior capsular structures and increased overlap of muscular and tendinous components of the rotator cuff, both of which can interfere with evaluation (2).

Patient comfort is important to consider prior to MR imaging. Simple measures can help minimize patient motion during the study so that better-quality images can be obtained. Taking a few moments to discuss the procedure with the patient prior to scanning and continuing communication during the scanning procedure can help decrease patient anxiety and may decrease patient motion and/or avoid the need for premedication in some patients. During the scan, supports placed beneath the patient's knees help decrease pressure on the lower back. Attention should be given to appropriate temperature control within the scanner bore. Blindfolding or prism glasses and audiovisual distracters can be helpful for alleviating claustrophobia in some patients. Patients who are extremely claustrophobic or anxious may require mild pharmacological sedation prior to imaging. Alternatively, such patients may be accommodated in large-bore, open-sided, or other less restrictive magnet designs.

Surface Coils

The use of surface coils is requisite for shoulder MR imaging. The higher signal-to-noise ratio produced by these coils allows for improved spatial resolution; both of these factors improve the diagnostic ability of MR exams. The most basic and commonly used coil is the *single-loop coil*. It is a linear coil in a curved configuration. Its main disadvantage is the sharp decrease in image homogeneity and signal-to-noise ratio with increasing distance from the center of the coil. A variant of the single-loop coil is the *Helmholtz pair*, which consists of a pair of flat circular surface coils. One coil is placed anterior and one posterior to the shoulder joint. The advantage of the Helmholtz pair is improved signal homogeneity across the field of view as compared to that obtained with a linear loop coil. Flexible coils are those that wrap around and conform to the anatomic area of interest. They offer improved patient comfort.

Surface coils based on quadrature and phased array technology provide further improvement in signal-to-noise ratio, which can be used to implement smaller fields of view, thinner slices, and higher-resolution matrices, all of which contribute to better spatial resolution. Quadrature coils generally provide approximately 40% increased signal-to-noise ratio as compared with a comparably sized linear coil. Multicoil or phased array coils consist of two or more resonating loops.

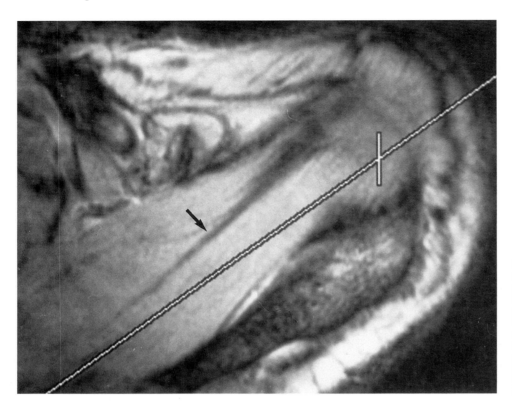

FIGURE 3.1. Coronal oblique coronal image slice prescription. Transaxial gradient echo image acquired through the superior aspect of the supraspinatous muscle and tendon is shown. A ray has been positioned along the long axis of the muscle and parallel to the angle of the glenohumeral joint. Note the divergence in angle between the axis of the tendon (*arrow*) and that of the muscle/joint.

They provide high signal-to-noise ratio and image homogeneity over a larger anatomic region, though they are somewhat more expensive and more demanding in terms of computer requirements. Surface coils should be positioned on the patient's shoulder in the coronal oblique plane in order to maximize signal-to-noise ratio in the region of the rotator cuff (3). It is important that the coil be centered over area of primary interest. Restraint bands should be used to restrict movement of the coil with respiratory or gross patient motion. Because the sensitive range of a surface coil is proportional to its diameter, coil size should be concordant with the size of the patient's shoulder (4).

Coil burnout refers to the excessively increased signal intensity of tissue that is located in very close proximity to the coil. This extremely high signal intensity can obscure subtle pathology. A small amount of foam padding inserted between the coil and the patient's shoulder helps minimize coil burnout. Image uniformity can also be improved with the use of certain postprocessing software algorithms that help normalize the signal intensity profile across the field of view.

Imaging Planes

Preliminary scout images are obtained in the coronal plane using short TR (repetition time) spin echo or gradient echo sequences. These images can be acquired using the body coil

or a surface coil with a large field of view. The primary purpose of these scout images is to serve as a localizer for subsequent pulse sequences.

The next set of images is acquired in the transaxial plane. Transaxial images should cover the area between the inferior glenoid fossa and the acromioclavicular joint. We routinely obtain 3-mm-thick multislice proton density–weighted spoiled gradient echo images. These images provide good visualization of the joint capsule, labrum, subscapularis muscle, and long head of the biceps. Proton density– and T2-weighted fast spin echo images are also acquired in patients with glenohumeral instability to further evaluate the biceps tendon, labrum, capsule, and glenohumeral ligaments. Additional indications for the use of transaxial T2-weighted images include suspected abnormalities of the glenohumeral joint space or associated bursae, osseous or soft-tissue masses, or injuries of the subscapularis muscle or tendon. Another purpose of transaxial images is to orient the appropriate plane for prescription of subsequent coronal oblique and sagittal oblique images.

Coronal oblique images are obtained in a plane parallel to the supraspinatus tendon. The course of the tendon is slightly oblique to the direction of the muscle fibers (Fig. 3.1), and it also diverges slightly from the plane of the glenohumeral joint. Coverage in the anterior-to-posterior direction should proceed from the subscapularis muscle and tendons anteriorly to the infraspinatus-teres minor muscles posteriorly. We routinely acquire coronal oblique images using proton density– and T2-weighted fast spin echo sequences with fat saturation. These images are the primary means of evaluation of the rotator cuff for potential tears or other abnormalities and for assessing the amount of retraction in patients with full-thickness rotator cuff tears. Coronal oblique images are also helpful for assessing the superior and inferior portions of the fibrocartilaginous glenoid labrum and the subscapularis notch (5,6).

Finally, sagittal oblique images are obtained in a plane perpendicular to that of the supraspinatus tendon. Coverage should extend from the glenoid fossa medially to the cortex of the humerus laterally. T1- and T2-weighted fast spin echo sequences are obtained at our institution, with a short echo train length used to minimize blurring. These images are useful adjuncts to the coronal oblique images for the evaluation of the rotator cuff pathology and surrounding structures. T1-weighted images permit visualization of acromial abnormalities and evaluation of alterations in site and signal intensity of the rotator cuff musculature. T2- and proton density–weighted sagittal oblique images help confirm the presence of small rotator cuff tears and to determine their extent.

Pulse Sequences

Conventional spin echo, fast spin echo, and gradient echo pulse sequences are widely used for shoulder MR imaging. Fast spin echo has replaced conventional spin echo pulse sequences in many centers. Each of these pulse sequences is discussed here, in addition to other imaging options that are available to improve image quality and/or diagnostic capability. Faster imaging sequences such as rapid/turbo/snapshot gradient echo and echo planar imaging have not yet been demonstrated to have utility in routine shoulder MR imaging. Despite the significantly shorter scanning times these sequences provide, they are often limited by relatively poor image quality due to artifacts and low spatial resolution, rendering them inadequate for thorough evaluation of the shoulder.

Conventional Spin Echo

Conventional spin echo sequences are commonly used in shoulder imaging due to their established efficacy, widespread availability, and familiarity with their use. Imaging parameters are selected in order to maximize signal-to-noise ratio, tissue contrast, and spatial resolution, while keeping artifacts and imaging times to a practical minimum. Short TR/TE T1-weighted images provide the general anatomic information and clearly depict abnormalities related to the marrow space and peribursal fat planes. These images are also used for MR arthrography. Typical parameters for T1-weighted images include TR of 400 to 600 ms, TE of 8 to 20 ms, and two to four signal averages.

Proton density–weighted images provide high signal-to-noise ratio due to the combined use of a relatively long TR and short TE. They provide high sensitivity for detection of injury to the rotator cuff and glenoid labrum-capsular complex. T2-weighted images utilize relatively long TR and TE and contribute high specificity regarding rotator cuff and other pathology. They have poor signal-to-noise ratio but are essential for visualizing soft-tissue edema, fluid collections, and for characterizing signal intensity alterations within the rotator cuff. Representative parameters for proton density– and T2-weighted images include TR of 2,200 to 3,000 ms, TE of 20 to 30 ms (first echo, proton density–weighted image) and 70 to 80 ms (second echo, T2-weighted image), and one to two signal averages.

A slice thickness of 3 to 4 mm with a 0.5- to 1-mm interslice gap is typically used. The field of view is adjusted for patient size. However, a smaller field of view has been shown to produce significant improvement in MR sensitivity for diagnosing rotator cuff tears. Therefore, the field of view should typically be 12 to 14 cm but should not exceed 16 cm at high field or 18 cm at low field. A matrix size of 192×256 is commonly prescribed, though higher-resolution matrices of up to 224×512 can be used for portions of the exam.

Fast Spin Echo

In fast spin echo imaging, the initial 90-degree excitation pulse is followed by a series of separately phase encoded 180-degree radiofrequency refocusing pulses, each of which generates an echo. Imaging time is thus decreased proportional to the echo train length, which typically ranges from 4 to 16 for shoulder imaging. The substantial time reduction that is achieved can be used to improve signal-to-noise ratio by increasing number of signal averages or to increase spatial resolution by using higher-resolution matrices.

Fast spin echo images display similar tissue contrast to that seen on conventional spin echo images. However, small lesions can be obscured by decreased edge definition when short effective TE or long echo train length settings are used. Fat appears brighter on fast spin echo than on conventional spin echo images. This increased signal can obscure small lesions that are located adjacent to fat on T2-weighted fast spin echo images. Fat saturation techniques minimize this effect. Fast spin echo images have high sensitivity to depiction of fluid. Fast spin echo images have somewhat decreased sensitivity to magnetic susceptibility effects and generally display slightly less degradation from motion due to the rephasing effects of the multiple 180-degree pulses (7).

Typical imaging parameters for T2-weighted fast spin echo sequences include TR of 3,000 to 4,000 ms, effective TE of 70 to 80 ms, two to four signal averages, 256×256 or 512×224 matrix, and an echo train length of 12 to 16. T1- and proton density–weighted images are often acquired using a short echo train length of five or less.

Gradient Echo

Gradient echo sequences offer much shorter imaging times due to their use of short TR and gradient refocusing, while maintaining adequate signal-to-noise ratio due to their use of relatively small flip angles.

Tissue contrast in gradient echo imaging depends on a number of factors: TR, TE, flip angle, number of slices per acquisition, and steady state or spoiled sequences (8,9). In steady state sequences, residual transverse magnetization from previous excitations is utilized to produce images with T2*/T1 weighting. Examples of this technique are the GRASS and FISP sequences. In spoiled sequences, residual transverse magnetization is destroyed to produce more strongly T1-weighted images. Examples include spoiled GRASS and FLASH. Use of a long TR in either of these techniques produces primarily proton density–weighted images.

In comparison to conventional spin echo imaging, gradient echo images display increased artifact from magnetic field inhomogeneities since they lack a 180-degree radiofrequency refocusing pulse. Magnetic susceptibility artifacts appear as areas of signal void with or without associated peripheral hyperintensity. These effects are seen around foci of metal, air, or calcium and are accentuated at high field strength and with long TE. Bone marrow on gradient echo images obtained with long TE has a different appearance from spin echo images. Due to the many interfaces among bony trabeculae, fat, and cells contained in bone marrow, its signal becomes relatively hypointense on gradient echo images (10). Chemical shift phase cancellation artifact is seen as decreased signal intensity at interfaces between fat and water.

This occurs with use of a field strength-specific TE when fat and water protons are out of phase with each other. At 1.5 Tesla, for example, fat and water protons are of opposed phase at 2.1 ms and every 4.2 ms thereafter.

In multislice gradient echo imaging, more than one image is acquired per TR, producing higher signal-to-noise ratio images that are generally proton density weighted. In the shoulder, gradient echo images have been primarily used for evaluation of the glenoid labrum (Fig. 3.2) (7). Multislice spoiled gradient echo images are routinely obtained in the axial plane for evaluation of the labrum. Parameters used are TR of 300 ms, TE of 15 ms, flip angle of 30 degrees, 15-cm field of view, 256 × 192 matrix, and two excitations. Use of a later echo of 20 ms or greater may also be employed to achieve greater T2* weighting and fluid contrast. Due to their complex image contrast and accentuated susceptibility artifact, gradient echo sequences have not achieved wide use for evaluation of the rotator cuff.

Imaging Options

Fat Suppression

Fat suppression can be accomplished using radiofrequency fat saturation, short tau inversion recovery, and phase contrast methods. Fat saturation is a frequency-selective technique in which fat protons are subjected to radiofrequency saturation and gradient dephasing prior to signal acquisition. Fat saturation is routinely used in many centers in the acquisition of coronal and sagittal oblique proton density– and T2-weighted images. This may allow for increased

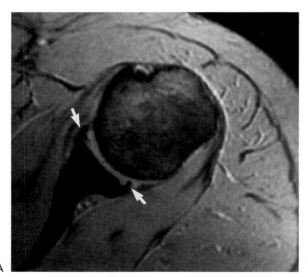
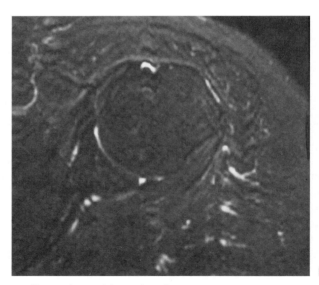

A   B

FIGURE 3.2. Comparison of labral appearance on gradient echo and fast spin echo sequences. Transaxial images depict the anterior and posterior labra. On the gradient echo image **(A)**, the labra (*arrows*) are clearly depicted as hypointense structures. They are contrasted by the high signal intensity of underlying hyaline cartilage. On the fast spin echo image **(B)**, it is difficult to identify the labra because they are isointense with surrounding structures and due to the paucity of joint fluid.

sensitivity in the detection of small amounts of fluid contained in small rotator cuff tears. The accuracy of detecting rotator cuff lesions with use of fat saturation has been reported to be 90% to 95% (11,12,13). In comparison to conventional spin echo imaging, use of fat saturation has been reported to increase the sensitivity for detecting partial tears from 67% to 92% (13).

Additional benefits of fat saturation include improved depiction of marrow abnormalities and differentiation of fluid and fat at their interface (14,15,16). It also helps minimize artifacts due to motion and chemical shift misregistration. Disadvantages of fat saturation are that it lengthens imaging time by limiting the number of slices that can be obtained in a given TR, produces unfamiliar tissue contrast, and may produce incomplete suppression of fat and/or inadvertent suppression of water-containing tissues. The effectiveness of fat saturation is decreased at low magnetic field strengths, and it is highly sensitive to local magnetic field inhomogeneities.

Short tau inversion recovery (STIR) sequences use an initial 180-degree radiofrequency inverting pulse followed by a specific inversion time selected so that fat protons recover to zero net magnetization. Following this, a standard spin echo pulse sequence is performed. In comparison to fat saturation, STIR requires longer imaging times to obtain an equivalent number of slices. However, this technique may produce more uniform fat suppression in the presence of a heterogeneous magnetic field or when imaging is performed on a low magnetic field strength system (17).

Artifact Suppression

Several imaging options are available for minimizing imaging artifacts when performing shoulder MRI. Respiratory ordered phase encoding reduces respiratory motion artifacts. A bellows device is used to monitor the patient's respiratory cycle during image acquisition. Phase encode data are retrospectively rearranged to simulate imaging during a single prolonged respiration. This technique does not significantly increase imaging time though it is not universally available. A practical strategy is to acquire relatively lengthy T2-weighted images early during the examination when the patient is most comfortable and less likely to move. One can repeat a specific sequence with the phase- and frequency-encoding gradients reoriented to verify whether observed signal alterations represent actual abnormalities or motion artifacts.

Spatial presaturation bands are useful for decreasing vascular pulsation artifacts. Radiofrequency pulses are applied outside the area of interest to decrease the signal intensity of protons flowing into the section. Gradient moment nulling or flow compensation is another technique that helps decrease vascular pulsation as well as respiratory motion artifacts. This method is primarily used in conjunction with T2-weighted sequences. Its effects are due to rephasing of moving spins at the time of echo collection.

Oversampling techniques are useful for eliminating aliasing artifacts from tissue that is located outside the prescribed field of view. Phase oversampling requires additional imaging time to acquire data from outside the field of view. No phase wrap is a method that produces similar results but does not require additional scan time. This method acquires twice the amount of data along the phase axis while simultaneously reducing the number of signal averages and discarding portions of the image located outside the field of view. It has no net effect on the signal-to-noise ratio, spatial resolution, or imaging time.

Chemical shift misregistration artifacts occur at fat–water interfaces. Low signal intensity is seen along one side of the interface and high signal intensity at the opposite margin. This artifact is observed along the frequency-encoding direction. It can be minimized when smaller voxels are used to increase resolution and with use of fat suppression techniques. Reorienting the phase and frequency encoding gradient directions displace such artifacts to another portion of the image.

Susceptibility artifacts are due to local heterogeneity in the magnetic field. These artifacts appear as signal voids, which may have increased peripheral high signal intensity. Use of fast spin echo sequences minimizes this artifact, whereas gradient echo sequences accentuate susceptibility artifact due to their lack of radiofrequency refocusing pulses.

Partial Fourier Transform

Partial Fourier reconstruction can be used to decrease imaging time by as much as 50%. With half-Fourier imaging, approximately one-half of the data lines are collected during the scan. Based on inherent data symmetry, the remaining data are then mathematically generated by a computer. This option maintains good image contrast and spatial resolution, through signal-to-noise ratio diminished by the square root of the percentage of reconstructed data (18). In addition, motion and data truncation artifacts become more prominent. This option is not routinely used in shoulder MR imaging.

Three-dimensional Fourier Transform

Three-dimensional Fourier transform can be used to acquire a volume of data that have thin slices with no interslice gap. Because phase encoding occurs along two axes, imaging time is prolonged considerably. Images can be reformatted in any orthogonal or oblique plane for better assessment of anatomy or pathology. Due to the additional phase encode steps and imaging time, motion artifact is accentuated. Therefore, this option is not routinely employed for shoulder MR imaging.

MR Arthrography

MR arthrography can be useful in the evaluation of the rotator cuff and capsulolabral complex (19). Baseline T1-

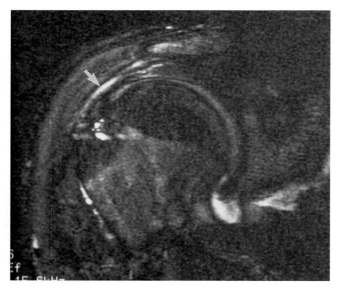

FIGURE 3.3. T2-weighted coronal oblique image obtained during MR arthrography. High signal intensity is seen in the joint space due to contrast injection. Bright signal is also appreciated in the subacromial-subdeltoid bursa (*arrow*), representing preexisting fluid, presumably relating to impingement syndrome and/or subacromial bursitis. The rotator cuff was demonstrated to be intact.

weighted images should be obtained prior to initiation of the procedure, unless fat suppression is used. Under fluoroscopy, a needle is placed into the glenohumeral joint, and a small amount of iodinated contrast is injected to verify intraarticular position. Approximately 12 to 20 ml of dilute gadopentate dimeglumine (2 ml in 250 ml saline) is injected, avoiding the introduction of air or overdistension of the joint. High-resolution T1-weighted images are then obtained in multiple imaging planes and are supplemented by T2-weighted images, usually acquired with a fast spin echo technique. Fat suppression should be used to facilitate distinction of extravasated contrast material from fatty tissue (20,21). Intraarticular saline injection followed by fast spin echo T2-weighted imaging with fat suppression is an alternative to use of paramagnetic contrast (Fig. 3.3) (20,21).

Rotator cuff tears are diagnosed on MR arthrography when contrast material is observed leaking outside the joint capsule into or through a cuff defect. In patients with a full-thickness rotator cuff tear, contrast will leak into the subacromial-subdeltoid bursa. Labral morphology can be appreciated with MR arthrography as contrast distends the joint space and outlines the fibrocartilaginous labrum.

MR arthrography is associated with increased cost, some patient discomfort, and the potential risks inherent to a mildly invasive procedure. Although it can improve depiction of some partial thickness rotator cuff tears, it is generally not utilized as a routine screening study for patients with rotator cuff symptoms. Instead, its use is reserved for patients with suspected rotator cuff tears and equivocal imag-

ing studies and for improving depiction of abnormalities related to the capsulolabral complex. It is also of benefit in evaluating patients after surgery.

Kinematic Imaging

Kinematic imaging involves acquisition of fast gradient echo images as the arm is rotated from maximal internal rotation to maximal external rotation in five to six increments. Images are obtained at each position through the superior, middle, and inferior portions of the shoulder joint. This technique allows for assessment of the anterior capsule and labrum as it is stretched taut during external rotation.

ANATOMIC VARIANTS AND DIAGNOSTIC PITFALLS

It is important to be familiar with the many common variations in shoulder anatomy that can be encountered on MR images in order to avoid diagnostic errors. Many of these variants can be mistaken for pathology if not recognized. Additionally, MR imaging techniques can be associated with technical artifacts that must also be differentiated from pathology.

Rotator Cuff

The appearance of most tendons on MR imaging is typically one of uniform hypointensity on all pulse sequences, with signal intensity similar to that of cortical bone. Foci of relatively increased signal intensity observed within the substance of such tendons are usually considered pathologic or indicative of injury (22,23). However, in the rotator cuff, areas of relative increased signal intensity are commonly observed in asymptomatic individuals and may represent normal variation and/or artifact as opposed to pathology (4,22, 24,25,26). Degenerative changes due to age, subclinical disease, partial volume averaging, and other artifacts can all contribute to foci of relative increased signal intensity within the rotator cuff.

The distal supraspinatus tendon often contains a discrete focus of relative increased signal intensity. This focus is observed in normal individuals of all ages and is located approximately 5 to 10 mm proximal to the insertion of the tendon on the greater tuberosity of the humerus (16,23). The morphology of this signal variation is round or oval with well-defined margins (Fig. 3.4). It is usually approximately 8 mm in diameter. This focus is most prominent on proton density– and T1-weighted images that are acquired in the coronal oblique plane (16). Its signal intensity is equivalent to that of skeletal muscle on all pulse sequences. Therefore, it appears relatively hypointense—though still slightly higher in signal intensity than surrounding tendon—on T2-weighted images. The appearance on T2-weighted images is

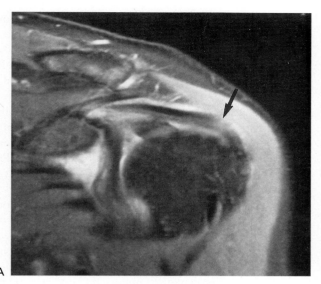
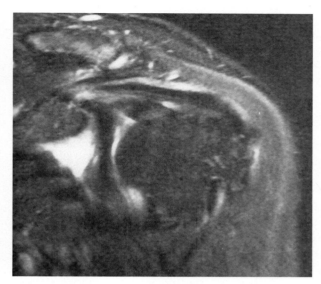

FIGURE 3.4. A: Fat-saturated proton density–weighted coronal oblique image demonstrates a focus of relative increased signal intensity within the distal supraspinatus tendon (*arrow*). **B:** The corresponding fat-saturated T2-weighted image shows reduced prominence of this focus, which is now barely perceptible.

important for distinguishing this normal variation from fluid that is bright on T2-weighted images. The presence of fluid within the rotator cuff tendons is a reliable indication of a rotator cuff tear.

Several explanations have been proposed to explain the above phenomenon. The location, size, and shape of the focus of relative increased signal intensity corresponds to that of the critical zone of the supraspinatus tendon. The critical zone is a microvascular watershed area of blood supply between branches of the anterior humeral circumflex and suprascapularis arteries (16). Therefore, this region is predisposed to low-level ischemic changes. It is thought that chronic ischemia and proximity to mechanical impingement in this region by the coracoacromial arch contribute to the high frequency of rotator cuff tears that occur in this region. The signal alteration in the critical zone may result from differences in vascularity of this area as compared with that of surrounding tendon or may be due to subclinical degenerative changes related to ischemia and/or impingement.

Another hypothesis for the signal alteration in the distal supraspinatus tendon is the "magic angle" phenomenon. When parallel collagen fibers are oriented at an angle of approximately 55 degrees relative to the main magnetic field, artifactually increased signal intensity is produced on short TE images (16). The fibers of the supraspinatus tendon begin to course anteriorly at approximately the location of observed increased signal intensity, making the magic angle theory plausible. In addition, Timins et al. have shown that the location of the foci of hyperintensity within the tendon can be changed by altering the position of the patient's arm, thereby changing the orientation of collagen fibers within the magnetic field (27).

Partial volume averaging is another explanation that has been offered to explain this focus of increased signal intensity in the supraspinatus tendon. Excessive external rotation of the arm produces partial volume averaging with fluid in the adjacent biceps tendon sheath or subscapularis bursa (1). On coronal oblique images, the resulting increased signal intensity may appear similar to that of a rotator cuff tear. T2-weighted sagittal oblique views help confirm that the high signal is actually located outside the cuff in the subscapularis bursa or biceps tendon sheath (1,28). Partial volume averaging with the infraspinatus muscle also produces relative increased signal intensity in the distal supraspinatus and/or posterior rotator cuff. Vahlensieck et al. demonstrated that partial volume averaging with such muscle is accentuated by internal rotation of the arm (29). In this position, the muscle belly of the infraspinatus is positioned superior and lateral to the supraspinatus tendon, potentially contributing to apparent increased signal within the supraspinatus tendon (1,16,17). Fat surrounding the subacromial-subdeltoid bursa can also contribute to partial volume averaging with the supraspinatus tendon. To avoid or resolve this situation, one may utilize fat suppression (11,16,23) or increase spatial resolution (11,12,13,17). Of course, nonuniform fat suppression may also contribute to foci of artifactually increased signal intensity in the region of the rotator cuff, as previously discussed.

Due to the potential for partial volume averaging to interfere with evaluation of the rotator cuff, the shoulder should be imaged with the arm in neutral or only slight external rotation. Isointensity of the observed signal focus with adjacent skeletal muscle should be observed on all pulse sequences, and T2-weighted images should be used to confirm that the focus does not demonstrate fluid intensity (16,23). Correlating findings with images acquired in alternate planes also helps avoid potential misdiagnosis (27,30).

Skeletal muscle can extend distally above or beneath the rotator cuff tendons. The relatively increased signal intensity of muscle may appear to represent diffusely increased signal intensity within the cuff tendons similar to the appearance of tendinosis (Fig. 3.5). This is most likely to occur when low spatial resolution images are acquired or when motion results in blurring and/or ghosting artifacts that obscure detail. Slips of skeletal muscle that extend distally can usually be traced back to their originating muscle belly, and their signal intensity should remain equivalent to that of skeletal muscle on all pulse sequences.

Motion artifacts that project over the rotator cuff tendons may generate alterations in signal intensity. Use of respiratory ordered phase encoding, spatial radiofrequency presaturation pulses, and gradient moment nulling can help minimize this artifact. A clue to distinction of motion artifacts from actual pathology is that the latter invariably project across the image along its phase encoding direction, and usually motion artifacts can be seen to extend beyond the confines of the rotator cuff tendons.

Muscle Tendon Junction

The musculotendinous junction of the supraspinatus is typically located superior to the apex of the humeral head on coronal oblique images. Proximal displacement of this junction provides evidence for retraction due to a full-thickness tear of the supraspinatus tendon (2,16,31). The transition between tendon and muscle is gradual, however, thereby accounting for some variation in position of the musculotendinous junction in normal subjects. Changes in arm positioning, such as increased abduction, may also cause the musculotendinous junction to be located more proximally. Typically, the musculotendinous junction is located between 11 and 1 o'clock in relation to the apex of the humerus. Regardless of arm position, it should not be located more than 15 degrees medial to the 12 o'clock position.

Although actual retraction of the musculotendinous junction is highly specific for a full-thickness rotator cuff tear, it is not very sensitive. A number of full-thickness tears—particularly smaller ones—do not demonstrate this finding, and partial thickness tears do not produce retraction (32). Therefore, musculotendinous retraction is a useful finding for the diagnosis of moderate to large full-thickness rotator cuff tears, but it is of limited usefulness in diagnosing smaller tears.

Muscle Atrophy

MR is useful for demonstrating muscle atrophy with associated fatty replacement that can result from chronic full-thickness rotator cuff tears (11). Neurological conditions such as impingement of the axillary or suprascapularis nerves

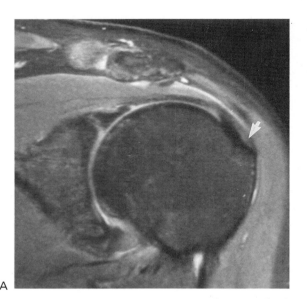
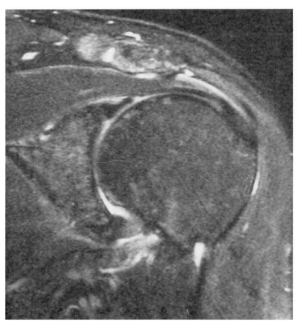

A   B

FIGURE 3.5. A: Fat-saturated proton density–weighted coronal oblique image demonstrates muscle fibers of the supraspinatus muscle (*arrow*) overlapping those of the corresponding tendon. This results in moderate signal intensity distal to the tendon at its insertion on the humerus. The corresponding fat-saturated T2-weighted image **(B)** shows continued isointensity of this signal to skeletal muscle.

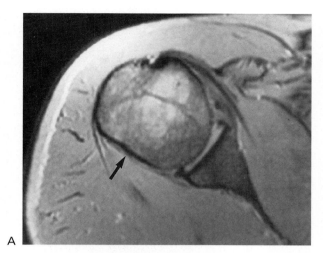 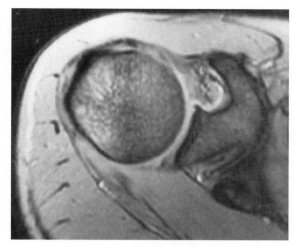

FIGURE 3.6. Proton density–weighted transaxial gradient echo image **(A)** demonstrates normal flattening of the posterolateral humeral head (*arrow*). At the level of the coracoid process **(B)**, the humeral head has a more rounded appearance.

by paralabral cysts or other masses, quadrilateral space syndrome, and neuritis can also produce atrophy of the rotator cuff musculature (2). Therefore, when atrophy of the rotator cuff muscles is observed, one must not automatically assume that it is secondary to rotator cuff tear. Instead, a careful search for other possible causes should be undertaken.

Bone and Marrow

Curvilinear low-intensity signal at the bony apophyses is observed in skeletally immature individuals (33). This could be mistaken for a fracture. Imaging of the opposite shoulder for comparison can be helpful in making the distinction in confusing cases. Curvilinear low-intensity signal is also apparent at the physeal plate on T1-weighted axial images. On T2-weighted images corresponding high signal intensity may be observed, reflecting the long T2 relaxation of hyaline cartilage and/or chemical shift misregistration at the fat–water interface (33).

Flattening of the posterolateral humeral head is a normal finding that may be confused with a Hill-Sachs impaction fracture. Normal flattening occurs just proximal to the insertion of the teres minor tendon (Fig. 3.6), and is encountered on transaxial images that are approximately 20 mm or more caudal to the proximal humeral head. Hill-Sachs lesions are more proximal in location, usually about 12 mm below the proximal humeral head (35). Depression of the humeral head at or above the level of the coracoid process should raise one's suspicion for a Hill-Sachs fracture, particularly if bone marrow edema is observed. Angular depression of the posterolateral humerus and abnormalities of the anteroinferior glenoid labrum further support a diagnosis of Hill-Sachs fracture.

Humeral head cysts are common and are characteristically located in the posterolateral humeral head in a location

similar to that of a Hill-Sachs fracture (36). A cyst at the insertion of the distal rotator cuff can also simulate a partial tear at the tendon insertion.

An anterior hooked (Type 3) acromion process has been shown to contribute to rotator cuff impingement. However, studies have shown limited correlation between the MR appearance and plain film appearance of the acromion (40). A great deal of interobserver variability exists in describing acromial morphology by MRI. The optimal plane for evaluation of the slope of the acromion process on MR images is the sagittal oblique view (41). A lateral downsloping acromion narrows the space between itself and the humerus, potentially contributing to impingement of the supraspinatus tendon (Fig. 3.7) (42). Subacromial osteophytes are also associated with rotator cuff impingement but are commonly observed in asymptomatic individuals (43). *Pseudospurs* refer to prominent fibrocartilaginous hypertrophy at the insertion of the coracoacromial ligament on the inferior portion of the acromion process (Figs. 3.7, 3.8) (2). On coronal oblique images, the inferior or superior tendon slips of the deltoid muscle can also appear similar to subacromial osteophytes (2,23). A mature osteophyte is identified by the presence of central high signal intensity marrow fat on T1-weighted images. Immature or sclerotic osteophytes may not demonstrate this finding. Accessory ossicles may be present at the superior apophysis of the glenoid or as an os acromiale (Fig. 3.9). An os acromiale is present in approximately 5% of the population as a normal variant and can contribute to impingement (2,34). Distinction of an os acromiale from the normal acromioclavicular joint is best accomplished on transaxial images that are acquired near the cephalad portion of the shoulder.

Residual hematopoietic marrow is frequently present within the glenoid and proximal humeral metaphysis of normal subjects (33,37). It produces foci of relative low signal

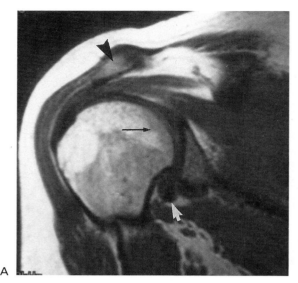 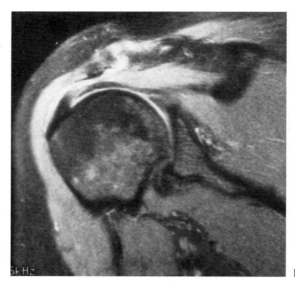

A   B

FIGURE 3.7. T1-weighted coronal oblique image **(A)** and corresponding fat-suppressed proton density–weighted image **(B)**. There is relative low signal intensity within the proximal humeral metaphysis and medial humeral epiphysis (*thin arrow*) on the T1-weighted image, representing residual hematopoietic marrow. Such marrow is mildly hyperintense on the fat-suppressed image. Also noted on these images are a laterally downsloping acromion process (*arrowhead*) and the rounded appearance of the axillary recess of the glenohumeral joint (*white arrow*).

intensity within the marrow space on T1-weighted images (Fig. 3.10). Residual hematopoietic marrow is more prominent in children, though reconverted hematopoietic marrow can be seen in adults with anemia and marrow replacement (38). Extension of hematopoietic marrow into the proximal humeral epiphysis occurs in many normal individuals. This commonly appears as a curvilinear band of relative decreased signal intensity along the medial subcortical humeral head on T1-weighted images. Less frequently, central, globular, or patchy foci of epiphyseal hematopoietic marrow are observed (33). Hematopoietic marrow should

be relatively symmetrical, hypointense relative to fatty marrow on T2-weighted images and contrast-enhanced T1-weighted images, and mildly hyperintense on T2-weighted fat saturation images (Fig. 3.7) (33,39). It should not be associated with any soft-tissue mass, cortical destruction, or medullary expansion.

Bursae and Joint Space

In normal subjects, the glenohumeral joint space usually contains 1 to 2 ml of synovial fluid (16,34,44,45) and nearly

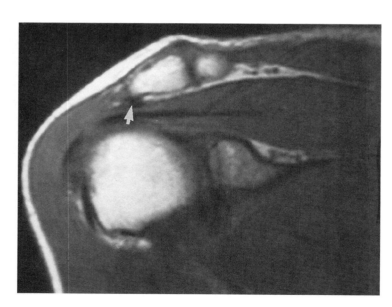

FIGURE 3.8. T1-weighted coronal oblique image demonstrates a low signal intensity structure (*arrow*) projecting from the inferior aspect of the lateral acromion. This represents a tendinous insertion, resulting in a "pseudospur" appearance.

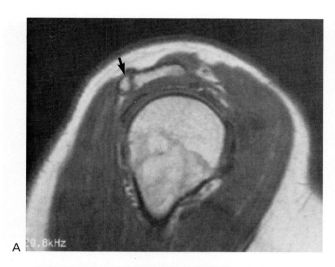

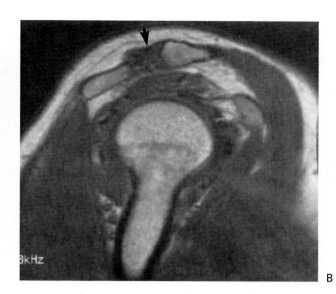

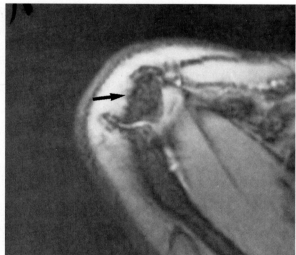

FIGURE 3.9. Sagittal oblique T1-weighted image **(A)** depicts an os acromiale (*arrow*). An adjacent lateral image **(B)** shows the normal acromioclavicular joint (*arrow*). The os acromiale (*arrow*) is well depicted on a transaxial gradient echo image **(C)** acquired near the top of the shoulder.

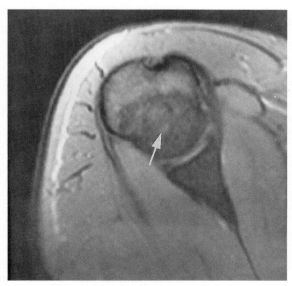

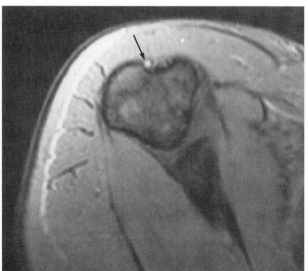

FIGURE 3.10. Transaxial proton density–weighted gradient echo image **(A)** demonstrates low-signal hematopoietic bone marrow in the humeral metaphysis (*white arrow*). An adjacent image **(B)** depicts bright signal lateral to the biceps tendon (*arrow*) representing blood flow in the humeral circumflex vessels.

always contains less than 5 ml of fluid. Distension of the ax-illary recess of the joint space indicates the presence of a joint effusion, which can be associated with a rotator cuff tear, osteoarthritis, or other inflammatory conditions (2,46). The glenohumeral joint space normally communicates with the subscapularis bursa between the superior and middle glenohumeral ligaments (26,47). The subscapularis bursa is present in 90% of individuals. The subacromial-subdeltoid bursa and the subcoracoid bursa communicate with one another. Therefore, the presence of contrast within the subacromial-subdeltoid bursa during MR arthrography may indicate a full-thickness rotator cuff tear (11,23,26), or alternatively they could be due to inadvertent injection of contrast material into the subcoracoid bursa (2). Additional bursae in the shoulder can occur as normal variants. Common locations are ventral to the subscapularis tendon and between the infraspinatus tendon and the joint capsule (2,23,26,34,47).

Fluid-filled bursae can simulate a cystic soft-tissue mass. Normally only a thin film of fluid is observed within most bursae. A small amount of fluid in the subacromial-subdeltoid bursa can be seen in normal individuals. Any significant effusion is abnormal. However, even large volumes of fluid within the subacromial-subdeltoid bursa are not specific for rotator cuff tear. Other potential etiologies include subacromial bursitis due to associated inflammation or infection (2). Bursal fluid collections are most sensitively observed on fat-suppressed T2-weighted images.

Biceps Tendon

The biceps tendon is best evaluated on axial T2-weighted fat saturation images, where it normally displays low signal intensity. Unusual variants of the biceps muscle include a third head in 12% of individuals and absence of the long head (48).

The biceps tendon sheath communicates with the gleno-humeral joint space (Fig. 3.11) (2,23). A small amount of fluid within the biceps tendon sheath is normal. In normal subjects, such fluid should be limited to the dependent portion of the sheath and should not be of sufficient volume to encircle the tendon (16,23,29,31,48). In the presence of excessive fluid, abnormalities such as tendon injury and/or inflammation should be suspected. Increased signal intensity within the lateral bicipital groove is frequently visualized on transaxial gradient echo images (Fig. 3.10) (23). This signal alteration should not be mistaken for a fluid collection or tendon injury. It is due to flow-related enhancement within the anterolateral branch of the anterior circumflex humeral artery and vein. Prominent suprascapular vessels may also exhibit flow-related signal enhancement that can mimic fluid collections. Magic angle phenomenon may cause increased signal intensity in the biceps tendon on T1- and proton density–weighted images (49) that can simulate bicipital tendinitis or partial thickness tears.

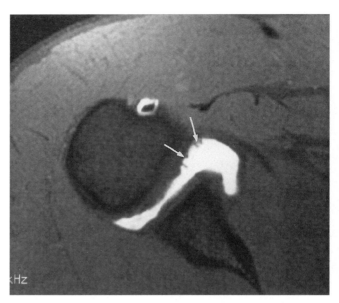

FIGURE 3.11. Transaxial fat-saturated proton density–weighted image obtained after intraarticular injection of gadolinium chelate solution demonstrates communication between the joint space and the biceps sheath. Small peripheral filling defects within the opacified joint space represent synovial folds (*arrows*).

Peribursal Fat

A peribursal fat plane parallels the subacromial-subdeltoid bursa. It appears as a curvilinear focus of increased signal intensity on T1-weighted images. Discontinuity of the fat plane can be associated with rotator cuff tears (11,23), but is also observed due to subacromial bursitis and in normal subjects (16,23,26). In rotator cuff tears, such interruption is thought to be due to edema and inflammation. However, in many normal subjects, the peribursal fat plane appears discontinuous on images acquired through its anterior extent.

Cartilage

MRI has not proven optimal for evaluation of hyaline cartilage thickness in the shoulder. Cadaver studies have revealed significant variation between observed and true cartilage thickness. It can also be difficult to distinguish hyaline cartilage from overlying muscle, particularly over the dorsal humerus where the musculotendinous junction of the infraspinatus abuts the articular surface (50).

Hyaline cartilage should appear continuous, smooth, and of uniform thickness as it parallels the bony glenoid (Fig. 3.12). Intraarticular air can mimic cartilage lesions by generating areas of signal void that are due to susceptibility artifact (51). Air may be present due to inadvertent intraarticular injection during MR arthrography or due to positioning of the arm in external rotation, which causes lower intraarticular pressure and causes dissolved blood gases to escape (51,52). Termed the *vacuum phenomenon,* this typically occurs at the

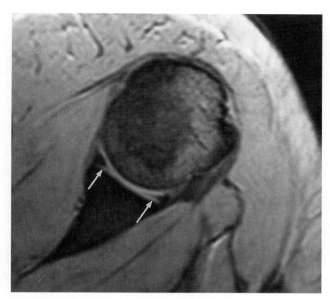

FIGURE 3.12. Transaxial gradient echo image demonstrates bright signal intensity representing hyaline cartilage (*arrows*) undercutting the relative low signal intensity fibrocartilaginous anterior and posterior labra.

superior glenohumeral joint. Such foci of air can simulate intraarticular loose bodies or chondrocalcinosis. They are not commonly seen in patients with joint effusions (52).

Labrum

The glenoid labrum is subject to considerable variation in morphology. The classically described triangular or wedge

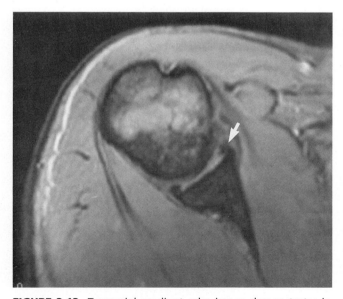

FIGURE 3.13. Transaxial gradient echo image demonstrates irregular (i.e., cleaved) morphology of the anterior labrum (*arrow*).

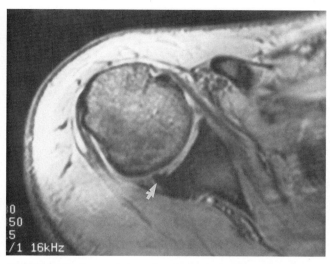

FIGURE 3.14. Transaxial gradient echo image depicts asymmetrical size of the anterior and posterior labra. In this patient, the posterior labrum (*arrow*) is larger than the anterior labrum.

shape is only seen in 45% of anterior labra and 78% of posterior labra (53). Asymptomatic individuals may demonstrate round, blunted, crescent-shaped, thin, or absent labra. Thin and absent labra may represent degenerative changes or may be secondary to recurrent subluxation or dislocation (54,55,56). Other less common variants are cleaved and notched shapes (Fig. 3.13) (53,54). Labral shape can also vary with humeral rotation. Labra also vary in size and are not always symmetrical bilaterally (Fig. 3.14) (53).

Labral tears often occur in the anterior labrum in close proximity to the insertion of the glenohumeral ligaments. A tear frequently appears as complete absence of a portion of the labrum or separation of the labrum from the underlying glenoid (57). An enlarged anterosuperior labrum that is retracted due to a tear is called the *glenoid labrum ovoid mass sign* (GLOM) (5,53, 54,57). Increased signal intensity extending through the labrum to its articular surface can also indicate a labral tear (5,36). Linear or globular foci of relative increased signal intensity within the substance of the labrum can be confused with labral tears, but they may represent normal variation or labral degeneration (58). In the absence of a tear, increased signal intensity within the labrum can also be the result from the magic angle phenomenon, particularly in the posterosuperior and anteroinferior labrum (53,54,57). This alteration is most prominent on proton density– and T1-weighted images. A spurious diagnosis of labral tear can be avoided by recognizing the characteristic location of this signal abnormality and by confirming its hypointensity on T2-weighted images (21,59).

The *Buford complex* refers to focal thickening of the middle glenohumeral ligament that attaches directly to the superior labrum just anterior to the biceps tendon (Fig. 3.15). This variant is associated with an absent anterosuperior labrum (60). The middle glenohumeral ligament can be very

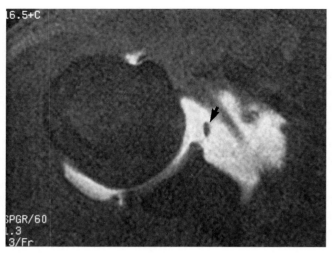

FIGURE 3.15. Transaxial fat-saturated proton density–weighted image obtained during MR arthrography demonstrates a thickened middle glenohumeral ligament (*arrow*) in a patient with the Buford complex. Note absence of the anterior labrum.

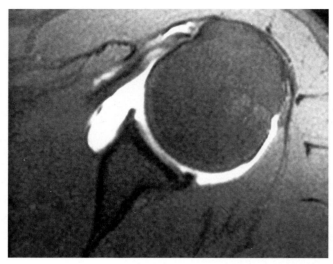

FIGURE 3.16. Transaxial fat-saturated proton density–weighted image obtained during MR arthrography demonstrates relatively medial insertion of the joint capsule on the scapular neck.

prominent and simulate a torn labral fragment (61). A dislocated biceps tendon that abuts the anterior labrum can also mimic a labral tear (57,62). Sublabral foramina where the anterosuperior labrum is focally detached are present in 8% to 12% of individuals and should not be mistaken for a tear (61). Hyaline cartilage extending beneath the labrum, often referred to as *hyaline cartilage undercutting*, is sometimes confused with changes from a labral tear due to its relatively high signal intensity (Fig. 3.12) (54,57).

Capsule

On standard MR images, the posterior capsule inserts at the tip of the labrum. In normal individuals, the posterior capsule has been demonstrated to insert at the base of the labrum using MR arthrography (47,53,56). Insertion of the anterior capsule is more variable and is classified according to its capsular attachment site on the glenoid (53,56,63). Transaxial images are optimal for visualizing the attachment site. Type 1 capsules insert at the tip of the labrum or near its base. Type 2 capsules insert more medially, but no more than 1 cm proximal to the labrum on the scapular neck. Type 3 capsules insert more than 1 cm proximally (6, 47) and may not be distinguishable from congenital or acquired anterior capsular pouches or from healed anterior capsular stripping (Fig. 3.16) (56). Type 3 capsules are generally associated with glenohumeral instability. However, a recent prospective MR arthrography series showed no correlation between joint instability and capsular insertion site (56).

Ligaments

The three glenohumeral ligaments are bands of thickened capsular tissue. The inferior and middle glenohumeral liga-

ments are the main stabilizers of the shoulder. Several normal variations are associated with the glenohumeral ligaments. For example, up to 30% of normal individuals have an absent or attenuated middle glenohumeral ligament (56). On conventional spin echo images, the glenohumeral ligaments are not easily separable from the subscapularis tendon. The superior glenohumeral ligament is seen in only 30% of conventional MR images, though it is more consistently seen on MR arthrograms (56) and in the presence of a joint effusion.

Iatrogenic Changes

Steroid or anesthetic injections produce transient increased T2 signal in the rotator cuff and adjacent soft tissues (Fig. 3.17) (64). Metal artifacts along arthroscopic tracts or related to surgical clips or sutures generate signal voids that can obscure structures or can be associated with foci of increased signal intensity in involved tissues (Fig. 3.18). Prior rotator cuff repair with tendon-to-tendon anastomosis produces increased signal intensity within the rotator cuff on proton density– and T2-weighted images and a bony trough in the humerus (28). On T2-weighted images, the increased signal intensity related to postoperative changes is usually not as high as that of fluid. Prior acromioplasty can result in flattening of the undersurface of the acromion process and decreased acromial marrow signal (26,28).

MR Arthrography

MR arthrography has improved the sensitivity and specificity of MRI for the detection of capsulolabral abnormalities (45,58,65,66). In people who have had prior surgery or reconstruction, it also provides improved diagnostic

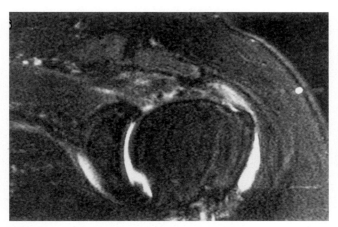

FIGURE 3.17. Fast spin echo fat-saturated T2-weighted image demonstrates abnormal foci of increased signal intensity involving the supraspinatus tendon, with fluid the overlying subacromial-subdeltoid bursa, in this patient who received local anesthetic and steroid injection 1 day earlier. Follow-up images (not shown) obtained 4 weeks later did not demonstrate any rotator cuff tear. (From Tsao LY, Mirowitz SA. MR imaging of the shoulder: imaging techniques, diagnostic pitfalls and normal variants. *Magn Reson Imaging Clin North Am* 1997;5:683–704, with permission.)

accuracy (45,64). MR arthrography is also a useful method for visualizing small articular surface partial-thickness rotator cuff tears (45,56,64,67) and allows improved depiction of the glenohumeral ligaments (45,58,65).

A sublabral foramen is observed in approximately 10% of normal individuals on MR arthrography (61,68). It is most commonly located at the base of the superior labrum and its junction with the biceps tendon, or at the base of the antero-superior labrum between the middle and superior gleno-

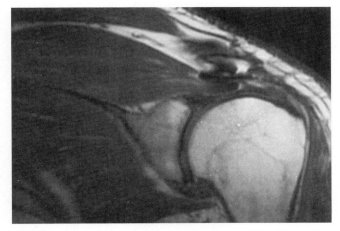

FIGURE 3.18. Multiple foci of signal void with surrounding hyperintensity are present in this patient with micrometallic fragments resulting from previous acromioplasty and rotator cuff repair. These artifacts obscure visualization of the rotator cuff and cause focal areas of increased signal intensity that can appear similar to that due to injury.

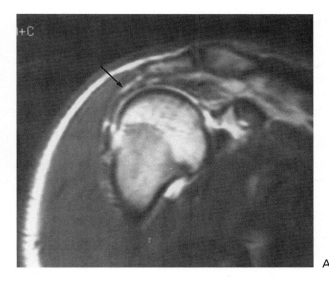

A

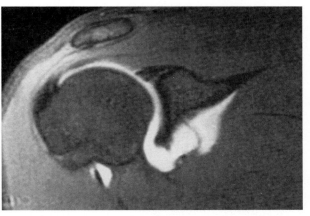

B

FIGURE 3.19. Proton density–weighted coronal oblique image **(A)** obtained after intraarticular injection of gadolinium chelate solution demonstrates high signal intensity within the joint space and in the peribursal region (*arrow*). A fat-saturated proton density–weighted image **(B)** in the oblique coronal plane demonstrates suppression of the bright signal outside the cuff, confirming that it represents peribursal fat plane rather than extravasated contrast solution due to a rotator cuff tear.

humeral ligaments. Sublabral foramina can accumulate contrast material and mimic a labral tear. Increased signal intensity can be observed at the insertion site of the inferior glenohumeral ligament due to partial volume averaging with adjacent contrast material.

Peribursal fat planes and extravasated contrast material have similar signal intensity (Fig. 3.19). Therefore, on non-fat-suppressed T1-weighted images, it may be difficult to distinguish peribursal fat from contrast that has leaked through a full-thickness rotator cuff tear. Use of fat saturation techniques allows for differentiation between these entities (69). Synovial folds may appear similar to intraarticular loose bodies (Fig. 3.11), though the former structures should be small and of uniform size (56).

REFERENCES

1. Davis SJ, Teresi LM, Bradley WG, et al. Effect of arm rotation on MR imaging of the rotator cuff. *Radiology* 1991;181:265–268.
2. Stoller DW, Wolf EM. The shoulder. In Stoller DW, ed. *Magnetic resonance imaging in orthopaedics & sports medicine.* Philadelphia: Lippincott–Raven, 1993, 511–632.
3. Glickstein MF. MR imaging of the shoulder: optimizing surface coil positioning [Letter]. *AJR* 1989;153:431–432.
4. Mirowitz SA. *Pitfalls, variants and artifacts in body MR imaging.* St. Louis: Mosby–Year Book, 1996;317–343.
5. Legan JM, Burkhard TK, Goff WE II, et al. Tears of the glenoid labrum: MR imaging of 88 arthroscopically confirmed cases. *Radiology* 1991;179:241–246.
6. Legan JM, Burkhard TK, Goff WE II, et al. Tears of the glenoid labrum: MR imaging of 88 arthroscopically confirmed cases. *Radiology* 1991;179:241–246.
7. Zlatkin MB, Bjorkengren AG, Gylys-Morin V, et al. Cross sectional imaging of the capsular mechanism of the glenohumeral joint. *AJR* 1988;150:151–158.
8. Constable RT, Anderson AW, Zhong J, et al. Factors influencing contrast in fast spin echo MR imaging. *Magn Reson Imaging* 1992;10:497–511.
9. Elster AD. Gradient-echo MR imaging: techniques and acronyms. *Radiology* 1993;186:1–8.
10. Resendes M, Helms CA, Eddy R, et al. Double-echo MPGR imaging of the rotator cuff. *J Comput Assist Tomogr* 1991;15:1077–1079.
11. Sebag GH, Moore SG. Effect of trabecular bone on the appearance of marrow in gradient-echo imaging of the appendicular skeleton. *Radiology* 1990;174:855–859.
12. Quinn SF, Sheley RC, Demlow TA, et al. Rotator cuff tendon tears: evaluation with fat-suppressed MR imaging with arthroscopic correlation in 100 patients. *Radiology* 1995;195:497–500.
13. Reinus WR, Shady KL, Mirowitz SA, et al. MR diagnosis of rotator cuff tears of the shoulder: value of using T2-weighted fat-saturated images. *AJR* 1995;164:1451–1455.
14. Songson RD, Hoang T, Dan S, et al. MR evaluation of rotator cuff pathology using T2-weighted fast spin-echo technique with and without fat suppression. *AJR* 1996;166:1061–1065.
15. Harned EM, Mitchell DG, Burk DL Jr, et al. Bone marrow findings on magnetic resonance images of the knee: accentuation by fat suppression. *Magn Reson Imaging* 1990;8:27–31.
16. Mirowitz SA, Apicella P, Reinus WR, et al. MR imaging of bone marrow lesions: relative conspicuousness on T1-weighted, fat suppressed T2-weighted, and STIR images. *AJR* 1994;162:215–221.
17. Mirowitz SA. Normal rotator cuff: MR imaging with conventional and fat-suppression techniques. *Radiology* 1991;180:735–740.
18. Tsai JC, Zlatkin MB. Magnetic resonance imaging of the shoulder. *Radiol Clin North Am* 1990;28:279–291.
19. Haacke EM, Mitchell J, Lee D. Improved contrast at 1.5 Tesla using half Fourier imaging: application to spin-echo and angiographic imaging. *Magn Reson Imaging* 1990;8:79–90.
20. Flannigan B, Kursunoglu-Brahme S, Snyder S, et al. MR arthrography of the shoulder: comparison with conventional MR imaging. *AJR* 1990;155:829–832.
21. Fritz RC, Stoller DW. Fat-suppression MR arthrography of the shoulder [Letter]. *Radiology* 1992;185:614–615.
22. Loredo R, Longo C, Salonen D, et al. Glenoid labrum: MR imaging with histologic correlation. *Radiology* 1995;196:33–41.
23. Iannotti JP, Zlatkin MB, Esterhai JL, et al. Magnetic resonance imaging of the shoulder. Sensitivity, specificity, and predictive value. *J Bone Joint Surg Am* 1991;73:17–29.
24. Kaplan PA, Bryans KC, Davick JE, et al. MR imaging of the normal shoulder: variants and pitfalls. *Radiology* 1992;184:519–524.
25. Kieft GJ, Bloem JL, Obermann WR, et al. Normal shoulder: MR imaging. *Radiology* 1986;159:741–745.
26. Zlatkin MB, Iannotti JP, Roberts MC, et al. Rotator cuff tears: diagnostic performance of MR imaging. *Radiology* 1989;172:223–229.
27. Zlatkin ME, Reicher MA, Kellerhouse LE, et al. The painful shoulder: MR imaging of the glenohumeral joint. *J Comput Assist Tomogr* 1988;12:995–1001.
28. Timins ME, Erickson SJ, Estkowski LD, et al. Increased signal in the normal supraspinatus tendon on MR imaging: diagnostic pitfall caused by the magic-angle effect. *AJR* 1995;165:109–114.
29. Owen RS, Ianotti JP, Kneeland JB, et al. Shoulder after surgery: MR imaging with surgical validation. *Radiology* 1993;186:443–447.
30. Vahlensieck M, Pollack M, Lang P, et al. Two segments of the supraspinatus muscle: cause of high signal intensity at MR imaging? *Radiology* 1993;186:449–453.
31. Tsao LY, Mirowitz SA. MR imaging of the shoulder: imaging techniques, diagnostic pitfalls and normal variants. *Magn Reson Imaging Clin North Am* 1997;5:683–704.
32. Neumann CH, Holt RG, Steinbach LS, et al. MR imaging of the shoulder: appearance of the supraspinatus tendon in asymptomatic volunteers. *AJR* 1992;158:1281–1287.
33. Rafii M, Firooznia H, Sherman O, et al. Rotator cuff lesions: signal patterns at MR imaging. *Radiology* 1990;177:817–823.
34. Mirowitz SA. Hematopoietic bone marrow within the proximal humeral epiphysis in normal adults: investigation with MR imaging. *Radiology* 1993;188:689–693.
35. Bergman RA, Thompson SA, Afifi AK, et al. *Compendium of human anatomic variation: text, atlas, and world literature.* Baltimore: Urban & Schwarzenberg, 1988:206.
36. Richards RD, Sartoris DJ, Pathria MN, et al. Hill-Sachs lesion and normal humeral groove: MR imaging features allowing their differentiation. *Radiology* 1994;190:665–668.
37. Gudinchet F, Naggar L, Ginalski JM, et al. Magnetic resonance imaging of nontraumatic shoulder instability in children. *Skeletal Radiol* 1992;21:19–21.
38. Mirowitz SA. Hematopoietic bone marrow within the proximal humeral epiphysis in normal adults: investigation with MR imaging. *Radiology* 1992;188:689–693.
39. Maniatis A, Tavassoli M, Crosby WH. Factors affecting the conversion of yellow to red marrow. *Blood* 1971;37:581–586.
40. Richardson ML, Patten RM. Age related changes in marrow distribution in the shoulder: MR imaging findings. *Radiology* 1994;192:209–215.
41. Epstein RE, Schweitzer ME, Frieman BG, et al. Hooked acromion: prevalence on MR images of painful shoulders. *Radiology* 1993;187:479–481.
42. Peh WCG, Farmer THR, Totty WG. Acromial arch shape: assessment with MR imaging. *Radiology* 1995;195:501–505.
43. Ozaki J, Fujimoto S, Nakagawa Y, et al. Tears of the rotator cuff of the shoulder associated with pathological changes in the acromion: a study in cadavers. *J Bone Joint Surg Am* 1998;70:1224–1230.
44. Needell SD, Zlatkin MB, Sher JS, et al. MR imaging of the rotator cuff: peritendinous and bone abnormalities in an asymptomatic population. *AJR* 1996;166:863–867.
45. Chandnani V, Ho C, Gerharter J, et al. MR findings in asymptomatic shoulders: a blind analysis using symptomatic shoulders as controls. *Clin Imaging* 1992;16:25–30.
46. Tirman PFJ, Bost FW, Steinbach LS, et al. MR arthrographic depiction of tears of the rotator cuff: benefit of abduction and external rotation of the arm. *Radiology* 1994;192:851–856.

47. Schweitzer ME, Magbalon MJ, Fenlin JM, et al. Effusion criteria and clinical importance of glenohumeral joint fluid: MR imaging evaluation. *Radiology* 1995;194:821–824.
48. Rafii M, Firooznia H, Golimbu C, et al. CT arthrography of capsular structures of the shoulder. *AJR* 1987;146:361–367.
49. Erickson SJ, Fitzgerald SW, Quinn SF, et al. Long bicipital tendon of the shoulder: normal anatomy and pathologic findings on MR imaging. *AJR* 1992;158:1091–1096.
50. Erickson SJ, Cox IH, Hyde JS, et al. Effect of tendon orientation on MR imaging signal intensity: a manifestation of the "magic angle" phenomenon. *Radiology* 1991;181:389–392.
51. Hodler J, Loredo RA, Longo C, et al. Assessment of articular cartilage on the humeral head: MR anatomic correlation in cadavers. *AJR* 1995;165:615–620.
52. Shogry MEC, Pope TL Jr. Vacuum phenomenon simulating meniscal or cartilaginous injury of the knee at MR imaging. *Radiology* 1991;180:513–515.
53. Patten RM. Vacuum Phenomenon: a potential pitfall in the interpretation of gradient-recalled-echo MR imaging of the shoulder. *AJR* 1994;162:1383–1386.
54. Neumann CH, Peterson SA, Jahnke AH. MR imaging of the labral-capsular complex: normal variations. *AJR* 1991;157:1015–1021.
55. McNiesh LM, Callaghan JJ. CT arthrography of the shoulder: variations of the glenoid labrum. *AJR* 1987;149:963–966.
56. Rafii M, Firooznia H. Variations of normal glenoid labrum [Letter]. *AJR* 1989;152:201–202.
57. Massengill AD, Seeger LL, Yao L, et al. Labrocapsular ligamentous complex of the shoulder: normal anatomy, anatomic variation, and pitfalls of MR imaging and MR arthrography. *Radiographics* 1994;14:1211–1223.
58. McCauley TR, Pope CF, Jokl P. Normal and abnormal glenoid labrum: assessment with multiplanar gradient-echo MR imaging. *Radiology* 1992;183:35–37.
59. Liou JTS, Wilson AJ, Totty WG, et al. The normal shoulder: common variations that simulate pathologic conditions at MR imaging. *Radiology* 1993;186:435–441.
60. Monu JUV, Pope TL, Chabon SJ, et al. MR diagnosis of the superior labral anterior posterior (SLAP) injuries of the glenoid labrum: value of routine imaging without intraarticular injection of contrast material. *AJR* 1994;163:1425–1429.
61. Williams MM, Snyder SJ, Buford D Jr. The Buford complex- the "cord-like" middle glenohumeral ligament and absent anterosuperior labrum complex: a normal anatomic capsulolabral variant. *Arthroscopy* 1994;10:241-247.
62. Tuite MJ, De Smet AA, Norris MA, et al. MR diagnosis of labral tears of the shoulder: value of T2*-weighted gradient-recalled-echo images made in external rotation. *AJR* 1995;164:941–944.
63. Patten RM. Tears of the anterior portion of the rotator cuff (the subscapularis tendon): MR imaging findings. *AJR* 1994;162:351–354.
64. Zlatkin MB, Dalinka MK, Kressel HY. Magnetic resonance imaging of the shoulder. *Magn Reson Q* 1989;5:3–22.
65. Hodler J, Kursunoglu-Brahme S, Snyder S, et al. Rotator cuff disease: assessment with MR arthrography versus standard MR imaging in 36 patients with arthroscopic confirmation. *Radiology* 1992;182:431–436.
66. Chandnani VP, Gagliardi JA, Murnane TG, et al. Glenohumeral ligaments and shoulder capsular mechanism: evaluation with MR arthrography. *Radiology* 1995;196:27–32.
67. Palmer WE, Caslowitz PL. Anterior shoulder instability: diagnostic criteria determined from prospective analysis of 121 arthrograms. *Radiology* 1995;197:819–825.
68. Palmer WE, Caslowitz PL, Chew FS. MR arthrography of the shoulder: normal intra-articular structures and common abnormalities. *AJR* 1995;164:141–146.
69. Vahlensieck M, Peterfy CG, Wischer T, et al. Indirect MR arthrography: optimization and clinical applications. *Radiology* 1996;200:249–254.
70. Palmer WE, Brown JH, Rosenthal DI. Rotator cuff: evaluation with fat-suppressed MR arthrography. *Radiology* 1993,188:683–687.

CLINICAL EVALUATION OF THE PAINFUL SHOULDER

BRIAN D. CAMERON
JOSEPH P. IANNOTTI

The prospects for successful treatment of the patient with shoulder pain are dependent on making the correct clinical diagnosis. The clinician should begin with a complete history and physical examination. The ensuing clinical evaluation should focus on identifying a mechanical problem associated with the shoulder. Once a mechanical problem has been determined, further diagnostic testing may be needed to confirm the diagnosis and define the extent of the pathology. An appropriate treatment plan can then be implemented. In most cases, this will initially consist of nonoperative measures. Immediate surgical intervention will be indicated for a narrow spectrum of patients. It will also become a reasonable treatment alternative among patients who have failed an appropriate course of conservative management. Lack of an identifiable mechanical problem will often render an unreliable surgical result (1).

Magnetic resonance imaging (MRI) has evolved into a highly useful adjunct in the clinical evaluation of the patient with shoulder pain. The exceptional contrast resolution afforded by magnetic resonance allows extensive noninvasive evaluation of the soft tissues (2). These images provide reliable diagnostic information regarding rotator cuff pathology, including the size of the tear, extent of retraction, and amount of muscle atrophy (3). This information contributes significantly to surgical planning. MRI has found significant application in identifying other pathological entities, including ganglion cysts, labral injuries, and biceps tendon lesions. The addition of MR arthrography to conventional MRI may provide more accurate information regarding labral pathology and internal glenoid impingement (4).

Despite the many benefits afforded by MRI, the potential exists for overuse and abuse (3). The clinician should be keenly aware of the inherent sensitivity and specificity of MRI in detecting occult or incidental anatomic abnormalities that are not associated with clinically significant pathology and must therefore resist the temptation to rely exclusively on the information that it provides (5,6). Instead, this data should be integrated with the patient's history and correlative physical examination (2,6). Identification of various MRI abnormalities may be of little consequence in the absence of clinical symptoms. It is appropriately ordered when it provides information that is not available from plain radiographs and clinical examination, and when this information will affect patient management (3).

COMMON DISORDERS OF THE SHOULDER

Although rotator cuff disease and glenohumeral instability comprise a large proportion of the patient population, many other discrete disease states also result in shoulder pain. Table 4.1 lists, by anatomic region, the most common causes of shoulder girdle pain. The causes of shoulder pain in a specific patient can often be attributed to more than one of these problems.

The normal function of the shoulder girdle is based on the interrelationship of its various parts. The shoulder girdle is composed of three diarthrodial joints (glenohumeral, acromioclavicular, and sternoclavicular), two bursal articulations (scapulothoracic and acromiohumeral), four major muscle groups (scapulothoracic, thoracohumeral, scapulohumeral, and claviculohumeral), and four sets of ligaments (glenohumeral, acromioclavicular, coracoclavicular, and sternoclavicular). The pathological interrelationship of these component parts of the shoulder can result in complex causes of shoulder pain. The complexity arises when a primary disorder secondarily results in pathomechanics or pathology in other structures. These secondary abnormalities will often contribute symptoms to the pain syndrome. The overall presentation of the painful shoulder can therefore be complex.

Recurrent and frequent episodes of glenohumeral instability can often result in pain from secondary rotator cuff tendonitis or rotator cuff tears (7). Chronic rotator cuff disease can often result in loss of glenohumeral motion, thereby mimicking the clinical findings of adhesive capsulitis. Less commonly, chronic rotator cuff tears can result in pain secondary to glenohumeral arthropathy. In addition, rotator cuff problems are often associated with clinically significant acromioclavicular joint (AC) joint arthropathy and/or biceps tendonitis, biceps degeneration, or rupture (8). Adhesive capsulitis as one cause of decreased shoulder motion (frozen shoulder) can also present with clinical findings of rotator cuff tendonitis. Chronic cervical radiculopathy or brachial plexus injury can often result in abnormalities of

TABLE 4.1. COMMON CAUSES OF SHOULDER PAIN

I. GLENOHUMERAL ARTICULATION AND CAPSULE
  Recurrent instability
  Multidirectional
  Voluntary
  Involuntary traumatic
  Involuntary atraumatic
  Articular cartilage degeneration
  Rheumatoid arthritis
  Osteoarthritis
  Post-traumatic
  Recurrent instability
  Crystal-induced arthropathy
  Neuropathic
  Septic
  SLAP lesions
  Biceps tendon
    Tendinitis
    Instability
  Osteonecrosis
  Adhesive capsulitis and frozen shoulder syndromes
  Proximal humeral fractures
II. ROTATOR CUFF
  Tendinitis
    Rotator cuff tears
      Partial and complete
    Internal glenoid impingement
    Coracoid impingement
    Calcific tendinopathies
III. ACROMIOCLAVICULAR JOINT
  Dislocations; distal clavicle fractures and nonunions
  Degenerative joint disease
  Os acromiale
IV. SCAPULA
  Fractures; nonunion; malunion
  Osteochondroma
  Snapping scapula syndrome
V. BRACHIAL PLEXUS & CERVICAL SPINE
  Cervical degenerative disc disease
  Thoracic outlet syndrome
  Traumatic and viral brachial plexus injuries
  Isolated entrapment neuropathies
    Suprascapular
    Ganglion cyst
    Axillary
VI. STERNOCLAVICULAR JOINT
  Instability
  Degenerative joint disease
  Clavicular fractures and growth plate injuries

the synchronized scapulothoracic and glenohumeral motion that occurs during elevation of the arm (9). These abnormalities of shoulder kinematics can result in scapular lag and secondary rotator cuff tendonitis.

A complete understanding of the etiology of a patient's shoulder pain can only come from an understanding of the complex normal anatomic and kinematic relationships of the component parts of the shoulder girdle and the interrelationship of the pathological conditions that alter these relationships. The complete diagnosis of an individual's shoulder pain comes from the integrated use of a careful history and physical examination and the careful interpretation of the anatomic and pathological findings of the diagnostic studies. It is also important from a clinical standpoint to understand the anatomic changes that often occur with the aging process or subsequent to prior surgical intervention. These secondary changes may not play a significant role in an individual patient's pain; therefore, their clinical relevance must be placed into perspective.

ETIOLOGY AND PATHOLOGY OF ROTATOR CUFF DISEASE

Disorders of the rotator cuff are the most common causes of a painful shoulder (10). These disorders include impingement, partial- and full-thickness rotator cuff tears, calcific tendinitis, and coracoid impingement. The pathomorphological changes of the rotator cuff are probably multifactorial, including intrinsic and extrinsic factors. Important etiologic considerations include age-related degeneration, acute trauma, repetitive microtrauma, anatomic impingement, and secondary impingement associated with either glenohumeral instability or capsular contracture. Other pathologic entities that may represent additional sources of pain in association with rotator cuff pathology include acromioclavicular arthropathy, biceps tendinitis, and frank rupture of the long head of the biceps tendon. Pain related to nerve root, brachial plexus, or peripheral nerve lesions should be thoroughly evaluated and differentiated from primary shoulder pathology.

The natural history of progression from tendinitis to partial- and full-thickness rotator cuff tears is controversial and incompletely understood. Most studies reveal that the pathology associated with overuse or microtrauma is fairly age related and may represent progression of the disease (5, 11,12). Tendinitis or tendinosis is generally seen among patients under the age of 40 (13). Partial-thickness rotator cuff tears are predominantly seen in the fifth and sixth decades, while full-thickness rotator cuff tears generally appear in the population over 60 years old. Partial-thickness rotator cuff tears, whether due to repetitive motion, trauma, or age-related degeneration, are most commonly seen on the articular surface of the tendon (13–17). Although some of these partial-thickness rotator cuff tears may have the potential to heal, more than 50% will continue to enlarge over time, and almost 30% will progress to become full-thickness cuff tears after 1 year (13,18). It is uncertain whether this progression becomes clinically apparent.

The severity of rotator cuff pathology is variable. The impingement syndrome as described by Neer is not a singular condition, but rather a progressive continuum of pathologic changes. Most authors divide these pathologic changes into three stages (8,19,20). The most mild changes (Stage I) are associated with inflammation of the rotator cuff tendons and overlying bursa. The second stage includes fibrosis and degenerative changes of the cuff tendons. The third stage includes rotator cuff tear, biceps tendon rupture, and bone changes. The supraspinatus tendon is especially susceptible to anatomic and age-related degenerative factors that may result in tearing of the tendon. In each of these three stages, the supraspinatus tendon is most commonly and severely affected. Full-thickness tears of the supraspinatus tendon are most commonly a result of degenerative changes. Similar stages of disease can occur in the long head of the biceps tendon and are usually related to the same underlying pathologic condition that causes the rotator cuff pathology (21,22).

Microvascular injection studies reveal a hypovascular critical zone in the supraspinatus tendon near its insertion site to the greater tuberosity (13,21,23,24). The vascularity in this region also appears to diminish with age. Relative hypoperfusion of this area has been demonstrated with the arm in the adducted position as well as while lifting a 1-kg weight above shoulder level, indicating that the vascular compromise may be transient and dynamic as related to daily functional activities of the shoulder (24). The articular surface of the cuff is hypovascular relative to the bursal surface, resulting in a higher incidence of partial-thickness rotator cuff tears on the articular surface of the cuff (24,25). Histological studies reveal diminished tendon cellularity, loss of cellular staining, and collagen fragmentation in conjunction with advanced age (10,26). Further studies show that a thinner, less uniform arrangement of collagen bundles near the articular surface leads to an ultimate strength that is half that of

the bursal portion of the tendon. This may also predispose the tendon to a higher incidence of articular surface partial thickness tears (13,27).

Many authors attribute rotator cuff injury to extrinsic anatomic factors such as coracoacromial arch narrowing (20, 24,28). The components of the osteoligamentous arch are the acromion, coracoacromial ligament, and the coracoid process. The acromion has been classified into three distinct morphological shapes (Fig. 4.1): Type I, flat; Type II, curved; Type III, hooked. These types form a continuum from flat to hooked, and in many cases a significant amount of interobserver variability exists (29). Impingement lesions and rotator cuff tears are more commonly associated with a curved or hooked acromion (24). Age-related proliferative spur formation on the undersurface of the acromion and AC joint results in narrowing of the rigid boundaries within which the supraspinatus tendon resides. There is a strong correlation between degenerative hypertrophic spur formation and the incidence of full-thickness rotator cuff tears (24). Histological changes on the bursal surface of the acromion have been detected in association with bursal side rotator cuff tears, suggesting that bursal side tears are related to subacromial spurs (13). Other authors feel that a lower resistance to shear stresses on the articular layer of the cuff in association with coracoacromial arch narrowing can result in either bursal or articular side rotator cuff tears (13). Although there is a strong correlation between hypertrophic spur formation and rotator cuff tearing, debate persists on whether the hypertrophic changes are the cause or the result of the rotator cuff lesion (24). The coracoacromial (CA) ligament is generally not felt to be a primary cause of the impingement syndrome, although thickening and fraying of the CA ligament precedes bony spur formation, and pathologic changes in the CA ligament are associated with the early stages of the impingement syndrome.

Variations in the acromial angle, or "acromial tilt," will affect the volume of the coracoacromial arch (Fig. 4.2) (28,30). A low-lying acromion has been shown to narrow the coracoacromial outlet and has been related to a higher incidence of impingement lesions and rotator cuff tears

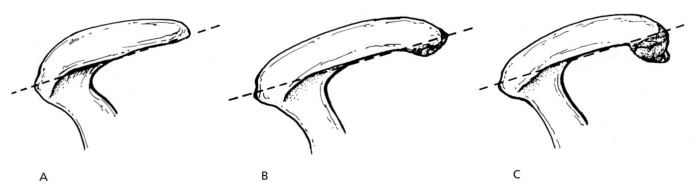

A   B   C

FIGURE 4.1. Types of acromial morphology. **A:** Type I, or flat acromion; **B:** Type II, or curved acromion; **C:** Type III, or hooked acromion. (Redrawn from McConville OR, Iannotti JP. Partial thickness rotator-cuff tears. *JAAOS* 1999;7[1]:32–43.)

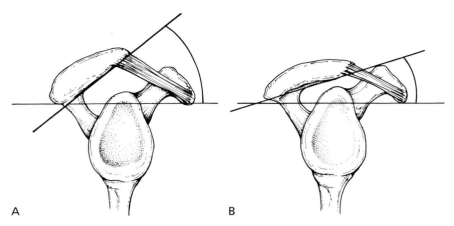

FIGURE 4.2. Variations in acromial tilt. **A:** An acromion with increased inclination, or tilt, will result in a larger subacromial outlet. **B:** An acromion with decreased tilt will result in a decreased subacromial outlet. (Redrawn from Herzog RJ. Magnetic resonance of the shoulder. *J Bone Joint Surg* 1997;79A[6]: 934–953.)

(24). A developmental failure of one of the acromial centers of ossification to fuse will result in an os acromiale (Fig. 4.3). This developmental abnormality occurs in 2% of the population and is seen bilaterally 60% of the time. The unfused segment, with its proliferation of fibrocartilage on the undersurface, is pulled downward by the deltoid. The coracoacromial outlet is thus effectively narrowed, leading to attritional changes in the rotator cuff (24).

The anatomic morphology of the coracoid process may occasionally be such that the tip extends lateral to the plane of the glenohumeral joint. With the arm in extreme adduction and internal rotation, the biceps and subscapularis tendons may become mechanically irritated due to this "coracoid impingement" (24).

Overuse syndromes occur in overhead-throwing athletes, swimmers, and overhead laborers. This repetitive microtrauma results in rotator cuff tendinopathy (11). Repetitive overhead activities bring the greater tuberosity and supraspinatus tendon into close proximity with the coracoacromial arch. Arm position, loading conditions, number of repetitions, and duration of activity are interrelated factors that may contribute to tendon pathology. These repetitive overhead factors probably act in concert with preexisting disease, such as supraspinatus outlet narrowing and age-related

tendon degeneration, to lead to the development of symptomatic subacromial impingement.

Tensile overload of the rotator cuff may follow acute trauma as well as repetitive microtrauma. First-time traumatic anterior dislocators over 40 years old have a 40% to 60% incidence of acute rotator cuff tears (24). Acute tearing of the rotator cuff in older individuals often occurs in the presence of tendon degeneration and may extend through a previously asymptomatic rotator cuff tear (12). Acute lesions in younger individuals often occur following a violent traumatic episode in otherwise normal tendon tissue. Trauma more often leads to articular surface tears than bursal surface tears (13,31).

Impingement may be secondary to a dynamic mechanism. Lesions affecting the muscular balance of either the rotator cuff or scapulothoracic articulation result in functional impingement syndrome and overuse of the rotator cuff musculature (24). Chronic symptoms of rotator cuff tendinitis in this patient population can result from inadequate strengthening, stretching, or biomechanics of the shoulder. Among patients with impingement syndrome, there is increased superior translation of the humeral head with active forward elevation of the arm. This may be attributed to poorly conditioned dynamic stabilizers. In throwing athletes,

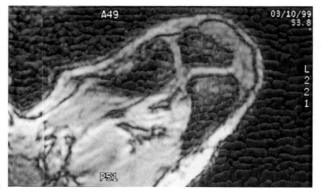
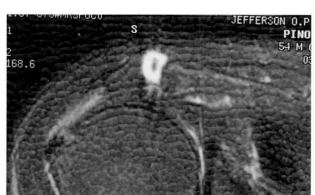

FIGURE 4.3. Meso os acromiale **(A)** with an associated rotator cuff tear **(B)**.

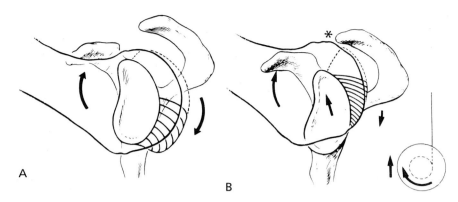

A

B

FIGURE 4.4. A: Normal capsular laxity allows the humeral head to remain centered during forward elevation of the arm. **B:** Posterior capsular tightness leads to obligate superior translation during forward elevation of the arm, similar to the climbing effect of a yo-yo. (From Matsen FA III, Arntz CT. Subacromial impingement. In: Rockwood CA Jr., Matsen FA III, eds. *The shoulder.* Philadelphia: WB Saunders, 1990, Vol. II:623–646, with permission.)

glenohumeral instability leads to traction stress on the rotator cuff, and this repetitive microtrauma leads to undersurface tearing of the rotator cuff (32,33). Alternatively, subtle anterior glenohumeral instability may lead to "internal impingement" between the articular surface of the supraspinatus tendon and the posterior superior glenoid margin (13,34, 35). On the other end of the spectrum, posterior capsular tightness can result in tendinitis of the rotator cuff (9). Posterior capsular contracture contributes to subacromial impingement by causing obligate anterosuperior translation of the humeral head during forward elevation of the arm (Fig. 4.4). This dynamic cephalad migration forces the humeral head against the anteroinferior acromion. Finally, scapulothoracic dysrythmia, or scapular lag, is evident when poor muscular control or paralysis of the scapular stabilizers prevents the acromion from rotating with the humerus (Fig. 4.5) (36). The resulting decrease in acromiohumeral distance produces mechanical impingement (24).

Calcific tendinitis, rheumatoid arthritis, and crystal induced synovitis can result in inflammatory conditions of the rotator cuff. Calcific tendinitis is a cell-mediated deposition of calcium into an area of fibrocartilaginous metaplasia of the tendon, generally the supraspinatus (24,37). During the avascular formative phase, the calcium salts are deposited within the substance of the tendon tissue. Edema, cellular proliferation, and increased vascularity accompany the resorptive phase. Increased intratendinous pressure quickly leads to the acute onset of severe pain. Large deposits of calcium and localized edema within the rotator cuff or subacromial bursa may also become a source of mechanical impingement.

Space-occupying material such as foreign bodies or surgical hardware may result in mechanical impingement. In addition, prominence of the greater tuberosity resulting from malunion of a proximal humerus fracture, or inferior placement of a humeral head prosthesis, will result in impingement. In these clinical situations, surgical correction of the mechanical impingement should address the specific etiologic factor associated with narrowing of the subacromial space.

Many causes for pathology are associated with the rotator cuff. Each of the different etiologies will result in a clinical presentation of rotator cuff–related pain associated with use of the arm at or above shoulder level. This clinical presentation is often termed the *impingement syndrome,* as it describes pain that is associated with positive impingement signs and a positive impingement test. It is critically important to understand that although all of the many causes of rotator cuff symptoms result in this clinical presentation, only a small number are associated with mechanical compromise and diminution of the space beneath the coracoacromial arch. It is only in these few etiologic entities that surgery to alter and decompress the coracoacromial arch is appropriate. Only in these specific instances with significant and chronic symptoms, which are refractory to nonoperative

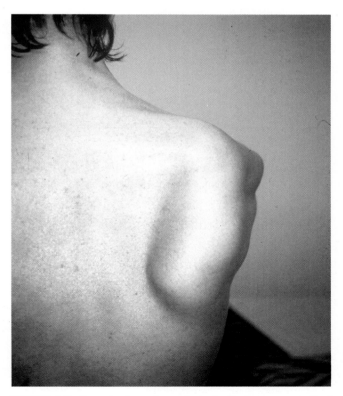

FIGURE 4.5. Scapular (serratus anterior) winging as a result of long thoracic nerve palsy.

TABLE 4.2. CAUSES OF ROTATOR CUFF DISEASE

I. TRAUMA
    Acute high velocity
    Acute rotator cuff tears
       Partial and complete
    Overuse related syndromes
       Athletic and work injuries
       Recurrent glenohumeral instability
    Acromioclavicular; coracoid
       Malunion
       Nonunion
       Separations
    Acute tendon rupture long head biceps

II. DEGENERATIVE
    Proliferative and degenerative changes
       Acromion
       AC joint
       Greater tuberosity
    Intrinsic degenerative and senescent changes
    Calcific tendinitis

III. INFLAMMATORY
    Rheumatoid arthritis
    Crystal arthropathy
    Calcific tendinitis

IV. DEVELOPMENTAL
    Os acromiale
    Coracoid malformation
    Type II and Type III acromion

V. SCAPULOTHORACIC DYSFUNCTION
    Long thoracic nerve palsy
    Spinal accessory nerve palsy
    Scapulofacial muscular dystrophy
    Chronic cervical spine disease

VI. SCAPULOHUMERAL NEUROMUSCULAR LESIONS
    Entrapment syndrome
    Suprascapular nerve
       Axillary nerve

VII. IATROGENIC OR ACQUIRED
    Hardware placement
    Foreign materials
    Inferior placement of humeral prosthesis

management, should surgery be recommended. Table 4.2 lists the various etiologies associated with rotator cuff disease.

DIAGNOSIS OF ROTATOR CUFF TENDONOPATHIES

Clinical Presentation and Symptoms

As is usually the case in medicine, a complete history sets the foundation for an accurate diagnosis. The patient age, activity level, location of pain, occupation, and history of acute or repetitive trauma are important variables that should be obtained.

Age is an etiologic factor in the development of the impingement syndrome and may help the clinician sort out the severity of pathology. Excluding the presence of repetitive motion or acute trauma, impingement is more commonly

seen after the third decade of life. Rotator cuff tears are uncommon in asymptomatic individuals under the age of 40, but they become more prevalent with increasing age. Asymptomatic partial-thickness rotator cuff tears are most predominant (24%) in patients between the ages of 40 and 60 years, while partial- and full-thickness rotator cuff tears are equally common (28%) in patients over the age of 60. When a symptomatic tear occurs in this elderly population, there is a 50% incidence of a contralateral full-thickness tear of the rotator cuff.

Pain is the predominant symptom associated with rotator cuff pathology and is usually located over the anterior, superior, and lateral aspects of the shoulder (24). The pain is often referred to the level of the deltoid tuberosity and is rarely associated with pain distal to the elbow. These symptoms may also be accompanied by fatigue, weakness, crepitus, and decreased range of motion. Pain is generally minimal with the arm at rest in a neutral and supported position. The pain is typically exacerbated with overhead reaching, especially when lifting against resistance. Night pain is commonly associated with rotator cuff pathology, often waking the patient from sleep or preventing the patient from sleeping on the affected side. In chronic conditions affecting the rotator cuff, pain in the area of the posterior deltoid and trapezius may occur. Crepitation, when present, is generally noted with elevation of the arm and is more commonly associated with full-thickness rotator cuff tears (24). Weakness may be a manifestation of either pain inhibition or muscular fatigue. True weakness will often present as an inability to raise the arm above the shoulder level. Decreased range of motion may be secondary to pain or weakness of the rotator cuff, but it also may be a manifestation of capsular contracture. A posterior capsular contracture of 10 to 15 degrees is common with the impingement syndrome and primary rotator cuff disease (24).

Axial neck pain is not commonly associated with isolated rotator cuff pathology. If periscapular pain is primarily related to rotator cuff pathology, it is exacerbated by motion of the shoulder but not the neck. Acromioclavicular and subacromial injection studies reveal that irritation of the AC joint produces pain over the joint itself, along the anterolateral neck, deltoid, and trapezius–supraspinatus region, whereas subacromial irritation produces pain in the lateral acromion, deltoid, and infrequently in the forearm or fingers (38). Pain below the level of the elbow, in association with symptoms of paresthesia or dysesthesia, is usually associated with cervical, brachial plexus, or peripheral nerve lesions and is not associated with isolated rotator cuff pathology.

Physical Findings

A directed but thorough physical examination of the shoulder and upper extremity is essential to making the proper diagnosis and instituting appropriate treatment methods (24). This evaluation begins with simple visual inspection of symmetry of the deltoid contour and posterior aspect of the shoulder.

The degree of muscular atrophy in the supraspinatus and infraspinatus fossae should be noted. Mild atrophy may be seen with chronic rotator cuff disease, while moderate to severe atrophy is usually associated with chronic, large rotator cuff tears, suprascapular nerve injury, or brachial plexus injury.

The severity of palpable tenderness may be variable, but it is usually commensurate with the degree of pain that the patient is experiencing. When acute tenderness is present in association with acute inflammation, swelling, or erythema, the clinician should begin to consider calcific tendinitis, infection, or an inflammatory soft-tissue process (24). Most patients with primary rotator cuff disease will have some degree of mechanical tenderness over the anterolateral aspect of the acromion, anterior aspect of the greater tuberosity, and bicipital groove. In chronic states, palpable crepitus over the superior aspect of the shoulder can usually be elicited by rotation of the shoulder with the arm in 90 degrees of elevation, and it is suggestive of a full-thickness tear of the rotator cuff. A palpable defect at the anterior aspect of the greater tuberosity occasionally is detectable in these individuals with a full-thickness rotator cuff tear (24). If clinically significant degenerative changes of the AC joint are associated with rotator cuff pathology, then tenderness can also be elicited over this area. (24) Tenderness over the acromioclavicular joint may also represent an isolated finding in the absence of rotator cuff pathology. Tenderness over the supraspinatus or infraspinatus muscle bellies may reflect a suprascapular nerve injury. Tenderness over the quadrangular space (bounded by the teres major, teres minor, long head of the triceps, and humeral shaft) may indicate an axillary nerve injury. Tenderness over the area of the trapezium, occiput, or medial scapula may represent a myofascial etiology rather than mechanical rotator cuff pathology.

Active and passive range of motion should be determined in all planes. The six positions that we record are forward elevation, external rotation at the side, internal and external rotation in 90 degrees of scapular abduction, cross body adduction, and internal rotation behind the back. Decreased active elevation of the arm, with normal passive range of motion, may indicate a massive tear of the rotator cuff or a nerve lesion. Occasionally, apparent weakness in external rotation or forward elevation may be related to pain inhibition rather than true weakness. A subacromial injection of 10 cc of lidocaine will often alleviate the pain and allow an accurate estimation of active motion.

Symmetrical loss of both active and passive rotation (in the absence of previous surgery) indicates adhesive capsulitis or capsular contracture. Posterior capsular contracture is a common manifestation of rotator cuff disease and results in a restriction of internal rotation both at 90 degrees of abduction and behind the back. There will also be a limitation of cross body adduction. A subacromial lidocaine injection may be required to differentiate true loss of motion from pain inhibition.

Lag Signs

The external rotation lag sign as described by Hertel et al. represents a mismatch of active and passive ranges of motion (Fig. 4.6) (39). The arm is passively brought into terminal passive external rotation with the elbow at the side. The examiner then asks the patient to actively maintain the arm in this position. Inability to maintain the arm in external rotation is highly suggestive of a full-thickness tear of either the supraspinatus tendon or the posterior cuff. The external rotation lag sign is almost always negative in the presence of tendinitis or a partial thickness rotator cuff tear.

The internal rotation lag sign assesses the integrity of the subscapularis. The patient's arm is internally rotated behind the back so that the hand rests on the ipsilateral lumbosacral area. The examiner then lifts the hand off of the patient's body, into maximal passive internal rotation. Inability to actively maintain the hand in this position constitutes a positive lift off sign. The subscapularis may alternatively be assessed using the abdominal compression test (Fig. 4.7), whereby the patient is asked to compress the abdomen with

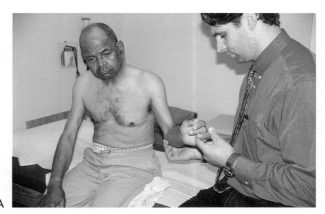
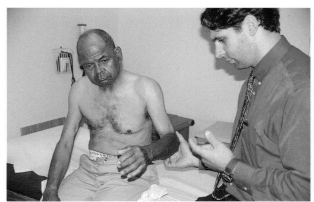

FIGURE 4.6. External rotation lag sign. The arm is passively externally rotated **(A)**. Failure to actively maintain full external rotation **(B)** is indicative of a large rotator cuff defect.

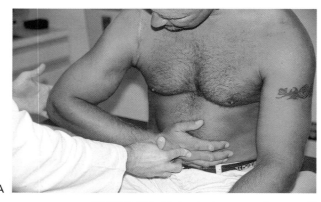
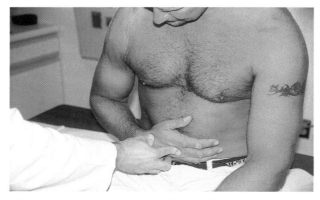

A   B

FIGURE 4.7. Abdominal compression test. The hand is placed on the abdomen with the elbow anterior to the coronal plane **(A)**. Inability to maintain the elbow anteriorly in the coronal plane **(B)** indicates subscapularis insufficiency.

an open palm, while bringing the elbow anterior to the coronal plane. Failure to maintain this posture denotes subscapularis insufficiency (Fig. 4.8).

A final lag sign that we incorporate to evaluate the posterior cuff is the Hornblower's sign (Fig. 4.9). The arm is passively brought into 90 degrees of abduction and full external rotation. While the examiner supports the elbow, the patient is asked to maintain maximal external rotation. Any loss of active external rotation represents weakness of the posterior rotator cuff. One caveat of the test is that if the arm is allowed to extend posterior to the scapular plane, the patient with mild external rotation weakness from a rotator cuff tear will be able to maintain external rotation by recruiting a larger contribution of muscle force from the posterior deltoid. This will give a falsely negative lag sign. All of the lag signs should be performed bilaterally to determine relative asymmetry.

Impingement Signs

Pain over the anterolateral and superior aspects of the shoulder can be elicited or exacerbated by the impingement signs.

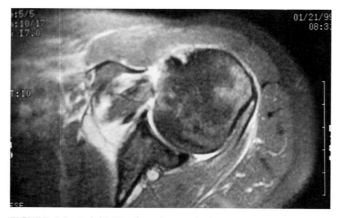

FIGURE 4.8. Axial MRI of a subscapularis tear.

Several impingement signs have been described (24,19). The classic impingement sign as described by Neer provokes pain as the arm is passively forward elevated in the sagittal plane (Fig. 4.10). When pain is elicited at the maximal extent of the flexion arc, the sign is considered positive. The Hawkins reinforcement test places the patients' shoulder in 90 degrees of abduction and 30 degrees of flexion (in the horizontal plane) (Fig. 4.11). Pain is provoked as the arm is then internally rotated to bring the greater tuberosity beneath the anterior aspect of the acromion. The classic Jobe sign places the outstretched arm in 90 degrees of scapular abduction and full internal rotation (Fig. 4.12). Pain that is elicited when downward resistance is applied to the arm represents rotator cuff disease. The cross body adduction test places the patient's shoulder in 90 degrees of abduction and 90 degrees of horizontal flexion. The examiner then further flexes the shoulder. If pain is elicited, the patient is questioned regarding the location of pain. Pain in the acromioclavicular region may represent arthropathy of this joint. Pain in the coracoid or biceps region may represent coracoid impingement. Pain in the posterior aspect of the shoulder may represent either posterior capsular contracture or posterior labral pathology.

The impingement test is performed by injection of 8 to 10 cc of lidocaine into the subacromial space (24). Use of corticosteroid is often injected with the impingement test as a means to decrease inflammation and provide long-term improvement of the symptoms. The impingement test is considered positive if there is at least a 50% improvement in the pain when the impingement signs are repeated (24). This improvement is noted within 5 to 10 minutes after injection of the local anesthetic. To perform this test properly, the examiner must carefully examine the patient both prior to and after injection, and he or she should make a specific effort to quantitate the pain associated with the impingement signs. The impingement test is always positive when pain is associated with the impingement signs and is secondary to clinically significant rotator cuff pathology. This assumes that the injection has been properly placed into the subacromial

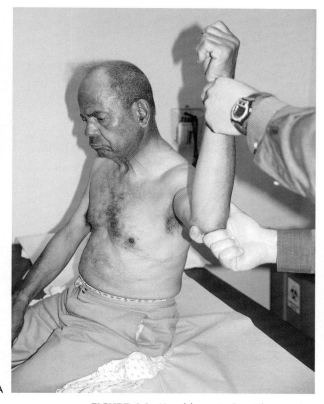
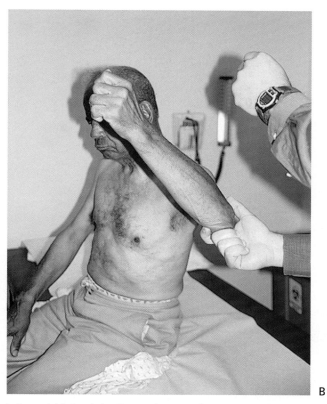

A   B

FIGURE 4.9. Hornblower's sign. The arm is passively brought into abduction and external rotation **(A)**. Failure to maintain full external rotation of the abducted arm **(B)** indicates a large posterior rotator cuff defect.

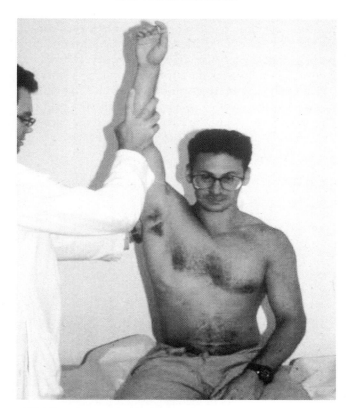

FIGURE 4.10. Neer impingement sign.

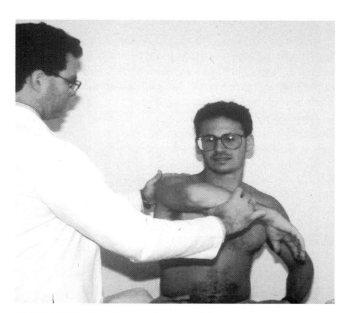

FIGURE 4.11. Hawkins reinforcement test.

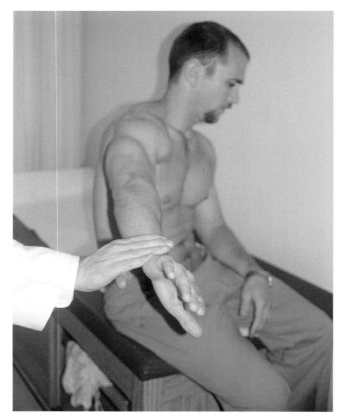

FIGURE 4.12. Jobe test will frequently elicit pain when rotator cuff pathology is present.

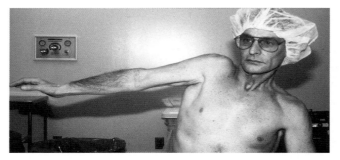

FIGURE 4.13. Shrug sign is seen with a large uncompensated or massive rotator cuff tear.

space. Of all the clinical tests available, the impingement test is the most specific in ascribing the shoulder pain to rotator cuff pathology. The impingement test is usually a predictor of the improvement in pain that will be afforded by subacromial decompression and rotator cuff repair (12).

Commonly associated findings with rotator cuff tears include weakness with abduction or external rotation. Weakness is most reliably tested in the nonimpingement arcs after partial improvement of the pain following lidocaine injection in the subacromial space (impingement test). Chronic large tears of the rotator cuff often present with atrophy in both the supra- and infraspinatus fossa. Some patients with large unbalanced tears of the rotator cuff will demonstrate the "drop arm sign," which is failure to actively resist gravity after the arm is passively forward elevated (24). The "shrug sign" is apparent in these patients because they are unable to initiate forward elevation of the arm (Fig. 4.13).

Associated Pathology

Evaluation of the biceps includes examination of the contour of the muscle belly in both a passive and contracted posture. Distal retraction is seen with frank rupture of the long head of the biceps. Rupture of the long head of the biceps tendon is commonly associated with the impingement syndrome

and concomitant rotator cuff pathology. Biceps tendon rupture under these conditions is usually associated with the older patient population, and it is usually secondary to attritional changes in the tendon. Pain originating from the long head of the biceps is usually relieved following rupture of the tendon and clinically appears as a "Popeye muscle," with distal retraction of the biceps toward the elbow (Fig. 4.14). Persistent shoulder pain in this patient population is usually related to the underlying rotator cuff disease. Bicipital tendinitis may present with palpable tenderness over the bicipital groove as well as positive provocative tests (22). The Speed test provokes pain with resisted elevation of the outstretched, supinated arm. The Yerguson's test should be performed with the arm externally rotated and the elbow slightly flexed (Fig. 4.15). Pain will then be elicited during resisted supination. The arm is then brought to the side, and the elbow is flexed to 90 degrees. Resisted supination in this position should not elicit any symptoms over the bicipital groove. If pain is noted, the test is equivocal.

Clinically symptomatic arthropathy of the acromioclavicular joint will generally manifest as tenderness to palpation directly over the joint. The pain is exacerbated by provocative tests, which axially load the joint. These maneuvers in-

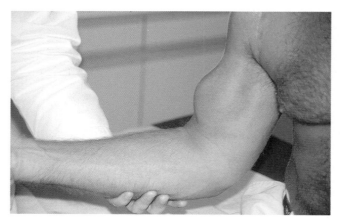

FIGURE 4.14. Rupture of the long head of the biceps presents as a "Popeye muscle."

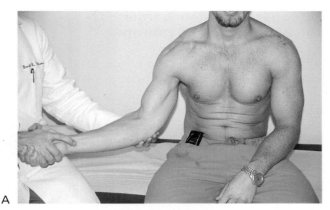
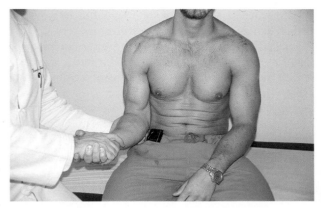

A   B

FIGURE 4.15. Biceps provocative testing. Pain with resisted supination in position 1 **(A)** will be relieved when retested in position 2 **(B)**.

clude cross body adduction of the arm and internal rotation of the arm behind the back. If pain and tenderness over the AC joint persist in the presence of a positive impingement test, then relief of pain following a local injection of lidocaine into the joint can document the presence of clinically significant acromioclavicular pathology (24).

Imaging

Initial imaging studies may be obtained in accordance with the history and specific physical findings. Plain radiographs should generally be the initial imaging studies of the shoulder. The anteroposterior (AP) view in the scapular plane is excellent for evaluation of glenohumeral arthritis. It may also reveal signs of advanced rotator cuff disease (24) such as sclerosis of the greater tuberosity and acromion, and cystic changes in the greater tuberosity. A decreased acromiohumeral interval (<7 mm) may indicate that a large unbalanced full-thickness rotator cuff tear is allowing proximal migration of the humeral head (Fig. 4.16) (40). The AP views with internal and

external rotation of the arm are often helpful in detecting a calcific deposit within the supraspinatus tendon (Fig. 4.17). The axillary view will also demonstrate glenohumeral arthritis, allowing evaluation of posterior glenoid erosion. Calcific tendinitis and an os acromiale will also be apparent on the axillary view.

Specialized views (24) depicting acromial morphology include the coronal AP view with 30 degrees of caudal tilt (Rockwood view) (41) and the supraspinatus outlet view (Figs. 4.18, 4.19). Degenerative changes of the acromioclavicular joint can best be evaluated with a coronal AP view or the AP view with 20 degrees of cephalic tilt (Fig. 4.20) (12). Plain films are excellent for the evaluation of osseous abnormalities or soft-tissue calcifications, but they do not provide direct information regarding soft tissue pathology, such as rotator cuff tears.

MRI has become the imaging study of choice for most clinicians in the evaluation of rotator cuff disease following the plain films (4,24). Magnetic resonance will demonstrate the above pathology quite clearly; however, its greatest utility

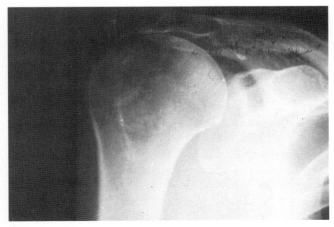

FIGURE 4.16. Superior humeral head migration in cuff tear arthropathy.

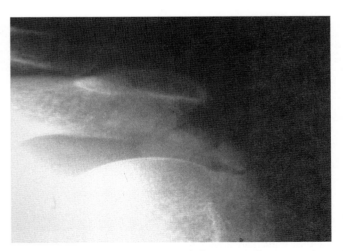

FIGURE 4.17. Calcific tendinitis of the supraspinatus tendon.

is realized when it is obtained for prognostic information and when determining a surgical treatment strategy.

From the foregoing description of the varied etiologies for the clinical presentation of rotator cuff–related pain syndromes, it is clear that careful scrutiny of all of the clinical data and diagnostic studies must be performed before an accurate diagnosis can be made and appropriate treatment offered.

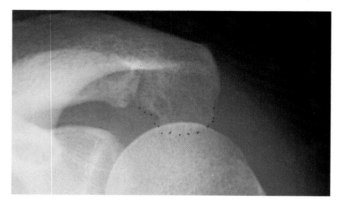

FIGURE 4.18. Rockwood tilt view shows the projection of the acromial spur anterior to the clavicle.

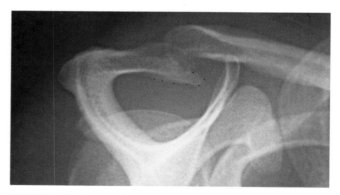

FIGURE 4.19. Supraspinatus outlet view demonstrates the anterior inferior projection of the acromial spur.

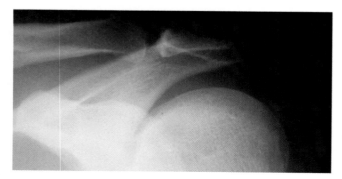

FIGURE 4.20. Zanca view (cephalic tilt) is useful in evaluating the acromioclavicular joint.

Nonoperative Management of the Impingement Syndrome

Although surgical treatment may be considered for subacromial impingement, subacromial decompression as an isolated procedure to treat nonoutlet rotator cuff tendinitis and symptoms of the impingement syndrome are likely to fail. The most effective treatment for overuse syndromes is rehabilitation, including capsular stretching, rotator cuff and scapulothoracic strengthening, and patient education (24). Counseling should include alteration of athletic participation, training techniques, and job modification. Patients with suspected impingement or partial-thickness rotator cuff tears are initially managed in a similar manner.

Mechanical impingement of the rotator cuff is exacerbated by repetitive overhead use of the arm. An important aspect of nonoperative management is modification of those work, sporting, and daily activities that promote or exacerbate this process. Nonoperative treatment includes physician and therapist directed education to achieve an understanding of the pathomechanics of this problem. In some cases, the athletic trainer, coach, and/or employer may need to understand these concepts. Use of oral anti-inflammatory medication (salicylates or nonsteroidal anti-inflammatory drugs) or local corticosteroid injections are useful in managing the inflammation associated with this problem. Corticosteroid injection, particularly if misdirected into the substance of the rotator cuff tendon, can lead to softening, fibrillation, and degenerative changes within the cuff (42). Subacromial injection to the bursa should be used on an infrequent basis, particularly in the young, active patient population. Other modalities to decrease inflammation include the use of ice, particularly after participation in a therapeutic exercise program, and cortisone phonophoresis or iontophoresis (24).

Chronic rotator cuff problems often lead to limitation of passive arcs of motion due to capsular contracture (9). This problem is best treated by a home stretching program, which emphasizes forward elevation, external rotation at the side, cross body adduction, and internal rotation behind the back. This program should stress active assisted arcs of motion performed in gravity-minimized positions through an arc of motion that minimizes pain. As the pain subsides and the patient regains normal and pain-free passive arcs of motion of the shoulder, strengthening exercises of the rotator cuff and supportive scapulothoracic musculature are initiated. Progressive resisted strengthening exercises initially utilize light weights, therapeutic elastic bands, or tubing. Progression of the strengthening exercise program should not exacerbate the inflammatory condition and must be individualized to the patient's needs and expectations.

Successful rehabilitation of the chronic rotator cuff impingement syndrome may require up to 6 to 12 months of treatment, particularly if the subsequent performance of strenuous activities is required. In some cases, after a full course of nonoperative treatment, residual symptoms remain that are minimal in comparison to the presenting symptoms. In this clinical setting, the patient's age, medical health, and expectations should be carefully evaluated prior to consideration for surgical treatment. In some cases, it may be best to advise permanent modification in sport and/or work activity rather than surgical intervention.

Many factors play a role in the decision to recommend surgical intervention for rotator cuff repair. Nonoperative management, if initially recommended, includes the same modalities, principles, and guidelines as discussed for the patient without a rotator cuff tear. The success rate of nonoperative management is significantly decreased in the presence of a rotator cuff tear, particularly in the younger, active patient. Small (1- to 3-cm) chronic rotator cuff tears in older, more sedentary patients with normal active arcs of motion and negative lag signs can be initially treated with nonoperative management. Young, active patients with acute tears and weakness should have early surgical repair. Patients that have activity levels between these extremes should be individualized into nonoperative or surgical treatment groups based on the clinician's best judgment.

MRI as a Preoperative Study

Studies demonstrate that there is a high prevalence of rotator cuff tears by MRI among asymptomatic individuals (3,6). The value of MRI as it relates to rotator cuff pathology depends on the impact of specific anatomic data, which affects surgical treatment and outcome. The indications for surgery depend on the patient's age, activity level, mechanism of injury, patient expectations, and the failure of an appropriate nonoperative treatment program (12). We will generally recommend obtaining an MRI when there has been no evidence of improvement in symptoms after 6 to 12 weeks of conservative treatment (24). If the clinical indications for surgical intervention exist, then MRI is often clinically helpful in both confirming the diagnosis and evaluating the extent of the pathology. This information is useful in planning the surgical procedure and in providing important prognostic treatment information. Patients who do not have the appropriate surgical indications rarely benefit from an MRI unless it reveals an etiology for shoulder pain that had not previously been entertained. This situation occurs in about 11% of patients having an MRI (3).

The advantages of MRI include the ability to determine the size and location of the rotator cuff tear, degree of tendon retraction, and the chronicity of the tear as defined by the degree of muscle atrophy (3,6). Rotator cuff tears may be partial or full thickness. Partial-thickness tears are depicted as focal defects that are either intratendinous or limited to one surface without disrupting the entire thickness of the tendon (6). Magnetic resonance is somewhat less reliable, but still quite useful, in detecting partial-thickness tears (13, 43,44). The sensitivity and specificity in diagnosing a partial-thickness cuff tear are 82% and 85%, respectively. The pre-

dictive value of a positive study is 82% and for a negative study, 85% (33). However, MRI is especially accurate in the detection of full-thickness rotator cuff tears, with a sensitivity of 100% and a specificity of 95% (3,4,33). The predictive value of a positive study is 92%; for a negative study, 100% (33).

Prognostic information that confers poorer functional results includes large tears involving the infraspinatus, teres minor, or subscapularis. Other poor prognostic indicators include chronic rupture of the long head of the biceps tendon, superior migration of the humeral head, degenerative changes of the glenohumeral joint, and moderate to severe atrophy of the rotator cuff musculature (12).

Associated pathological conditions that may be detected by MRI include glenohumeral arthritis, labral pathology, acromioclavicular joint and biceps pathology, and ganglion cysts (3). Ganglion cysts may mimic the clinical findings of a chronic full-thickness cuff tear.

The specific utility of MRI in preoperative planning also depends on the treatment options available to an individual surgeon. Currently available options include arthroscopic and open acromioplasty, arthroscopic or open acromioplasty and debridement of a partial-thickness rotator cuff tear, open acromioplasty with rotator cuff repair, arthroscopic acromioplasty with either miniopen or arthroscopic cuff repair, arthroscopic or open acromioplasty with debridement of a full-thickness rotator cuff tear, and local muscle transfer for a massive chronic rotator cuff defect. The use of MRI is optimized when ordered by an experienced clinician who understands the information afforded by the MRI and who can integrate this information into a treatment plan that considers the severity of the pathology as well as the best surgical option to treat it.

Surgical Management of the Impingement Syndrome

The factors influencing the decision to recommend surgical intervention for rotator cuff impingement syndrome include the patient's age, activity level, expectations, general medical condition, chronicity and severity of the disease, and willingness and ability to participate successfully in the postoperative rehabilitation program. An algorithm for evaluation and surgical decision making is shown in Figure 4.21. In the elderly patient population, associated proliferative degenerative changes occur on the undersurface of the acromion, acromioclavicular joint, and greater tuberosity. Developmental variations in acromial shape (Types II, III) can also be observed, particularly in the younger patient population (24,25). In patients with mechanical causes for chronic pain associated with the rotator cuff mechanism, the principles of surgery that will ultimately define clinical success include adequate decompression of the subacromial space, restoration of rotator cuff integrity and tissue tension, and preservation of deltoid function and attachment (24).

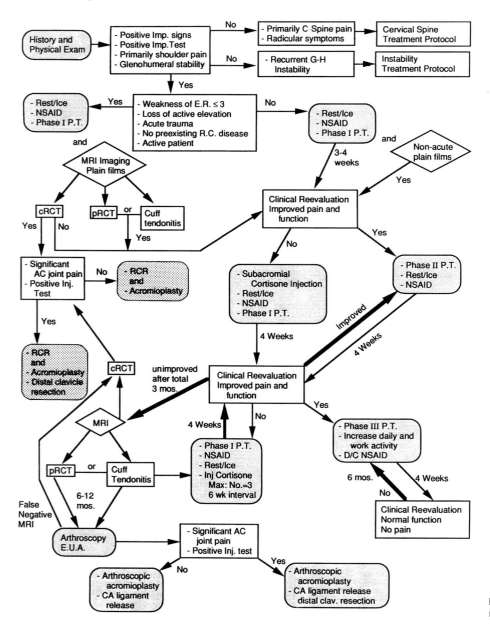

FIGURE 4.21. Algorithm for the treatment of rotator cuff disease.

The presence of an anterior acromial spur, in association with a favorable injection test, will usually confer a more favorable outcome following subacromial decompression (20,46).

Subacromial decompression may be performed through a standard open anterior-inferior acromioplasty, as described by Neer (20), or by arthroscopic acromioplasty. Nearly equal results are obtained following either open or arthroscopic acromioplasty (46,47). However, rehabilitation is usually accelerated after arthroscopic acromioplasty since the subacromial decompression is performed without detachment of the deltoid origin (48). Subacromial decompression is accomplished by removal of spurs from the anterior and anteroinferior aspects of the acromion, undersurface of the AC joint (or distal clavicle resection if specifically in-

dicated), and removal of osteophytes from the greater tuberosity. Among patients without tears of the rotator cuff, the success of subacromial decompression will largely depend on selection of those patients who have mechanical compromise of the subacromial space. This is identified by plain radiographs, which includes supraspinatus outlet or acromial tilt views, or by MRI. If complete rotator cuff tears are present as part of the impingement syndrome in physiologically young and active patients, it is recommended that these be repaired. Subacromial decompression, among patients with symptoms of impingement and unrecognized anterior glenohumeral instability, will result in adequate pain relief but will not allow athletes to return to their previous level of play (49).

Surgical Management of Partial Rotator Cuff Tears

Specific guidelines for the surgical management of partial rotator cuff tears are, at the present time, imprecise and lack satisfactory clinical data. Partial rotator cuff tears may occur on the bursal or articular surfaces of the tendon or within the tendon substance. Tears occurring within the substance are impossible to detect during arthroscopy but are frequently detected by MRI. Tears on the articular surface of the rotator cuff are best visualized and graded by arthroscopic examination. Classification of partial cuff tears considers the location, size, and depth of the tear. Grading depends on depth of the tear (16). Grade I tears are up to 3 mm in depth, Grade II tears have a depth of 3 to 6 mm, and Grade III tears are greater than 6 mm in depth (>50% of the tendon thickness).

We approach all partial thickness tears arthroscopically. This allows evaluation of both the bursal and articular surfaces of the tendon. It also allows identification of intraarticular lesions that may be overlooked when an open approach is used. Interestingly, concomitant pathology of the glenohumeral joint is found quite commonly. Surgical options for treatment of partial cuff tears in the clinical setting of impingement syndrome include arthroscopic subacromial decompression with or without arthroscopic debridement of the degenerative tissue of the tear for Grades I and II tears. Articular surface tears that are found incidentally at the time of arthroscopy may be treated with debridement alone, provided that no bursal pathology is identified (50,51). Subacromial decompression should be added in the presence of a bursal surface tear or impingement lesion (13,51,52). Alternatively, subacromial decompression may be combined with excision of the damaged tissue and formal repair of the resulting full-thickness defect. This appears to offer the best results in active patients with Grade III tears (17). It is our current practice to reserve this more aggressive procedure for acute traumatic partial tears that involve at least 50% of the thickness of the tendon tissue, which occur in active patients under 40 years of age. In all other patients, we perform subacromial decompression alone or in combination with debridement of the torn tendon tissue as the primary procedure. If the symptoms persist in active individuals with a large partial tear, we recommend a second procedure for formal cuff repair.

Partial thickness tears in the young, throwing athlete should be approached cautiously and closely examined for the presence of occult instability (32,47,49). This instability may lead to repetitive eccentric loading of the rotator cuff or to internal glenoid impingement. Acromioplasty is generally not indicated in this patient population unless bursal pathology is also seen. In most cases, open or arthroscopically assisted anterior capsulorrhaphy should be performed to alleviate the abnormal loading of the rotator cuff.

Management of Full-thickness Rotator Cuff Tears

Initial nonoperative management may be advised for patients who present with good strength and normal active arcs of shoulder motion (12). They should also have either a functional chronic rotator cuff tear or a small acute extension superimposed on a chronic tear. These patients usually have an intact posterior cuff (infraspinatus or teres minor) that is well balanced anteriorly and posteriorly. Nonoperative treatment in this setting is similar to that for patients with the impingement syndrome. If pain-related functional limitations persist despite an appropriate 3- to 6-month nonoperative treatment program, surgery may be recommended. Pain is the primary indication for surgery in the older patient with a full-thickness rotator cuff tear (24).

Early surgical treatment is recommended for patients who sustain acute trauma resulting in significant weakness of the rotator cuff. This includes an acute extension of a chronic rotator cuff tear that results in functional weakness. Young patients with higher functional demands who sustain an acute full-thickness rotator cuff tear should also have an early surgical repair in order to improve function and prevent propagation of the tear (12,24).

With complete rotator cuff tears, pain and function usually improve (85%–95%) following repair and successful rehabilitation of the rotator cuff (12,53–60). Results of acromioplasty and rotator cuff repair are superior to that of acromioplasty alone or in combination with debridement of the tendon defect (15,59,61). The methods of repair vary considerably and must be individualized to compensate for variations in tendon and bone quality, size of the tear, tendons involved, capsular contracture, and cuff retraction. Atrophy of the cuff musculature, cephalad migration of the humeral head, and acromioclavicular joint degenerative changes must all be considered as factors in the intraoperative decision-making process. The principles of rotator cuff repair include complete closure of the rotator cuff defect, without tension at the repair site when the arm is maintained in a neutral position. This can be achieved by a variety of means. The best means of repair, when technically feasible, is by directly suturing the rotator cuff tendon into bone (12). This may be facilitated by lysis of intraarticular and subacromial adhesions, release of the coracohumeral ligament, placement of relaxing incisions in the tendon, or muscle advancement. These secondary techniques should be performed only as necessary to achieve a tension-free repair (24).

Magnetic resonance has a significant impact on our surgical decision algorithm for full-thickness tears of the rotator cuff. Decisions are based on the size of the tear, degree of tendon retraction, location of the tear, and amount of muscular atrophy. We prefer to address a small (<3-cm) nonretracted tear of the supraspinatus tendon with arthroscopic acromioplasty and either miniopen (62–65) or arthroscopic rotator cuff repair. Larger (3- to 5-m) or moderately retracted tears with little atrophy are best managed with open acromioplasty and rotator cuff repair. Large chronic cuff defects with severe tendon retraction and muscle atrophy may be reconstructed with secondary tendon transfers. The pectoralis major or latissimus dorsi muscles may be used to reconstruct an irreparable subscapularis tear. The latissimus dorsi and teres major muscles may be transferred to reconstruct an irreparable tear of the supraspinatus and infraspinatus tendons (66). These tendon transfers are performed to improve functional deficits. Careful patient selection, meticulous surgical technique, and physician-supervised physiotherapy are critical in obtaining satisfactory results in these difficult and complex procedures. Inactive biological autogenous or allograft materials have been reported in a few clinical trials with variable success. Prosthetic materials should be considered experimental at this time. It is the authors' practice to avoid inactive biological or prosthetic materials as a means for tendon repair. In the case of severe weakness in association with irreparable cuff tears, we prefer to employ the technique of tendon–muscle transfers.

On an occasional basis, aggressive subacromial decompression in the setting of a massive irreparable rotator cuff tear can result in significant improvement of pain (67). In selected patients, this may provide enough improvement of pain and function to avoid more aggressive procedures requiring distant tendon transfers (12). Although these patients may be improved by tuberoplasty, bursectomy, subacromial decompression, and rotator cuff debridement, functional deficits in strength and endurance often persist. The best results of this procedure occur in older, more sedentary patients who demonstrate an intact portion of the posterior rotator cuff and good deltoid function (68). These patients generally have fair external rotation strength and are highly motivated with respect to their participation in the lengthy and aggressive postoperative rehabilitation program.

In the setting of a massive rotator cuff tear with a proximally migrated humeral head, preservation and repair of the coracoacromial ligament is advocated, and shortening of the normal AP diameter of the acromion should be avoided (12,69).

Management of Associated Pathology

Symptomatic os acromiale may require surgical intervention (70). In these circumstances, osteotomy and internal fixation and bone grafting may be required in addition to standard subacromial decompression and rotator cuff repair.

Advanced symptomatic degenerative AC joint disease unresponsive to rest, nonsteroidal anti-inflammatory medication, and intraarticular injection will require distal clavicle resection. This procedure may be performed either open or arthroscopically and should be performed at the time of concomitant acromioplasty or rotator cuff repair. The superior and posterior capsule should be preserved in order to maintain stability of the distal clavicle. Failure to address symptomatic AC arthropathy will lead to residual pain and an unsatisfactory result following acromioplasty or rotator cuff repair.

Coracoid impingement syndrome as described by Gerber et al. (71) and Dines et al. (72) may require surgical alteration of the coracoid shape by coracoid osteotomy.

Severe degeneration and fraying of the long head of the biceps tendon may be noted at the time of arthroscopic examination (22). We perform an open biceps tenodesis when these changes are found.

Postoperative Management

Postoperative treatment and rehabilitation must be individualized. It must consider the adequacy of the repair, the quality of the tissue, and the complexity of the procedure. In general, gentle passive range of motion exercises, in gravity-free arcs, are started immediately following surgery. Active range of motion, employing isometric and isotonic strengthening with weights or surgical tubing, is not started for at least 6 weeks; in some cases, it may be delayed up to 8 to 10 weeks following surgery (12,24). Larger tears and more tenuous repairs may require postoperative immobilization in a brace for up to 4 to 6 weeks before initiating a rehabilitation program (60).

Results of Surgery

Results of open and arthroscopic acromioplasty are similar in the presence of an intact rotator cuff (73). Following arthroscopic acromioplasty, no significant difference in results is found between patients with an intact cuff and those with a partial-thickness rotator cuff tear (15). Worse results are found among patients with workman's compensation claims (46,74,75). Worse results are also noted among patients with full-thickness rotator cuff tears (15,47).

Preoperative factors that are generally associated with less favorable surgical results following repair of a full-thickness cuff repair relate to tear size (53,55) and chronicity of the tear. These factors include significant muscular atrophy, weakness of external rotation of grade 3 or less, loss of active arcs of motion of greater than 30 degrees compared with passive arcs of motion, and passive elevation of less than 130 degrees, for a duration of greater than 6 months (53). Multiple steroid injections, rupture of the long head of the biceps tendon, cephalad migration of the humeral head, and physiological age over 65 years have also been correlated with less favorable results (Table 4.3) (1).

Intraoperative factors that are generally associated with less favorable results relate to the difficulty of repair. These factors include poor quality of the remaining tendon tissue, massive tears with severe loss of tendon substance, and severe tendon scarring and retraction. Tension at the repair site and incomplete cuff closure generally result in failure (Table 4.3).

TABLE 4.3. POOR PROGNOSTIC FACTORS IN ROTATOR CUFF REPAIR

I. PREOPERATIVE
   Weakness of external rotation
   Grade 3 or less
     Supraspinatus/infraspinatus/subscapularis muscle atrophy
   Active range of motion 30 degrees less than passive arcs
   Passive elevation less than 130 degrees
   Symptoms greater than six months duration with a large or
     massive cuff tear
   Multiple steroid injections
   Cephalad migration of the humeral head
   Physiologic age over 65 years
II. INTRAOPERATIVE
   Poor-quality tendon or bone
   Massive tears with loss of tendon substance
   Tears with severe scarring and retraction
   Tension at repair site
   Incomplete cuff closure
III. POSTOPERATIVE FACTORS
   Detachment of deltoid origin
   Axillary or suprascapular nerve injury
   Delay in early mobilization of the shoulder
   Premature advancement of active range of motion or
     strengthening exercises

Other surgical factors that may lead to a poor result include inadequate acromioplasty and unidentified symptomatic acromioclavicular arthritis (12).

Postoperative factors that are generally associated with poor results include failure of the repair, deltoid origin detachment, axillary nerve or suprascapular nerve injury, delay in early mobilization of the shoulder, or premature advancement to active range of motion or strengthening exercises (Table 4.3) (12,55,76).

Retrospective clinical evaluation following repair of complete rotator cuff tears demonstrate that 85% to 95% of all patients have significant improvement of both pain and shoulder function (12,20,59,77). Pain relief is directly correlated to the adequacy of subacromial decompression. Functional improvement is correlated to improvement in pain level as well as to the quality of the repair and eventual healing of the rotator cuff (55). If an early satisfactory result is obtained, the pain relief and functional restoration are generally long lasting (12,24,78). Better results are obtained in small (<3-cm.), acute tears in young patients. Larger tears have a higher propensity for postoperative weakness, fatigue symptoms, and recurrent cuff defects (1,55). The ability to return to competitive overhead throwing activities at the professional or collegiate level is less than 50% (79,80).

GLENOHUMERAL INSTABILITY

Glenohumeral instability is defined as an episode of pathological humeral translation that results in clinical symptoms of pain and functional limitation. There is a wide variability in the amount of normal joint translation among individuals. In the absence of clinical symptoms, significant capsular hyperlaxity and large joint translations do not constitute a diagnosis of glenohumeral instability (81). The diagnosis of instability is thus primarily based on clinical symptoms of pain and dysfunction, in conjunction with supportive findings on physical exam and imaging studies. A subluxation occurs when an episode of glenohumeral translation occurs that results in pain but no loss of articular contact. This is in contrast to a dislocation, in which there is complete loss of articular contact. Between these entities is a wide spectrum of clinically significant instability ranging from atraumatic multidirectional instability to traumatic unidirectional instability. Important pathological considerations include factors intrinsic and extrinsic to the glenohumeral joint, the inciting event, direction and degree of instability, and volition. Considerable overlap of these factors exists between individuals presenting with the clinical complaint of instability, emphasizing the importance of a thorough understanding of the etiologic factors, as well as the available treatment options.

Glenohumeral Stabilizers

Evaluation of glenohumeral instability requires a fundamental understanding of the biomechanics of shoulder stability. Static and dynamic factors both contribute to the maintenance of joint stability. In general terms, static stabilizers contribute to stability at the end ranges of motion, whereas dynamic factors play an important role in the midranges of motion.

Static Factors

Static factors that contribute to glenohumeral stability include glenoid and humeral version, articular congruity and depth, integrity of the labrum, negative intraarticular pressure, and capsuloligamentous structures (82). The normal glenoid articular surface faces superiorly about 5 degrees and ranges between 10 degrees of anteversion and 7 degrees of retroversion (83). The humeral head has a normal neck-shaft angle of 135 degrees and faces an average of 30 degrees posteriorly, relative to the transepicondylar axis of the elbow. The radii of curvature of the articular surfaces are nearly identical (84–86). However, much of the surface area of the humeral head is left uncovered due to the smaller diameter of the glenoid. The glenoid labrum is intimately attached to bone, below the equator of the glenoid. Above the equator, the labrum is more loosely approximated (87). The glenoid labrum deepens the glenoid concavity by up to 100%, to an average depth of 9 mm in the superior-inferior plane and 5 mm in the anteroposterior plane (88). Loss of the labrum decreases the force required for dislocation by up to 20% (89).

The glenohumeral joint is essentially a closed system and has a resting intraarticular pressure gradient of –42 cm of

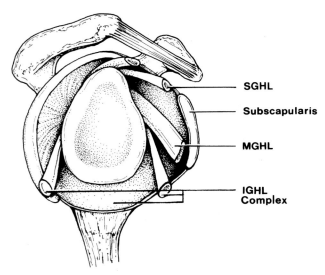

FIGURE 4.22. Glenohumeral ligaments: superior glenohumeral ligament (SGHL) and middle glenohumeral ligaments (MGHL). The inferior glenohumeral ligament complex (IGHL) is composed of the anterior and posterior bands, as well as the intervening axillary pouch.

water. Any attempt to pull the articular surfaces apart is countered by the vacuum effect provided by this negative intraarticular pressure. Venting of the capsule or an increase in joint fluid volume will eliminate this suction cup effect (90).

The shoulder capsule forms discrete structural glenohumeral ligaments (Fig. 4.22). They provide static stability that is dependent on arm position and direction of the applied force intended to displace the humeral head (91–93). The superior glenohumeral ligament and coracohumeral ligaments are described together because they combine to constitute the rotator interval. The rotator interval resists inferior translation of the humeral head and tightens when the arm is externally rotated at the side. It also restricts posterior translation when the arm is forward flexed and internally rotated. The long head of the biceps tendon also runs parallel to the rotator interval and resists inferior translation of the humeral head with the arm at the side (94).

The middle glenohumeral (Fig. 4.22) ligament is variably absent in 30% of cases (93). When present, it resists anterior translation of the humeral head when the arm is externally rotated between 60 and 90 degrees of abduction. It also assists in restricting inferior translation with the arm at the side. A morphological variant is the cordlike middle glenohumeral ligaments (MGHL). When present, there is a foraminal opening between it and the anterior band of the inferior glenohumeral ligament complex (IGHL), and the anterior superior glenoid labrum is notably absent (Fig. 4.23).

The inferior glenohumeral ligament complex is composed of the anterior band, posterior band, and an intervening axillary pouch (Fig. 4.22). It is more stout anteriorly and nearer the glenoid. The anterior portion of the inferior glenohumeral ligament tightens as the arm is abducted and exter-

nally rotated, effectively resisting anterior translation. Internal rotation of the adducted, forward-flexed arm tightens the posterior band, resisting posterior translation. Abduction of the arm tightens the axillary pouch, effectively resisting inferior translation with the arm in this position. The posterior capsule is quite thin and does not form any distinct ligamentous thickenings. However, it functions to resist posterior translation of the adducted, forward flexed, internally rotated arm.

Dynamic Factors

Dynamic stability of the glenohumeral joint is coordinated by active contraction of the rotator cuff, biceps, and scapulothoracic musculature (82,91,92,94). A well-balanced rotator cuff acts to compress the humeral head into the center of the glenoid concavity (95). An intact glenoid articular surface and labral complex are required to facilitate this concavity compression effect through different positions of rotation of the arm (89,95). A weak or poorly functioning rotator cuff allows greater translation of the humeral head during active rotation of the arm.

Intercalated, synchronous scapulothoracic, and glenohumeral motion is required to position the glenoid such that the forces placed on the humeral head are directed into the center of the glenoid concavity. Normal scapulothoracic rotation provides a stable glenoid base for the humeral head during arm rotation. Loss of scapulothoracic control is often manifest as scapular winging and may be attributable to serratus anterior or trapezius dysfunction. Failure to provide a stable glenoid base may increase the requirements placed on the static ligamentous stabilizers and lead to instability.

Pathoanatomy of Glenohumeral Instability

Traumatic Lesions

Instability is often the result of an acute traumatic event that exceeds the tensile strength of the capsule, ligaments, labrum, or bone. A traumatic anterior dislocation or subluxation often occurs following forced abduction and external rotation of the arm, leading to failure of the inferior glenohumeral ligamentous complex. Detachment of the inferior glenohumeral ligament from the anterior inferior glenoid (Bankart lesion) occurs most commonly (80% to 90% of the time) and may involve either the labrum or the anterior glenoid rim (96–98). Studies show that substantial midsubstance capsular stretching occurs prior to rupture (99,100). Other, less common sites of failure include capsular rupture and avulsion of the inferior glenohumeral ligament from its humeral attachment (96,101,102). Combinations of capsular stretching or rupture may coexist with glenoid or humeral ligament avulsions (99,103). A Hill-Sachs compression fracture of the posterolateral humeral head is commonly seen (over 80%) with traumatic anterior dislocations (96,104).

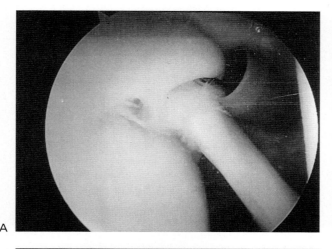

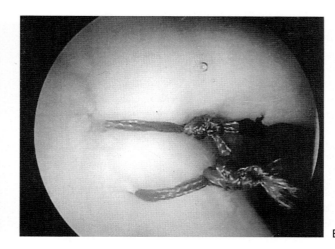

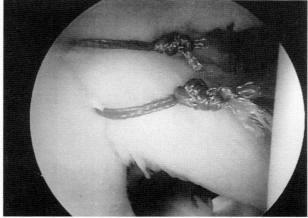

FIGURE 4.23. Cordlike middle glenohumeral ligament (Buford complex) is an infrequent normal variant **(A)**. Repair of the type II SLAP lesion should not include the MGHL **(B, C)**. Attachment of the MGHL to the anterior glenoid will severely restrict external rotation.

Traumatic posterior instability is usually the result of a posteriorly directed force on the arm, in a posture of forward flexion, internal rotation, and adduction. Detachment of the posterior inferior glenohumeral ligament may involve either the labrum or the posterior glenoid rim. This presumably occurs with stretching of the posterior capsule. We recently identified a previously unreported lesion: humeral avulsion of the posterior capsule (Fig. 4.24). An anteromedial compression fracture of the humeral head is seen with posterior dislocations.

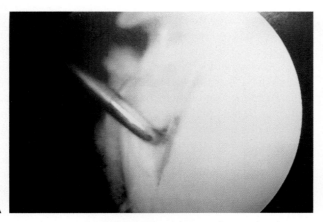

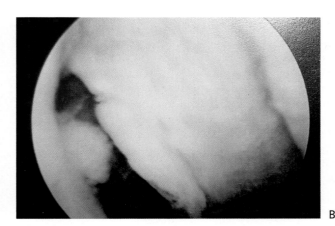

FIGURE 4.24. Arthroscopic examination reveals a small cleft in the posterior labrum **(A)** with a complete avulsion of the posterior humeral capsular attachment **(B)**.

Traumatic instability is generally unidirectional. In rare circumstances, the patient may exhibit symptoms and corresponding lesions of both anterior and posterior traumatic instability.

Infrequent causes of instability include glenoid hypoplasia or abnormal version of either the glenoid or humeral articular surfaces.

Capsular Laxity

Capsular laxity is a requisite for normal shoulder motion. The amount of capsular laxity is a variable characteristic among individuals. Excessive translation and hyperlaxity are not considered pathological entities unless associated with symptoms (81). Due to the wide variability in laxity, an overlap in joint translations exists between those patients with normal asymptomatic laxity and those with clinical instability (105). Although hyperlaxity usually exists without instability, it has been suggested that hyperlaxity is a risk factor for clinical instability. Obviously, excessive translation will occur in all planes in these individuals, but the direction of instability is described as that which elicits symptoms.

The coexistence of traumatic lesions and hyperlaxity frequently occurs. The spectrum of pathomechanical combinations is quite varied and includes unidirectional instability without hyperlaxity, unidirectional instability with hyperlaxity, multidirectional instability without generalized hyperlaxity, and multidirectional instability with hyperlaxity.

Classification, Mechanism of Injury, and Anatomic Findings

Many classifications for instability have been proposed and are based on the inciting mechanism and direction of instability. Important considerations in classifying instability include etiology, direction, degree, volition, and anatomic findings (Table 4.4). Based on these factors, five types of glenohumeral instability are recognized (106).

Involuntary unidirectional instability without hyperlaxity is secondary to a single traumatic event. These injuries usually result in anterior dislocation, occasionally in the posterior direction, and rarely in an inferior direction. In this group of patients, there is a high incidence (85% to 90%) of trauma-induced lesions. These lesions include glenoid labral tears, glenohumeral ligamentous or capsular disruption, rotator cuff tears, and glenoid and humeral tuberosity fractures. In the young, athletic population, the incidence of recurrent episodes of dislocation or subluxation approaches 90% (97,107–109). In the patient population over the age of 50 years, the incidence of rotator cuff tears associated with the first traumatic dislocation is reported to be 60% (110).

The second type of instability is multidirectional instability without hyperlaxity. It is a relatively rare pattern that may be secondary to a single inciting event or to two separate traumatic episodes (one anterior and the other posterior).

TABLE 4.4. CLASSIFICATION OF GLENOHUMERAL INSTABILITY

I. ETIOLOGY
Traumatic—Acute high-velocity trauma
  Primary
  Recurrent
Repetitive microtrauma
Atraumatic
Voluntary
II. DEGREE
Subluxation
Dislocation
Chronicity
III. DIRECTION
Unidirectional
Anterior or anterior/inferior
Posterior or posterior/inferior
Inferior
Multidirectional
IV. ANATOMIC FINDINGS
Labral or bony Bankart lesion
SLAP lesions
Capsular laxity or stretching
  Hill-Sachs lesion
Subscapularis rupture
  Abnormal glenoid or humeral version
Hypoplastic glenoid
Rotator interval and rotator cuff disruption
Articular cartilage degeneration
Rotator cuff partial tears and degeneration
V. TYPES OF INSTABILITY PATTERNS
Involuntary unidirectional traumatic
Involuntary bidirectional traumatic
Involuntary unidirectional atraumatic
Involuntary multidirectional
Voluntary (any direction)

Coexisting pathologic lesions of anterior and posterior instability are usually identified.

The third type of instability is involuntary, unidirectional instability with hyperlaxity. It is often secondary to repetitive trauma, usually occurring in swimming, diving, and overhead throwing sports. These injuries usually result in episodes of anterior subluxation, and occasionally dislocation (111). Posterior instability is seen less frequently. In most patients, the capsular volume is large. In addition, discrete labral pathology is frequently found and is usually mild. Hill-Sachs lesions and glenoid fractures are less common. Posterior instability is commonly positional. The patient may be able to demonstrate instability when the arm is placed in a particular position, but the underlying etiology is not truly voluntary.

The fourth type of instability is bilateral or multidirectional instability with hyperlaxity. The origin of instability is often atraumatic or follows a fairly minor injury. Bilateral capsular laxity is the hallmark in these patients, and most individuals exhibit generalized hyperlaxity in multiple joints. Multidirectional instability more often occurs bilaterally, and it always has a component of inferior subluxation (112,113). Incompetence of the rotator interval should be suspected with a history of inferior instability. Traumatic lesions such as glenoid labral tears, glenohumeral ligament tears, or Hill-Sachs lesions are rare.

The last type of instability may be unidirectional or multidirectional, but it is always voluntary in etiology (114). Instability may be bilateral and is often associated with psychological disorders or behavioral maladjustment in adolescent patients. Traumatic type anatomic lesions are rare.

Clinical Presentation: Symptoms and Physical Findings

A thorough inquiry regarding the circumstances surrounding the onset of symptoms will contribute to the correct diagnosis and classification of instability. This includes the arm position at the time of injury, the degree of trauma that caused the initial episode of instability, and direction and degree of instability (109). Acute traumatic dislocations often require medical attention for closed reduction and are associated with severe pain. Dislocations can have associated nerve palsy (generally neuropraxic types), most commonly affecting the axillary and musculocutaneous nerves. A violent dislocation that requires physician-assisted reduction has a high incidence of labral pathology. Patient age is the most important prognostic factor for recurrence. Traumatic dislocations in the young, athletic population are associated with a high recurrence rate. Athletic patients under the age of 20 have a recurrence rate approaching 95%. The recurrence rate decreases to 75% for patients 21 to 30 years old and drops to 15% for patients between 31 and 40 years of age (115). Recurrence is uncommon after age 40. However, dislocation in the elderly population (>60 years old) is associated with a high incidence of rotator cuff tears (110). Instability associated with generalized ligamentous laxity is much more prevalent in the younger population and becomes increasingly rare in the older population.

The frequency (recurrent vs. primary event), chronicity, degree (subluxation vs. dislocation), and direction are important clinical factors. An attempt should be made to recount the arm position and the direction of the applied force at the time of the inciting event (109). An arm position of abduction, external rotation, and extension usually indicates anterior instability, whereas forward flexion, adduction, and internal rotation suggests posterior instability.

The location of shoulder pain is helpful when it is placed in the context of arm position or performance of a particular activity. During episodes of subluxation, most patients describe pain and a sense of abnormal humeral translation associated with these positions or activities. If the amount of humeral translation is severe or traumatic in nature, pain may persist for many hours or days following the episode of subluxation. Acute anterior translation may present in the "dead arm syndrome" (111). These brief neurological symptoms usually occur in the postaxial border of the forearm or

ulnar digits of the hand. Anterior shoulder pain during the cocking phase of throwing suggests anterior instability. Pain in the superior or posterior aspect of the shoulder may indicate rotator cuff tendinitis, internal glenoid impingement, or osteoarthritis. Posterior shoulder pain associated with the follow-through phase of throwing suggests posterior instability. Inferior subluxation may occur when lifting heavy objects (e.g., a suitcase), with the arm at the side.

The activity level and functional impairment associated with instability are important when considering treatment recommendations. Clinical instability may present in an infrequent and subtle manner, or it may preclude the performance of normal activities of daily living. The high-performance throwing athlete who experiences symptoms in the provocative position should be considered separately from the recreational athlete who has minor symptoms related to a particular sport. The latter may wish to simply modify his or her sport rather than pursue surgical reconstruction if conservative management fails.

The clinician should be aware of the signs of voluntary instability. A patient who has a childhood history of dislocations or who readily dislocated to gain attention may exhibit voluntary instability. Such a patient may be unwilling to admit to any secondary gain from performing these "party tricks," and supplemental history from the family is helpful (109). Separating these patients from positional subluxators, who are able to demonstrate instability but do not have an underlying emotional disorder, may be difficult.

Physical Findings

We generally begin the examination on the contralateral, uninvolved side. The shoulders are compared with respect to laxity, range of motion, strength, and specialized provocative instability tests (116). When hyperlaxity of the shoulder is present, the clinician should look for signs of generalized ligamentous laxity (Fig. 4.25) such as hyperextension of the

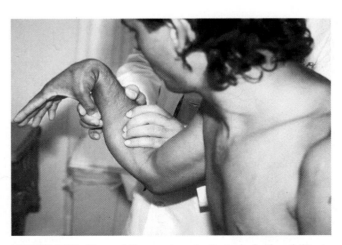

FIGURE 4.25. Signs of ligamentous laxity include the ability to oppose the thumb to the forearm.

elbows, knees or metacarophalangeal (MTP) joints, hypermobility of the patella, and the ability to abduct the thumb to the forearm.

Close inspection of scapulothoracic motion should be performed to detect scapular winging or dyskinesis (Fig. 4.26). Scapular winging will often be apparent by having the patient do wall push-ups, forward-elevate against resistance, and shrug the shoulders.

Strength is usually preserved unless a rotator cuff tear or nerve damage exists. Injury to the axillary nerve is associated with anterior dislocations and results in deltoid atrophy. A rotator cuff tear will present in the elderly patient and manifest as weakness in external rotation and atrophy of the supraspinatus and infraspinatus fossae.

Range of motion is usually full among patients with instability. Discomfort may be exhibited at the end range of motion and offers a clue to the direction of instability. Capsuloligamentous stretching or even a tear of the subscapularis tendon may present as increased external rotation of the arm at the side. A positive lift off test or abdominal compression test will confirm a subscapularis tendon tear.

Increased external rotation with the arm in 90 degrees of scapular abduction suggests stretching of the inferior glenohumeral ligamentous complex. Increased internal rotation with the arm in 90 degrees of scapular abduction suggests posterior capsular stretching. Patients who have undergone

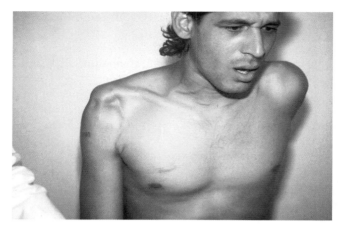

FIGURE 4.27. Sulcus sign.

previous instability repairs may have a restricted range of motion. Loss of external rotation at the side is occasionally seen following Putti-Platt or Magnuson Stack repairs. Pain in these patients may be due to recurrent instability or to glenohumeral arthritis (capsulorrhaphy arthropathy) from excessive anterior tightening.

Provocative Testing

Provocative instability testing is performed to evaluate the integrity of the static capsuloligamentous restraints at the end ranges of motion. The amount of humeral head translation is assessed and compared in both shoulders, and the reproduction of symptoms is noted.

The sulcus test is used to identify inferior instability (Fig. 4.27). Traction is placed on the arm as it rests at the side, and the sulcus below the acromion is quantified in terms of centimeters. The test is then repeated with the arm in full external rotation at the side. A competent rotator interval will lead to a significant decrease of the sulcus in external rotation. The test may also be repeated with the arm in scapular abduction to assess the integrity of the axillary pouch.

The anterior apprehension test is performed with the patient either supine or sitting. The arm is then brought into full abduction, external rotation, and extension. The examiner may additionally place an anteriorly directed force on the humeral head during the maneuver. Patients with anterior instability will experience true apprehension by expressing that the shoulder feels as though it is about to dislocate (Fig. 4.28). The test is very specific when true apprehension is elicited, and this should be differentiated from mere pain. Pain alone may indicate rotator cuff pathology or internal glenoid impingement. The posterior relocation test is then performed with the patient's arm in the same provocative position (Fig. 4.28). A posteriorly directed force is placed on the humeral head in order to reduce it into the glenoid. Relief of apprehension with this maneuver reinforces the diagnosis of anterior instability.

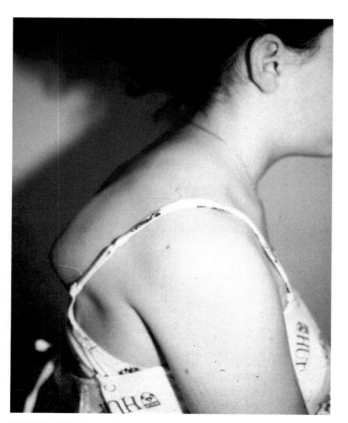

FIGURE 4.26. Scapular winging.

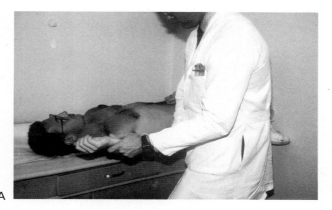
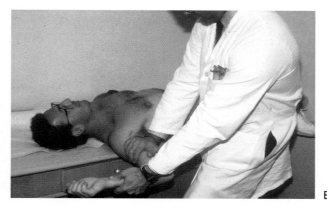

FIGURE 4.28. A: Apprehension with the arm in the provocative position (abduction, external rotation, extension) will often be relieved with a posteriorly directed force on the humeral head (**B,** relocation test).

Laxity is then assessed in the anterior and posterior directions. The load and shift test may be performed with the patient in the sitting position. The examiner stands behind the patient and stabilizes the scapula with one hand. The other hand grasps the humeral head and applies a medial centering force into the glenoid. Anterior and posterior translation is then assessed and compared to the opposite side (Fig. 4.29). Reproduction of symptoms should be noted in association with direction of the applied load.

The seated posterior stress test (Fig. 4.30) is performed with the examiner at the patient's side. One hand stabilizes the scapula while the other hand places a posteriorly directed force on the patient's flexed, adducted, internally rotated arm. The maneuver should be performed with the arm in both internal and external rotation, keeping in mind that the magnitude of posterior translation should normally decrease as the arm is internally rotated.

We prefer to perform the load and shift test with the patient supine (Fig. 4.31). The arm is brought into 40 to 60 degrees of scapular abduction and neutral rotation. Anterior and posterior forces are then applied to the humeral head, and the resulting translation is compared to the opposite side. The arm is then brought into 90 degrees of scapular abduction. An anteriorly directed force is placed on the humeral head to determine the amount of anterior translation that is present. Grade I translation occurs when the diameter of the humeral head rides onto the glenoid rim. Grade II translation occurs when the head is dislocated over the rim but spontaneously reduces. Grade III translation occurs when the dislocated head fails to spontaneously reduce. The testing is then repeated with the arm in progressively increasing external rotation. The degree of external rotation required to obliterate the anterior translation reflects the functional laxity of the inferior glenohumeral complex. The examiner compares these findings to the normal shoulder to determine a side-to-side difference in the integrity of the inferior glenohumeral ligament.

We perform the posterior load and shift test in a similar manner. The arm is brought into 90 degrees of scapular abduction, and a posteriorly directed force is applied. The amount of internal rotation required to tighten the posterior

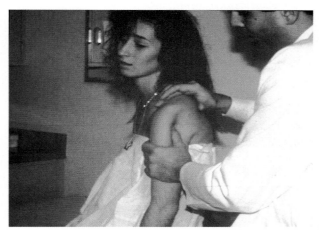
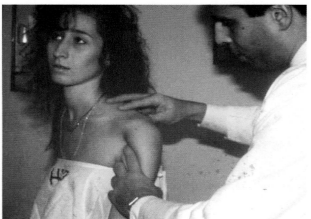

FIGURE 4.29. Anterior (**A**) and posterior (**B**) load and shift tests.

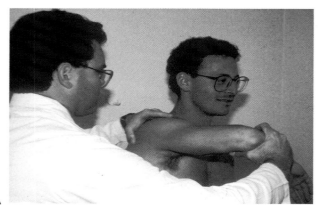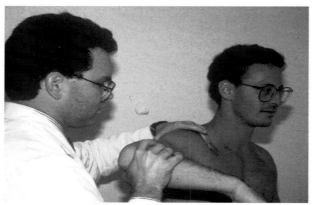

A   B

FIGURE 4.30. Posterior stress test. Posterior instability may be demonstrated with the arm in forward elevation, adduction, and internal rotation **(A)**. The joint will reduce when the arm is brought into the coronal plane **(B)**.

capsule and obliterate the posterior translation is recorded and compared to the opposite side.

Anterior or posterior translation of the humeral head over the glenoid rim can sometimes be elicited during physical examination of the awake but relaxed patient. Examination of both shoulders under anesthesia is the most reproducible clinical setting for performing these maneuvers.

Imaging Studies

Initial plain films of the shoulder should include a true AP, scapular lateral, and axillary views. Specialized views will contribute additional information regarding osseous abnormalities of the glenoid or humeral head. The West point and Apical oblique (Garth) views (117) visualize the anteroinferior glenoid rim and will often detect a bony Bankart lesion (Fig. 4.32). The Stryker notch view (Fig. 4.33) as well as an AP in internal rotation are useful for detecting a Hill-Sachs lesion of the humeral head. Computerized tomography is occasionally employed to evaluate osseous abnormalities of glenoid version, erosion, hypoplasia, and humeral defects (Fig. 4.34).

Nonosseous Bankart lesions and other capsulolabral pathology cannot be detected by plain radiography. Magnetic resonance imaging is superior to other imaging modalities at defining labral and capsuloligamentous pathology, accurately identifying labral lesions in over 90% of cases. Anterior labral tears seem to be easier to identify than posterior lesions (6). Occasionally, normal anatomical variants may be mistaken for labral tears. Also, abutment of the capsule against the labrum may simulate a labral tear in the undistended joint. Magnetic resonance arthrography is more accurate than noncontrast MR in the detection of capsulolabral abnormalities. Placing the arm in the provocative position during the study may further improve the ability to detect these lesions (6).

The impact of MRI on clinical decision making for glenohumeral instability is similar to that for rotator cuff tears. Before ordering the study, the clinician should know how it assists in making the diagnosis or altering the course of treatment. We base our decision to obtain an MRI on a careful history, physical examination, plain films, and the result of nonoperative measures. In many cases, the clinical di-

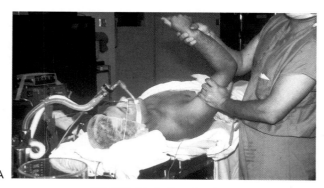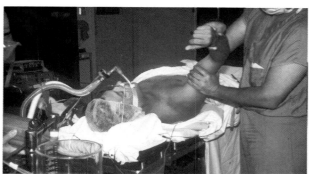

A   B

FIGURE 4.31. Examination under anesthesia includes the supine load and shift test. Humeral translation is assessed with the arm in abduction and neutral rotation **(A)**. The amount of external rotation required to obliterate the translation **(B)** indicates the integrity of the anteroinferior capsular structures and should be compared to the opposite side.

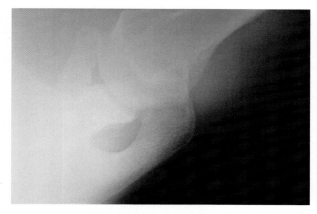

A

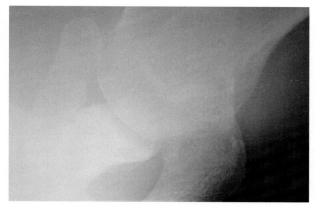

B

FIGURE 4.32. Garth **(A)** and West point axillary **(B)** views reveal bone loss of the anterior inferior glenoid rim.

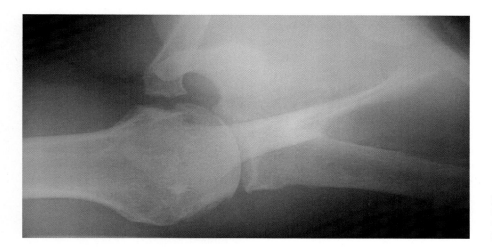

FIGURE 4.33. Stryker notch view will reveal a Hill-Sachs defect and allow evaluation of the base of the coracoid process.

agnosis may be clearly established by clinical examination and plain radiography. In this case, an MRI will not alter the diagnosis or treatment plan. Accordingly, patients with primary or recurrent unidirectional instability who have plain films displaying traumatic lesions of instability do not need further imaging studies. We reserve MRI for patients with a suspected, but unconfirmed, clinical diagnosis of instability that cannot be adequately defined by plain radiographs.

When a rotator cuff tear is suspected after glenohumeral dislocation, an MRI is helpful.

Nonoperative Management

The success of nonoperative treatment is dependent on the type and direction of instability, the patient's age and activity level, and the anatomic pathology. Most patients who sustain a primary traumatic anterior dislocation can be treated effectively by closed reduction and 2 to 3 weeks of immobilization, followed by a specific rehabilitation program to condition the dynamic stabilizers of the rotator cuff and scapula. Young, athletically active patients, sustaining a trau-

matic anterior dislocation associated with a Bankart lesion, have a high rate of recurrent instability despite appropriate nonoperative management. Patients with recurrent traumatic unidirectional glenohumeral instability will often require surgical intervention.

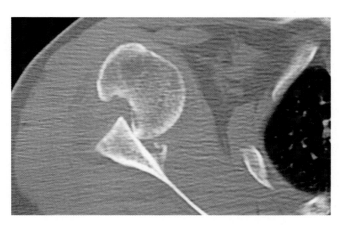

FIGURE 4.34. CT scan of a chronic anterior dislocation and large Hill-Sachs defect.

In contrast, a greater tuberosity fracture following traumatic anterior dislocation results in a marked decrease in the incidence of recurrent instability. Greater tuberosity fractures associated with traumatic dislocations require near anatomic position (0.5 to 1 cm of displacement) following closed reduction to achieve a good clinical result. If this degree of reduction is not obtained by closed means, then open reduction and internal fixation are required.

Most authors recommend nonoperative treatment as the initial treatment for posterior instability. This includes strengthening of the rotator cuff, deltoid, and scapular stabilizing muscles. Activity modification emphasizes avoidance of the provocative position of forward elevation, adduction, and internal rotation. Among patients with scapular dyskinesis, scapular rehabilitation is crucial to restoring synchronous scapular motion. Nonoperative treatment is successful in 80% of cases and should be exhausted before considering surgical alternatives. Currently, the results of surgery for posterior instability are much improved from earlier reports, approaching a 90% success rate.

In patients with atraumatic unidirectional instability without a Bankart lesion or patients with multidirectional instability, the preferred initial treatment is nonoperative.

This approach would include avoidance of precipitating athletic activities and participation in a strengthening program to optimize rotator cuff balance and endurance. Strengthening of the deltoid and periscapular musculature is also recommended. Rehabilitation of the serratus anterior, trapezius, and levator scapulae will allow proper positioning of the glenoid during arm rotation and will facilitate glenohumeral stability. Many patients in these two groups will have significant improvement of their symptoms of instability following 4 to 6 months of participation in these strengthening exercises. Nonoperative treatment is successful in 80% to 90% of cases. Patients who fail nonoperative treatment and have recurrent symptoms of instability become candidates for surgical intervention.

Voluntary instability should be treated with patient education and avoidance of voluntary episodes of instability. In some cases, formal psychiatric or psychological treatment is required. In those patients with significant underlying psychiatric problems, physiotherapy is often unsuccessful. In either clinical situation, surgical intervention should be avoided.

Surgical Management

Many operative procedures have been described for treatment of recurrent instability of the shoulder. Capsular reefing procedures such as the Putti-Platt are based on the concept of imbrication or shortening of the anterior capsule and subscapularis tendon (32). Capsular reattachment procedures as described by DuToit (118) as well as Bankart reattach the torn labrum and capsule to the glenoid rim (119, 120). Muscular sling procedures such as the Magnuson-

Stack (121) or modified Bristow procedures (122) are based on the transfer of a muscle tendon complex to achieve a dynamic sling effect when the arm is placed in an abducted and externally rotated position. Capsular shift procedures are designed to specifically reduce the inferior capsular recess and are most useful in patients without a glenoid labral or capsular defect. As a single and isolated procedure, this is best reserved for those patients with a large redundant capsule and multidirectional instability. Bone block procedures place a bone graft at the margin of the glenoid rim to extend and widen the glenoid cavity. A glenoid osteotomy (123) for the treatment of posterior instability is designed to decrease glenoid retroversion. A humeral osteotomy (124,125) procedure is designed to increase humeral retroversion and is recommended by its proponents for recurrent anterior instability in association with very large Hill-Sachs lesions (126).

Our indication for surgery is the proven recurrence of glenohumeral instability despite an extensive course of nonsurgical treatment. We first examine the shoulder under anesthesia, carefully noting any side-to-side difference in translation and integrity of the capsular constraints. We follow this with an arthroscopic evaluation of the shoulder. Arthroscopic evaluation of the unstable glenohumeral joint has allowed a more precise understanding of the pathologic findings associated with the various patterns of glenohumeral instability. Diagnostic arthroscopy along with examination of both shoulders under anesthesia and a careful preoperative history will allow for a clear understanding of the extent, direction, and anatomic findings associated with the instability pattern of the individual patient.

The nature of the surgery incorporates the etiology, direction of instability, MRI findings, results of examination under anesthesia, and arthroscopic findings to determine the surgical treatment. In most cases, repair of the Bankart lesion and reduction of excessive capsular laxity is the preferred treatment, regardless of whether it is performed open or arthroscopically.

Surgery for Traumatic Instability

Patients with recurrent traumatic anterior instability should have an anatomic repair of the capsular ligaments to the glenoid rim (Bankart repair). Humeral avulsion of the capsule or inferior glenohumeral ligament should also be repaired anatomically.

We will also perform an early Bankart repair in the young athletic individual who wishes to return to his or her previous level of athletic activity. This procedure may be performed either open or arthroscopically (Fig. 4.35). We will generally recommend the open procedure for patients who wish to return to contact sports such as football, hockey, or basketball. The best candidates for arthroscopic repair are first-time dislocators with a nonosseous Bankart lesion (127).

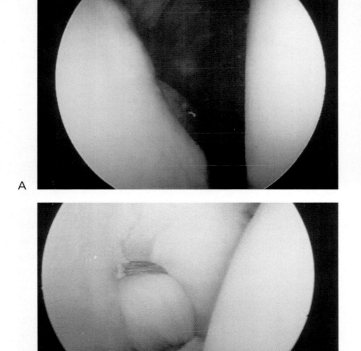

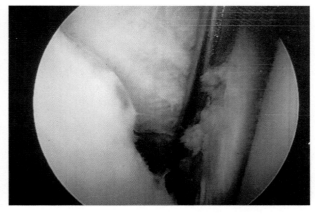

FIGURE 4.35. Arthroscopic Bankart repair. The Bankart lesion has healed medially and the anterior-inferior labrum is not visible **(A)**. The labrum is mobilized **(B)** and repaired to the glenoid rim **(C)**.

In this patient population, glenoid fracture is associated with a less favorable prognosis (128). In some patients, there are associated redundancy and stretching of the anterior capsule and inferior capsular recess. In these patients, a Bankart procedure is supplemented with a capsular shift to reduce the capsular redundancy (129). If the Bankart repair is performed arthroscopically in a patient with a patulous capsule or stretching due to recurrent anterior instability, then thermal capsulorrhaphy may be added to decrease the capsular redundancy. Instability patterns with only capsular redundancy (without a torn labrum or capsule) have a higher incidence of failure following arthroscopic stabilization.

Surgery for traumatic posterior instability should focus on repair of the posterior labral pathology. A posterior capsulorrhaphy may also be performed to reduce capsular redundancy. A combined approach may be needed to address coexisting lesions of traumatic anterior and posterior instability. All of the pathology should be addressed at the time of initial surgery.

In those patients without labral or capsular detachment from the glenoid rim, the capsular shift procedure is performed. Procedures requiring bone block, osteotomy, or coracoid transfer are reserved for those few patients with very specific indications relating to severe bone loss or significant abnormalities of glenoid version.

Surgery for Atraumatic Instability

The surgical approach to correcting multidirectional instability must be individualized. A determination should be made regarding the direction of instability and the degree of side-to-side difference in translation and capsular incompetency. The inferior capsular shift procedure is designed to decrease capsular volume, thickening the capsule on the side of the approach, and tensioning the capsule on the inferior and opposite sides (130,131). Neer also described tightening or closing the rotator internal in order to resist inferior subluxation (113).

Although some authors advocate an anterior approach in all cases, we prefer to approach the shoulder from the side of greatest instability because the overlapping capsule will reinforce the most unstable side. The opposite side will be tensioned by virtue of the shift itself.

Occasionally, a patient with multidirectional instability and hyperlaxity will display clinical signs of instability but lacks a clinical side-to-side difference in translation or evidence of traumatic capsulolabral lesions. We have performed localized arthroscopic thermal capsulorrhaphy in an attempt to tighten selectively the capsular restraints and improve clinical symptoms of instability. Early results with this technique have been encouraging. These patients are immobilized for at least 3 to 4 weeks. The ultimate success of these procedures for ideally suited patients will require further study.

Results of Surgery

Most retrospective clinical studies of the Bankart, capsular shift, Putti-Platt, modified Bristow, and Magnuson-Stack procedures report failure rates between 3% and 6%. Currently reported failure rates for arthroscopic stabilization within the first 2 years after surgery are reported to be between 5% and 40% (127,132,133). Those procedures using staples or screws have an associated risk of hardware migration or malposition. These problems can result in severe degeneration of the joint surface. The Putti Platt, Bristow, and Magnuson-Stack procedures can often result in significant limitation of external rotation (135). Limitation of external rotation can limit the patient's ability to return to overhead-throwing sports. All capsular shift procedures can result in these same limitations if the capsule is made excessively tight. The extent of capsular advancement is best judged at the time of surgical intervention. Potential neurovascular complications of anterior shoulder reconstruction include injury to the axillary and musculocutaneous nerves, and axillary and anterior humeral circumflex vessels.

Overall, the recurrence rate following surgery is 5% or less. The patient's ability to return to functional sport activity requires a long period of therapeutic exercises for stretching and strengthening. Contact sports are discouraged for a 6- to 12-month period following successful surgical intervention.

SHOULDER PAIN IN THE OVERHEAD ATHLETE

Individuals who participate in highly competitive overhead activities will place demands on the shoulder that may exceed the physiological limits of the tissues. Repetitive microtrauma associated with throwing, swimming, or tennis will lead to attenuation of the capsule, resulting in subtle degrees of instability. These patients frequently exhibit an underlying constitutional hyperlaxity that allows them to excel at their sport but predisposes them to instability. The overhead athlete with acquired damage to the static stabilizers most commonly exhibits anterior/inferior instability but may also demonstrate posterior/inferior or multidirectional instability. Alternatively, some patients may present with pain, weakness, clicking, or impingement symptoms and detect no sensation of actual instability. These patients present a di-

agnostic and therapeutic challenge. MRI is useful when plain radiographs are noncontributory. It is also helpful when the athlete presents with a high clinical suspicion of instability, but without a strong indication for surgery unless a specific and significant labral lesion can be identified. The goal of treatment for overhead athletes is not only elimination of pain but also return to their preinjury activity level.

Anterior Instability

Impingement symptoms in the overhead athlete are usually secondary to altered shoulder biomechanics, rather than age-related tendon degeneration and proliferative spur formation. The overhead athlete is generally young, and the impingement symptoms are due to subtle anterior glenohumeral instability. Scapular lag may also contribute to the painful symptoms. Although these patients have positive impingement signs, they also demonstrate apprehension and a positive relocation test. Load and shift testing may confirm capsuloligamentous laxity. Pathologic findings include minor labral clefts or fraying, capsuloligamentous stretching, and articular surface rotator cuff tears. Most patients will improve following nonoperative management incorporating rotator cuff, deltoid, and scapular conditioning. Failure of 6 months of conservative treatment is an indication for surgical repair of the anterior capsulolabral structures. Open capsulorrhaphy often risks overtightening the shoulder, which will preclude return to the original level of competition. Failure to recognize glenohumeral instability as the source of impingement symptoms frequently results in an acromioplasty as the surgical treatment. Isolated acromioplasty in the overhead athlete with anterior glenohumeral instability is not indicated and is cited as a reason for failure to return to a competitive level of athletic activity.

Internal Glenoid Impingement

Cadaveric studies show that the rotator cuff may be compressed between the greater tuberosity and the posterior superior glenoid rim when the arm is placed in maximum abduction and external rotation (Fig. 4.36) (136). This is referred to as *internal glenoid impingement* (35,137,138). The concept of internal glenoid impingement requires an advanced understanding of shoulder biomechanics. In the normal shoulder, the anterior capsulolabral structures become taut at the end range of abduction and external rotation. This occurs during the late cocking or early acceleration phase of throwing. Tightening of the anterior structures leads to 3 to 4 mm of obligate posterior translation of the humeral head on the glenoid (139). This posterior translation facilitates several more degrees of external rotation of the arm before the greater tuberosity forces the rotator cuff against the posterior superior glenoid rim. Repetitive throwing may lead to attenuation of the inferior glenohumeral ligament and an-

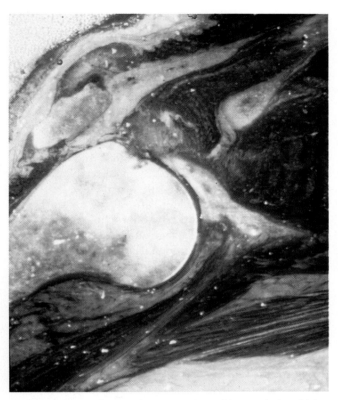

FIGURE 4.36. Cadaveric demonstration of internal glenoid impingement. Placing the arm in the extreme of abduction, external rotation, and extension pinches the posterior rotator cuff between the greater tuberosity and the glenoid rim.

terior capsule. Acquired damage to these structures leads to loss of obligate posterior translation during abduction and external rotation and will often lead to anterior glenohumeral translation. Anterior translation of the humeral head reduces the amount of external rotation available before the articular cartilage of the head ends and the rotator cuff contacts the glenoid rim.

Pain is usually associated with the throwing motion and is localized posteriorly and superiorly. The patient complains of *pain* rather than true *apprehension* during the load and shift test. This pain is alleviated with the relocation test (140). Magnetic resonance arthrography of the shoulder will demonstrate internal glenoid impingement and should be performed with the arm in the abducted, externally rotated position. Arthroscopic examination reveals fraying of the posterior aspect of the supraspinatus tendon as well as the corresponding posterior superior glenoid labrum (137). A rehabilitation program emphasizing strengthening of the rotator cuff, deltoid, and scapular muscles will be successful 80% of the time. Surgical management should include repair of the anterior capsulolabral structures. Isolated debridement of the partial thickness rotator cuff tear without capsulorrhaphy will often be insufficient to allow the athlete to return to his level of activity if anterior instability is present. (34)

SLAP LESIONS AND BICEPS TENDON PATHOLOGY

The exact role of the long head of the biceps remains controversial but pathology of the tendon and the superior labrum may become clinically significant and result in loss of normal shoulder function (141). Disorders of the biceps tendon and superior labrum include biceps tendinitis, subluxation, dislocation, frank rupture of the long head of the biceps, and SLAP lesions.

Biceps Tendinitis

The long head of the biceps lies within the impingement zone and is susceptible to the same mechanical compression as occurs with the rotator cuff tendons. Biceps tendinitis is most often an age-related phenomenon that occurs in conjunction with the impingement syndrome. Synovitis of the long head of the biceps is usually most apparent within the proximal portion of the bicipital groove, beneath the rigid transverse humeral ligament. Osteophytes can develop in this area and may contribute to mechanical compression of the tendon. Continued impingement leads to a chronic inflammatory response and hypertrophy of the tendon. Late rupture of the biceps tendon may occur and is usually associated with a full-thickness tear of the rotator cuff. Primary biceps tendinitis may occur in the absence of rotator cuff pathology, but it is seen less frequently.

Pain emanating from the biceps tendon may be located anteriorly in the biceps groove and will occasionally radiate down the belly of the muscle. The pain is exacerbated with repetitive overhead activities within the impingement zone. It is often difficult to distinguish biceps pain from rotator cuff tendinitis since they usually occur together.

Tenderness can usually be elicited over the intertubercular groove, which is located 7 cm distal to the acromion and is directed anteriorly when the arm is in 10 degrees of internal rotation. Biceps provocative signs, as described earlier, are usually positive. If the rotator cuff is intact, an impingement test may not relieve the biceps pain, owing to the fact that the biceps tendon is an intraarticular structure. A second injection may need to be placed either into the glenohumeral joint or directly into the biceps tendon sheath. When properly administered, a corticosteroid–lidocaine injection should provide significant relief of diagnostic and therapeutic value.

An MRI of the shoulder should not be performed for the diagnosis of isolated biceps tendinitis. When the MRI is obtained to evaluate a partial or full thickness rotator cuff tear, biceps tendinitis or tenosynovitis may be suspected if fluid is present surrounding the biceps tendon. Morphological alterations reflecting degenerative changes of the tendon may be noted as well.

Nonoperative management is directed at treatment of the impingement syndrome. An additional injection into the glenohumeral joint or biceps tendon sheath will result in significant improvement in symptoms. In the absence of rotator cuff tears or biceps tendon instability, the success of nonoperative treatment parallels that for the impingement syndrome. Frank rupture of the long head of the biceps tendon usually results in immediate relief of pain. Surgery is not warranted since the patient will not sustain any notable loss of function.

Biceps tendinitis that is recalcitrant to conservative care warrants an arthroscopic examination. An arthroscopic acromioplasty is usually performed to decompress the subacromial space, and any associated rotator cuff pathology should be addressed as discussed previously. The intraarticular portion of the biceps tendon should be examined. In addition, the extraarticular portion of the tendon that resides in the groove may be pulled into the joint using an Alice clamp that is placed through an anterior portal (spaghetti test). Open tenodesis of the tendon is performed if more than 25% of the tendon is degenerative or if there is evidence of instability of the tendon over the medial wall of the bicipital groove. Results demonstrate excellent pain relief and return to function.

Biceps Instability

The biceps tendon may sublux either medially or laterally depending on arm position. The etiology of biceps instability may be related to its anatomic course in the bicipital groove.

Most commonly, a medial displacement force is placed on the tendon when the arm is in external rotation and abduction. The tendon is then compressed against the medial wall of the groove. In the presence of a shallow groove or incompetence of the medial buttress, the tendon may displace medially. The primary restraint to medial displacement is the rotator interval. Tearing of either the supraspinatus or subscapularis tendons may lead to loss of this restraint. A full-thickness tear of the supraspinatus tendon and rotator interval will allow the biceps tendon to sublux medially *over* the subscapularis tendon. Conversely, tearing of the deep fibers of the subscapularis will allow the biceps tendon to dislocate medially *deep* to the subscapularis tendon. This so-called hidden lesion is often occult to detection during an open approach to the rotator cuff (142). Medial dislocation of the tendon will also occur in the presence of a complete tear of the subscapularis tendon.

Biceps instability often presents as a painful clicking sensation in the young overhead athlete. Gross instability of the biceps tendon often occurs in conjunction with a full thickness rotator cuff tear.

Physical examination includes biceps provocative testing. Assessment of rotator cuff integrity is imperative and should include the abdominal compression test, internal rotation lift off test, and side-to-side comparison of external rotation with the elbow at the side, in order to identify damage to the subscapularis tendon.

MRI is especially useful in detecting full-thickness tears of the rotator cuff as well as tearing of the deep surface of the subscapularis tendon. An empty bicipital groove, with medial translation of the biceps tendon, denoting biceps dislocation, is best appreciated on the axial views.

Nonoperative treatment is appropriate for subtle biceps instability in the absence of acute full-thickness rotator cuff tears. This includes rest, ice, anti-inflammatory medication, and injections into the tendon sheath or glenohumeral joint. Surgical treatment is indicated for recalcitrant biceps instability. Early surgical intervention should be employed in the young patient who presents with weakness and an acute traumatic full-thickness rotator cuff tear. We routinely perform diagnostic arthroscopy to confirm the presence of a hidden lesion, assess the damage to the biceps tendon, and evaluate the rotator cuff tendons and capsulolabral structures. In the absence of traumatic lesions of the biceps tendon, we will repair the rotator cuff and rotator interval. If the biceps tendon is damaged or remains unstable, a biceps tenodesis is performed.

SLAP Lesions

Lesions of the superior labrum have only recently been described as a clinically significant pathologic entity (143,144). The postulated mechanisms of injury include direct compression of the superior labrum resulting from a fall, a traumatic traction injury, and repetitive traction associated with overhead athletic activities. Clinical symptoms are believed to emerge as a result of anterosuperior or posterosuperior instability of the glenohumeral joint. Alternatively, symptoms may occur as a result of displacement of the unstable labrum into the joint. Four types of SLAP (superior labrum anterior and posterior) lesions have been described (Fig. 4.37) (144). Degenerative fraying of the superior labrum is a Type I lesion. The biceps and labrum remain firmly attached to the glenoid and are stable when probed. A Type II lesion is most common (144). The biceps and labrum are avulsed from the glenoid and can be displaced into the joint with a probe (Fig. 4.38). These tears should not be confused with a meniscoid labrum, which represents a normal anatomic variant. A type III lesion is a bucket handle tear of the superior labrum in which the biceps anchor remains firmly attached. A similar tear, which includes a portion of the biceps tendon, is a type IV lesion (Fig. 4.38). A recently described avulsion fracture of the supraglenoid tubercle represents a variation of the SLAP pathology (145).

Patients will present with nonspecific shoulder pain that is frequently associated with mechanical symptoms of "popping" or "catching." O'Brien's test (Fig. 4.39) (141) for the diagnosis of SLAP lesions places the patient's outstretched arm into forward elevation, adduction, and internal rotation (thumb down). The patient is then asked to resist the examiner's downward force on the arm. The test is repeated with the arm in full supination (thumb up). A positive test occurs

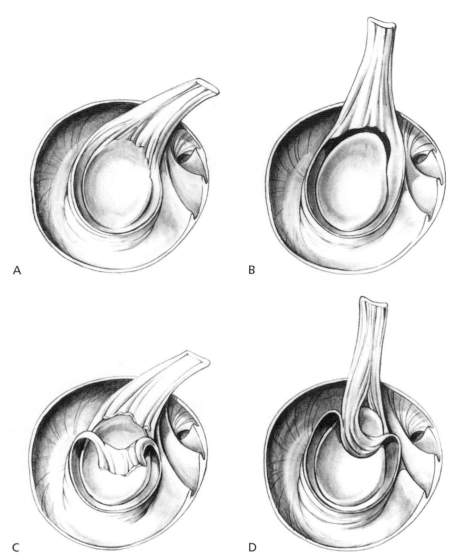

FIGURE 4.37. Classification of SLAP lesions. **A:** Type I is fraying of the superior labrum. **B:** Type II is complete detachment of the biceps anchor and labrum as a single complex. **C:** Type III is a bucket handle tear of the superior labrum with an intact biceps anchor. **D:** Type IV is a bucket handle tear of the superior labrum that extends along the biceps tendon. (From Snyder SJ, Karzel RP, Del Pizzo W, et al. SLAP lesions of the shoulder. *Arthroscopy* 1990;6[4]:274–279, with permission.)

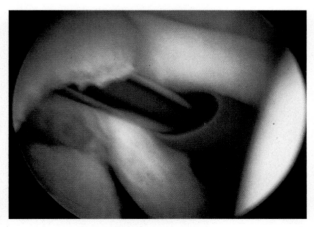
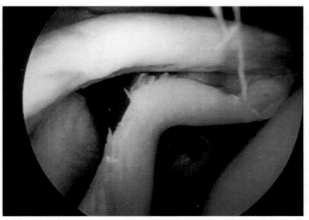

FIGURE 4.38. Arthroscopic demonstration of Type II **(A)** and Type IV **(B)** SLAP lesions.

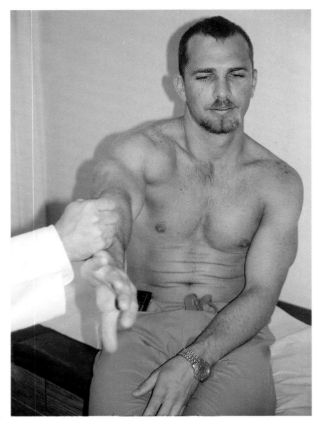
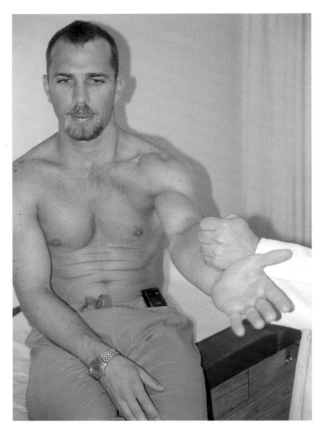

A   B

FIGURE 4.39. O'Brien's test. **A:** A downward directed force will result in pain with the arm in the "thumb down" position. A similarly directed force should be pain free in the "thumb up" position in order to constitute a positive test **(B)**.

when pain is elicited during the first maneuver and is diminished or alleviated with the second maneuver. Occasionally, there will be a popping or catching sensation during the test. The examiner should remember that adduction of the arm will exacerbate AC joint pain and should not confuse this with a positive O'Brien's test. A second test places the patient's hand at the hip with the thumb pointing posteriorly. Force is applied to the elbow in an attempt to sublux the shoulder anteriorly and superiorly. Anterior shoulder pain with or without a painful click constitutes a positive test and will detect a SLAP lesion in 78% of cases.

Nonspecific physical examination findings that are commonly seen in association with a SLAP lesion include a positive impingement test, rotator cuff signs, biceps provocative signs, and anterior instability. Patients will have concomitant partial or full-thickness rotator cuff tears in 40% of cases, and nearly 25% will have an anterior Bankart lesion (146).

A ganglion cyst may be present in either the suprascapular or spinoglenoid notch (147). These cysts arise from extraarticular extravasation of joint fluid through the superior labral tear (Fig. 4.40) in a similar manner as the development of a meniscal cyst of the knee. Compression of the suprascapular nerve will lead to pain and weakness of external rotation. This may clinically be confused with a large chronic rotator cuff tear.

The literature is scant regarding the natural history of the untreated SLAP lesion. Nonoperative management begins with ice, rest, anti-inflammatory medication, and treatment of associated conditions such as impingement. We do not believe that a strengthening or stretching program will eliminate the symptoms associated with a SLAP lesion.

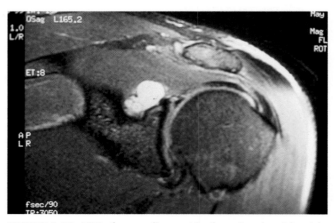

FIGURE 4.40. MRI of a ganglion cyst in the spinoglenoid notch. These are frequently associated with SLAP lesions.

The role of MRI in the diagnosis of SLAP lesions is not clearly defined. The accuracy of MRI in detecting superior labral tears varies, currently approaching 90%. The addition of contrast may improve these results. We will generally obtain an MRI, not only to evaluate the superior labrum but, more importantly, to define the associated pathology such as rotator cuff tears and ganglion cysts (3,147).

The nature of the surgery is dependent on the type of pathology found during arthroscopic examination of the shoulder (144,146,148). Type I lesions are debrided. Type II lesions are debrided and repaired to the superior glenoid using arthroscopic anchors. The bucket handle component of a Type III lesion is excised. The Type IV lesions are repaired or excised if <50% of the biceps tendon is torn. Otherwise, a biceps tenodesis is performed. We will generally attempt to decompress a ganglion cyst arthroscopically (147). Repair of the superior labrum will then prevent the recurrence of the cyst. An MRI is obtained 4 to 6 weeks postoperatively to confirm that the cyst has been fully decompressed. Successful results of operative treatment have been shown in 74% to 83% of patients with isolated symptomatic superior labral lesions (148,149).

CONCLUSION

The painful shoulder frequently presents a diagnostic and therapeutic challenge. Central to the effective management of these conditions is a thorough history and physical examination. Additional diagnostic studies are often useful and should be obtained under appropriate circumstances. They are not a substitute for the clinical examination.

Magnetic resonance imaging of the shoulder is considered unnecessary when the clinical diagnosis is clearly unrelated to mechanical shoulder pathology (cervical spine, peripheral nerve lesions) and when the surgical indications do not exist to warrant obtaining an MRI (atraumatic shoulder injury with incomplete rehabilitation). When the diagnosis is clearly established by clinical criteria, an MRI will not alter the treatment plan (traumatic anterior instability). Magnetic resonance is also of limited diagnostic value when evaluating patients with an isolated diagnosis of adhesive capsulitis, glenohumeral arthritis, acromioclavicular arthritis, or brachial plexopathy (3).

At our institution, MRI has its greatest impact as a preoperative study for patients with rotator cuff disease who have failed an adequate course of nonoperative treatment, and in patients who present with significant rotator cuff weakness following acute trauma. This information is important in identifying an appropriate surgical candidate, aiding surgical planning, and predicting outcome. An MRI is valuable as a diagnostic tool in patients with chronic shoulder pain who have failed nonoperative treatment and have a history and physical examination that do provide a clear anatomic source of shoulder pain. It is also helpful in the athlete with

a strong suspicion of clinical instability, but without firm surgical indications unless a significant labral lesion is identified.

The role of MRI continues to evolve as its ability to detect pathologic lesions improves. However, the principles guiding the decision to obtain an MRI remain the same. Magnetic resonance imaging is most valuable and cost-effective when the information that it contains will be used by an experienced clinician to influence the further management of the patient.

REFERENCES

1. Matsen FA III, Lippitt S, Sidles JA. *Practical evaluation and management of the shoulder.* Philadelphia: WB Saunders, 1994,151–219.
2. Williams GR, Iannotti JP, Rosenthal A, et al. Anatomic, histologic, and magnetic resonance imaginer abnormalities of the shoulder. *Clin Orthop* 1996;330:66–74.
3. Sher JS, Iannotti JP, Williams GR et al. The effect of shoulder magnetic resonance imaging on clinical decision making. *J Shoulder Elbow Surg* 1998;7(3):205–209.
4. Boorstein JM, Kneeland J, Dalinka MK, et al. Magnetic resonance imaging of the shoulder. *Current Prob Diag Rad* 1992;21 (1).
5. Sher J, Uribe J, Posada A, et al. Abnormal findings on magnetic resonance images of symptomatic shoulders. *J Bone Joint Surg* 1995;77A:10–15.
6. Herzog, RJ. Magnetic resonance of the shoulder. *J Bone Joint Surg* 1997;79-A(6):934–953.
7. Jobe FW. Painful athletic injuries of the shoulder. *Clin Orthop* 1983;173:117–124.
8. Neer CS. Impingement lesions. *Clin Orthop* 1983;173:71–77.
9. Matsen F, Artnz C. Subacromial impingement. In: Rockwood C, Matsen F, eds. *The shoulder.* Philadelphia: WB Saunders, 1990, 623–648.
10. Uhthoff HK, Sarker K. An algorithm for shoulder pain caused by soft tissue disorders. *Clin Orthol* 1990;254:121–127.
11. Cohen RB, Williams GR. Impingement syndrome and rotator cuff disease as repetitive motion disorders. *Clin Orthop* 1998;351: 95–101.
12. Iannotti, J. Full-thickness rotator cuff tears: factors affecting surgical outcome. *J Acad Orthop Surg* 1994;2:87–95.
13. McConville OR, Iannotti, JP. Partial thickness rotator-cuff tears. *JAAOS* 1999;7(1):32–43.
14. Gartsman GM. Arthroscopic treatment of rotator cuff disease. *J Shoulder Elbow Surg* 1995;4(3):228–241.
15. Gartsman GM. Arthroscopic acromioplasty for lesions of the rotator cuff. *J Bone Joint Surg* 1990;72A:169–180.
16. Ellman H. Diagnosis and treatment of incomplete rotator cuff tears. *Clin Orthop* 1990;254:64–74.
17. Weber SC. Arthroscopic debridement and acromioplasty versus mini-open repair in the management of significant partial-thickness tears of the rotator cuff. *Orthop Clin North Am* 1997; 28(1):79–82.
18. Yamanaka K, Matsumoto T. The joint side tear of the rotator cuff: a follow-up study by arthrography. *Clin Orthop* 1994;304:68–73.
19. Hawkins RJ, Abrams JS. Impingement syndrome in the absence of rotator cuff tear (Stages I and 2). *Orthop Clin North Am* 1987; 18(3):373–382.
20. Neer CS, II. Anterior acromioplasty for the chronic impingement syndrome in the shoulder: a preliminary report. *J Bone Joint Surg* 1972;54A:41–50.
21. Rathbun JB, Macnab, I. The microvascular pattern of the rotator cuff. *J Bone Joint Surg* 1970;52B(3):540–553.

22. Neviaser TJ. The role of the biceps tendon in the impingement syndrome. *Orthop Clin North Am* 1987;18(3):383–386.
23. Moseley HF, Goldie I. The arterial pattern of the rotator cuff of the shoulder. *J Bone Joint Surg* 1963;45B:780.
24. Iannotti JP. *Rotator cuff disorders: evaluation and treatment.* AA OS Monograph Series. 1991.
25. Lohr JF, Uhthoff HK. The microvascular pattern of the supraspinatus tendon. *Clin Orthop* 1990;254:35–38.
26. Brewer BJ. Aging of the rotator cuff. *Am J Sports Med* 1979; 17:102–110.
27. Clark JM, Harryman DT, II. Tendons, ligaments, and capsule of the rotator cuff. *J Bone Joint Surg* 1992;74A(5):713–725.
28. Zuckerman JD, Kummer FJ, Cuomo F, et al. The influence of coracoacromial arch anatomy on rotator cuff tears. *J Shoulder Elbow Surg* 1992;1(1):4–14.
29. Jacobson SR, Speer KP, Janda DH, et al. Reliability of radiographic assessment of acromial morphology. *J Shoulder Elbow Surg* 1995;4:449–453.
30. Aoki M, Ishii S, Usui M. *Clinical application for measuring the slope of the acromion.* St. Louis: Mosby–Year Book, 1990:200–203.
31. Itoi E, Tabata S. Incomplete rotator cuff tears: results of operative treatment. *Clin Orthop* 1992;284:128–135.
32. Paulos LE, Franklin JL. Arthroscopic shoulder decompression development and application: a five year experience. *Am J Sports Med* 1990;18(3):235–244.
33. Iannotti JP, Zlatkin MB, Esterhai JL, et al. Magnetic resonance imaging of the shoulder: sensitivity, specificity and predictive value. *J Bone Joint Surg* 1991;73A:17–29.
34. Walch G, Boileau P, Noel E, et al. Impingement of the deep surface of the supraspinatus tendon on the posterosuperior glenoid rim: an arthroscopic study. *J Shoulder Elbow Surg* 1992;1:238–245.
35. Jobe CM. Superior glenoid impingement. *Orthop Clin North Am* 1997;28:137–143.
36. Warner JJP, Micheli LJ, Arslanian LE, et al. Scapulothoracic motion in normal shoulders and shoulders with glenohumeral instability and impingement syndrome. *Clin Orthop* 1992;285:191–199.
37. Uhthoff HK. Calcifying tendinitis, an active cell-mediated calcification. *Virchows Archiv A, Pathol Anatom Histol* 1975;366(1):51–58.
38. Gerber C, Galantay RV, Hersche O. The pattern of pain produced by irritation of the acromioclavicular joint and the subacromial space. *J Shoulder Elbow Surg* 1998;7(4):352–355.
39. Hertel R, Ballmer FT, Lombert SM, et al. Lag signs in the diagnosis of rotator cuff rupture. *J Shoulder Elbow Surg* 1996;5(4):307–313.
40. Weiner DS, MacNab I. Ruptures of the rotator cuff: follow-up evaluation of operative repairs. *Can J Surg* 1970;13:219–227.
41. Ono K, Yamamuro T, Rockwood CA. Use of a thirty-degree caudal tilt radiograph in the shoulder impingement syndrome. *J Shoulder Elbow Surg* 1992;1(5):246–252.
42. Watson M. Major ruptures of the rotator cuff: the results of surgical repair in 89 patients. *J Bone Joint Surg* 1985;6713:618–624.
43. Gartsman GM, Milne JC. Articular surface partial-thickness rotator cuff tears. *J Shoulder Elbow Surg* 1995;4(6):409–415.
44. Wright SA, Cofield RH. Management of partial-thickness rotator cuff tears. *J Shoulder Elbow Surg* 1996;5(6):458–466.
45. Bigliani LU, Morrison D, April EW. The morphology of the acromion and its relationship to rotator cuff tears. *Orthop Trans* 1986; 1:228.
46. Lazarus M, Chansky H, Misra S, et al. Comparison of open and arthroscopic subacromial decompression. *J Shoulder Elbow Surg* 1994;3:1–11.
47. Altchek DW, Warren RF, Wickiewicz TL, et al. Arthroscopic acromioplasty: techniques and results. *J Bone Joint Surg* 1990;72A:1198–1207.
48. Norlin R. Arthroscopic subacromial decompression versus open acromioplasty. *Arthroscopy* 1989;5:321–323.
49. Tibone JE, Jobe FW, Kerlan RK, et al. Shoulder impingement syndrome in athletes treated by an anterior acromioplasty. *Clin Orthop* 1985;198:134–140.
50. Andrews J, Broussard T, Carson, W. Arthroscopy of the shoulder in the management of partial tears of the rotator cuff: a preliminary report. *Arthroscopy* 1985;1:117–122.
51. Snyder S, Pachelli A, Pizzo W, et al. Partial thickness rotator cuff tears: results of arthroscopic treatment. *Arthroscopy* 1991;7:1–7.
52. Ryu RKN. Arthroscopic subacromial decompression. *Arthroscopy* 1992;8:141–147.
53. Iannotti JP, Bernot MP, Kuhlman JR, et al. Postoperative assessment of shoulder function: a prospective study of full-thickness rotator cuff tears. *J Shoulder Elbow Surg* 1996;5(6):449–457.
54. Gupta R, Leggin BG, Iannotti, JP. Results of surgical repair of full-thickness tears of the rotator cuff. *Ortho Clin North Am* 1997;28(2):241–248.
55. Harryman DT, Mack LA, Wang KY, et al. Repairs of the rotator cuff: correlation of functional results with integrity of the cuff. *J Bone Joint Surgery* 1991;73A(7):982–989.
56. Iannotti J, Bernot M, Kuhlman J, et al. Prospective evaluation of rotator cuff repair. *J Shoulder Elbow Surg* 1993;2:S9.
57. Gore D, Murray M, Sepic S, et al. Shoulder-muscle strength and range of motion following surgical repair of full thickness rotator cuff tears. *J Bone Joint Surg* 1986;68A:266–272.
58. Ellman H, Hanker G, Bayer M. Repair of the rotator cuff: end-result study of factors influencing reconstruction. *J Bone Joint Surg* 1986;68A:1136–1144.
59. Hawkins RJ, Misamore GW, Hobeika PE. Surgery for full thickness rotator cuff tears. *J Bone Joint Surg* 1985;67A(9):1349–1355.
60. Bigliani LU, Cordasco FA, McIlveen SJ, et al. Operative repair of massive rotator cuff tears: long term results. *J Shoulder Elbow Surg* 1992;1:120–130.
61. Montgomery TJ, Yerger B, Savoie FH. Management of rotator cuff tears: a comparison of arthroscopic debridement and surgical repair. *J Shoulder Elbow Surg* 1994;3(2):70–78.
62. Warner JJP, Goitz RJ, Ingang JJ, et al. Arthroscopic-assisted rotator cuff repair: patient selection and treatment outcome. *J Shoulder Elbow Surg* 1997;6(5):463–472.
63. Liu SH. Arthroscopically assisted rotator cuff repair. *J Bone Joint Surg* 1994;76B:592–595.
64. Blevins FT, Warren RF, Cavo C, et al. Arthroscopic assisted rotator cuff repair: results using a mini-open deltoid splitting approach. *Arthroscopy* 1996;12(1):50–59.
65. Paulos LE, Kody MH. Arthroscopically enhanced "miniapproach" to rotator cuff repair. *Am J Sports Med* 1994;22(1):19–25.
66. Gerber C. Latissimus dorsi transfer for the treatment of irreparable tears of the rotator cuff. *Clin Orthop* 1993;275:152–160.
67. Rockwood CA, Jr., Williams GR, Jr., Burkhead WZ, Jr. Debridement of degenerative, irreparable lesions of the rotator cuff. *J Bone Joint Surg* 1995;77A(6):857–866.
68. Burkhart S. Arthroscopic treatment of massive rotator cuff tears. *Clin Orthop* 1991;267:45–56.
69. Wiley AM. Superior humeral dislocation: a complication following decompression and debridement for rotator cuff tears. *Clin Orthop* 1991;(263):135–141.
70. Bigliani LU, Norris TR, Fischer J. The relationship between the unfused acromial epiphysis and subacromial impingement lesions. *Orthop Trans* 1983;7(1):138.
71. Gerber C, Terrier FM, Ganz R. The role of the coracoid process in the chronic impingement syndrome. *J Bone Joint Surg* 1985;67B(5):703–708.
72. Dines DM, Warren RF, Inglis AE, et al. The coracoid impingement syndrome. *J Bone Joint Surg* 1990;72B:314–316.
73. Gartsman G, Blair M, Noble P, et al. Arthroscopic subacromial decompression: an anatomical study. *Am J Sports Med* 1988;16:48–50.

74. Ogilvie-Harris D, Wiley A, Sattarian J. Failed acromioplasty for impingement syndrome. *J Bone Joint Surg* 1990;72B:1070–1072.

75. Hawkins RJ, Brock RM, Abrams JS, et al. Acromioplasty for impingement with an intact rotator cuff. *J Bone Joint Surg* 1988;70B(5):795–797.

76. Groh G, Simoni M, Rolla P, et al. Loss of the deltoid after shoulder operations: an operative disaster. *J Shoulder Elbow Surg* 1994;3:243–253.

77. Cofield RH. Tears of rotator cuff. *Instr Course Lect* 1981;30:258–273.

78. Adamson GJ, Tibone JE. Ten year assessment of primary rotator cuff repairs. *J Shoulder Elbow Surg* 1993;2:57–65.

79. Tibone JE, Elrod B, Jobe FW, et al. Surgical treatment of tears of the rotator cuff in athletes. *J Bone Joint Surg* 1986;68A:887–891.

80. Tibone J, Jobe F, Kerlan R, et al. Shoulder impingement syndrome in athletes treated by an anterior acromioplasty. *Clin Orthop.* 1985;198:134–140

81. Harryman DT, II, Sidles JA, Harris S, et al. Laxity of the normal glenohumeral joint: a quantitative *in vivo* assessment. *J Shoulder Elbow Surg* 1992;1(2):66–76.

82. Pagnani MJ, Warren RF. Stabilizers of the glenohumeral joint. *J Shoulder Elbow Surg* 1994;3:173–190.

83. Saha AK. Dynamic stability of the glenohumeral joint. *Acta Orthop Scand* 1971;42:491–505.

84. Flatow EL, Soslowsky LJ, Ateshian GA, et al. Shoulder joint anatomy and the effect of subluxations and size mismatch on patterns of glenohumeral contact. *Orthop Trans* 1991;15:803–804.

85. Soslowsky LJ, Flatow EL, Bigliani LU, et al. Articular geometry of the glenohumeral joint. *Clin Orthop* 1992;285:181–190.

86. Iannotti JP, Gabriel JP, Schneck SL, et al. The normal glenohumeral relationships. *J Bone Joint Surg* 1992;74A(4):491–500.

87. Cooper DE, Arnoczky SP, O'Brien SJ, et al. Anatomy, histology, and vascularity of the glenoid labrum. *J Bone Joint Surg* 1992;74A(1):46–52.

88. Howell SM, Galinat BJ. The glenoid-labral socket: a constrained articular surface. *Clin Orthop* 1989;243:122–125.

89. Lippitt SB, Vanderhooft JE, Harris SL, et al. Glenohumeral stability from concavity-compression: a quantitative analysis. *J Shoulder Elbow Surg* 1993;2(1):27–35.

90. Gibb TD, Sidles JA, Harryman DT, II, et al. The effect of capsular venting on glenohumeral laxity. *Clin Orthop* 1991;268:120–127.

91. Blasier RB, Guldberg RE, Rothman ED. Anterior shoulder stability: contributions of rotator cuff forces and the capsular ligaments in a cadaver model. *J Shoulder Elbow Surg* 1992;1(3):140–150.

92. Warner JJP, Caborn DNM, Berger R, et al. Dynamic capsuloligamentous anatomy of the glenohumeral joint. *J Shoulder Elbow Surg* 1993;2:115–133.

93. DePalma AF, Gallery G, Bennett CA. Variational anatomy and degenerative lesions of the shoulder joint. In: Blount W, ed. *American Academy of Orthopaedic Surgeons instructional course lectures.* Vol. VI. Ann Arbor, MI: JW Edwards, 1949:255–281.

94. Soslowsky LJ, Malicky DM, Blasier RB. Active and passive factors in inferior glenohumeral stabilization: a biomechanical model. *J Shoulder Elbow Surg* 1997;6(4):371–379.

95. Poppen NK, Walker PS. Normal and abnormal motion of the shoulder. *J Bone Joint Surg* 1976;5 8A(2):195–201.

96. Taylor DC, Arciero RA. Pathologic changes associated with shoulder dislocations. *Am J Sports Med* 1997;25(3):306–311.

97. Thomas SC, Matsen FA. An approach to the repair of avulsion of the glenohumeral ligaments in the management of traumatic anterior glenohumeral instability. *J Bone Joint Surg* 1989;71A:506–513.

98. Bankart, ASB. The pathology and treatment of recurrent dislocation of the shoulder joint. *Br J Surg* 1938;26:23–29.

99. Speer KP, Deng X, Borrero S, et al. Biomechanical evaluation of a simulated Bankart lesion. *J Bone Joint Surg* 1994;76A:1819–1826.

100. Bigliani LU, Pollock RG, Soslowsky LJ, et al. Tensile properties of the inferior glenohumeral ligament. *J Orthop Res* 1992;10(2):187–197.

101. Nicola T. Anterior dislocation of the shoulder. *J Bone Joint Surg* 1942;24(3):614–616.

102. Wolf EM, Cheng JC, Dickson K. Humeral avulsion of glenohumeral ligaments as a cause of anterior shoulder instability. *Arthroscopy* 1995;11(5):600–607.

103. Field LD, Bokor DJ, Savoie FH, III. Humeral and glenoid detachment of the anterior inferior glenohumeral ligament: a cause of anterior shoulder instability. *J Shoulder Elbow Surg* 1997;6(1):6–10.

104. Hill HA, Sachs MD. The grooved defect in the humeral head: a frequently unrecognized complication of dislocations of the shoulder joint. *Radiology* 1940;35:690–700.

105. Lippitt SB, Harris SL, Douglas T, et al. In vivo quantification of the laxity of normal and unstable glenohumeral joints. *J Shoulder Elbow Surg* 1994;3:215–223.

106. Gerber C. Observations on the classification of instability. In: Warner JJP, Iannotti JP, Gerber C, eds. *Complex and revision problems in shoulder surgery.* Philadelphia: Lippincott–Raven, 1997:9–18.

107. Hovelius L, Eriksson K, Fridin H, et al. Recurrences after initial dislocation of the shoulder. *dBJS* 1983;65A(3):343–349.

108. McLaughlin HL, MacLellan DI. Recurrent anterior dislocation of the shoulder: a comparative study. *J Trauma* 1967;7:191–201.

109. Bigliani LU. *The unstable shoulder.* AAOS Monograph Series. 1996.

110. Hawkins RJ, Bell RH, Hawkins RH, et al. Anterior dislocation of the shoulder in the older patient. *Clin Orthop* 1986;206:192.

111. Rowe CR, Zarins B. Recurrent transient subluxation of the shoulder. *J Bone Joint Surg* 1981;63A(6):863–872.

112. Neer CS, II. Involuntary inferior and multidirectional instability of the shoulder: etiology, recognition and treatment. *Instr Cour Lect* 1985;34:232–238.

113. Neer CS, II, Foster CS. Inferior capsular shift for involuntary inferior and multidirectional instability of the shoulder. *J Bone Joint Surg* 1980;62A(6):897–908.

114. Rowe CR, Pierce DS, Clark JG. Voluntary dislocation of the shoulder: a preliminary report on a clinical, electromyographic, and psychiatric study of 26 patients. *J Bone Joint Surg* 1973;55A(3):445–460.

115. Simonet WT, Cofield RH. Prognosis in anterior shoulder dislocation. *Am J Sports Med* 1984;12(1):19–24.

116. Matthews LS, Pavlovich LJ. Anterior and anteroinferior instability: diagnosis and treatment. In: Iannotti JP, Williams GR, eds. *Disorders of the shoulder: diagnosis and treatment.* Philadelphia: Lippincott Williams & Wilkins, 1999:251–294.

117. Garth VT, Slappey CE, Ochs CW. Roentgenographic demonstration of instability of the shoulder: the apical oblique projection. *J Bone Joint Surg* 1984;66A(9):1450–1453.

118. DuToit GT, Roux D. Recurrent dislocation of the shoulder: a 24-year study of the Johannesburg stapling operation. *J Bone Joint Surg* 1956;38A:1–12.

119. Bankart ASB. The pathology and treatment of recurrent dislocation of the shoulder joint. *Br J Surg* 1939;26:23–29.

120. Rowe CR, Patel D, et al. The Bankart procedure: a long-term end-result study. *J Bone Joint Surg* 1978;60A(1):1–16.

121. Magnuson PB, Stack IK. Recurrent dislocation of the shoulder. *JAMA* 1943;123:889–892.

122. Helfet AJ. Coracoid transplantation for recurring dislocation of the shoulder. *J Bone Joint Surg* 195 8;40B(2):198–202.

123. Scott DJJ. Treatment of recurrent posterior dislocations of the shoulder by glenoplasty. *J Bone Joint Surg* 1967;49A:471.

124. Brostrom LA, Kronberg M, Soderlund V. Surgical and methodologic aspects of proximal humeral osteotomy for

stabilization of the shoulder joint. *J Shoulder Elbow Surg* 1993; 2(2):93–98.

125. Weber BG, Simpson LA, Hardegger F. Rotational humeral osteotomy for recurrent anterior dislocations of the shoulder associated with a large Hill-Sachs lesion. *J Bone Joint Surg* 1984;66A: 1443.

126. Kronberg M, Brostrom LA. Humeral head retroversion in patients with unstable humeroscapular joints. *Clin Orthop* 1990; (260):207–211.

127. Arciero RA, Wheeler JH, Ryan JB et al. Arthroscopic Bankart repair versus nonoperative treatment for acute, initial anterior shoulder dislocations. *Am J Sports Med* 1994;22(5):589–594.

128. Walch G, Boileau P, Levigne C, et al. Arthroscopic stabilization for recurrent anterior shoulder dislocation: results of 59 cases. *Arthroscopy* 1995;11(2):173–179.

129. Bigliani LU, Kurzweil PR, Schwartzbach CC, et al. Inferior capsular shift procedure for anterior-inferior shoulder instability in athletes. *Am J Sports Med* 1994;22(5):578–584.

130. Cooper RA, Brems JJ. The inferior capsular shift procedure for multidirectional instability of the shoulder. *J Bone Joint Surg* 1992;74A:1516–1529.

131. Wirth MA, Groh GI, Rockwood CA. Capsulorrhaphy through an anterior approach for the treatment of atraumatic posterior glenohumeral instability with multidirectional laxity of the shoulder. *J Bone Joint Surg* 1998;80–A(I 1) :1570–1578.

132. Green MR, Christensen KP. Arthroscopic versus open Bankart procedures: a comparison of early morbidity and complications. *Arthroscopy* 1993;9(4):371–374.

133. Warner JJ, Miller MD, Marks P, et al. Arthroscopic Bankart repair with the Suretac device. Part 1: Clinical observations. *Arthroscopy* 1995;11(1):2–13.

134. Zuckerman JD, Matsen FA. Complications about the glenohumeral joint related to the use of screws and staples. *J Bone Joint Surg* 1984;66A:175.

135. Angelo RL, Hawkins RL. Osteoarthritis following an excessively tight Putti-Platt repair. In *American Shoulder and Elbow Surgeons 4th Open Meeting,* Atlanta, 1988.

136. Jobe CM, Sidles J. Evidence for a superior glenoid impingement upon the rotator cuff: anatomic, kinesiologic, MRI & arthroscopic findings. In: *5th International Conference on Surgery of the Shoulder,* Paris, France, 1992.

137. Davidson PA, Elattrache NS, Jobe CM, et al. Rotator cuff and posterior-superior glenoid labrum injury associated with increased glenohumeral motion: a new site of impingement. *J Shoulder Elbow Surg* 1995;4(5):384–390.

138. Jobe CM. Superior glenoid impingement: current concepts. *Clin Orthop* 1996;(330):98–107.

139. Howell SM, Galinat BJ, Renzi AJ, et al. Normal and abnormal mechanics of the glenohumeral joint in the horizontal plane. *J Bone Joint Surg* 1988;70A(2):227–232.

140. Speer KP, Hannafin JA, Altchek DW, et al. An evaluation of the shoulder relocation test. *J Shoulder Elbow Surg* 1994;3:53.

141. Yamaguchi K, Bindra R. Disorders of the biceps tendon. In: Iannotti JP, Williams GR, eds. *Disorder of the shoulder: diagnosis and treatment.* Philadelphia: Lippincott Williams & Wilkins, 1999:159–190.

142. Walch G, Nove-Josserland L, Levigne C, et al. Tears of the supraspinatus associated with hidden lesions of the rotator interval. *J Shoulder Elbow Surg* 1994;3:353–360.

143. Andrews JR, Carson WG, McLeod WD. Glenoid labrum tears related to the long head of the biceps. *Am J Sports Med* 1985; 13(5):337–341.

144. Snyder SJ, Karzel RP, Del Pizzo W, et al. SLAP lesions of the shoulder. *Arthroscopy* 1990;6(4):274–279.

145. Iannotti JP, Wang ED. Avulsion fracture of the supraglenoid tubercle: a variation of the SLAP lesion. *J Shoulder Elbow Surg* 1992;1(1):26–30.

146. Snyder AJ, Banas MP, Karzel RP. An analysis of 140 injuries to the superior glenoid labrum. *J Shoulder Elbow Surg* 1995;4(4):243–248.

147. Iannotti JP, Ramsey ML. Arthroscopic decompression of a ganglion cyst causing suprascapular nerve decompression. *Arthroscopy* 1996;12:739–745.

148. Resch H, Golser K, Thoeni H, et al. Arthroscopic repair of superior glenoid labral detachment. *J Shoulder Elbow Surg* 1993; 2(3):147–155.

149. Stetson WP, Snyder SE, Karzel RP, et al. Long-term clinical follow-up of isolated SLAP lesions of the shoulder. In: *64th Annual Meeting of the AAOS,* Feb. 13–17, 1997.

CHAPTER 5

SHOULDER ANATOMY

MICHAEL B. ZLATKIN
CARY J. HOFFMAN
STEVEN NEEDELL

GENERAL SHOULDER ANATOMY

The shoulder enjoys a greater range of motion than any other joint in the body. In fact, it is not just a single joint but the synergistic action of four separate articulations: the glenohumeral, acromioclavicular, sternoclavicular, and scapulothoracic joints (Figs. 5.1–5.7).

The glenohumeral joint is a multiaxial ball-and-socket joint lying between the roughly hemispheric humeral head and the shallow glenoid fossa of the scapula (1). The glenoid fossa is essentially a pear-shaped cavity with dimensions approximately one-fourth the size of the humeral head (2). The glenoid is covered by articular cartilage that is thinner centrally. The humeral head is also covered with articular cartilage that thins slightly at the periphery to accentuate glenohumeral joint congruity (3). This anatomy permits a wider range of motion than is possible at any other joint. The shoulder is capable of flexion-extension, abduction-adduction, circumduction, and medial and lateral rotation (1). This anatomy provides mobility but renders the joint relatively unstable and therefore prone to subluxation and dislocation. This is because of the small size of the glenoid fossa compared to the humeral head and also because of the relative laxity of the joint capsule. These movements and the associated inherent instability of the glenohumeral joint have also recently been felt to be important conceptually with regard to understanding internal impingement in the overhand athlete. Cadaveric research has demonstrated pinching of the rotator cuff against the posterosuperior glenoid rim when the shoulder is positioned in maximum external rotation and abduction (4). This simulates the position of the late cocking phase of throwing and such, because the greater tuberosity appears to force the rotator cuff and glenoid abrum against the glenoid rim. Thus, repetitive throwing with fatigue of the shoulder musculature may represent one way that secondary restraints may fail to protect the rotator cuff against internal impingement.

The proximal end of the humerus consists of the head and greater and lesser tuberosities. The humeral head is nor-mally retroverted approximately 30° with the arm in anatomic position. The articular surface is directed superiorly, medially, and posteriorly with an axis angled 130° to 150° relative to the humeral shaft (3). The anatomic neck of the humerus lies at the base of the articular surface at the proximal end of the bone. The neck is the site of attachment of the inferior aspect of the joint capsule. The greater tuberosity is located on the lateral aspect of the proximal humerus and is the site of insertion of the supraspinatus, infraspinatus, and teres minor tendons (Fig. 5.1). The supraspinatus tendon inserts on the highest point of the greater tuberosity (Fig. 5.1). The infraspinatus and teres minor tendons localize, respectively, to the middle and lower thirds of the greater tuberosity and lie somewhat more posteriorly than the supraspinatus tendon insertion. The lesser tuberosity is situated on the anterior portion of the proximal humerus, medial to the greater tuberosity. The subscapularis tendon inserts here in a broad band (Fig. 5.1).

The intertubercular (bicipital) groove is located between the greater and lesser tuberosities. The transverse humeral ligament stretches between the two tuberosities, forming the roof of the intertubercular groove. The tendon of the long head of the biceps brachii muscle passes through here, surrounded by a synovial sheath (Fig. 5.3). The width of the groove can be variable in size; if it is shallow, this may predispose it to impingement. Below the greater and lessor tuberosities, the humerus tapers to a region referred to as the *surgical neck*. The intertubercular groove at this level normally then becomes more shallow, and its medial lip provides the insertion site for the latissimus dorsi and teres major tendons; its lateral lip provides the insertion site for the pectoralis major (3). The deltoid inserts along the deltoid tuberosity, a smooth, broad bony prominence on the midportion of the diaphysis. The coracobrachialis also inserts at this level along the medial border of the humerus. The long head of the triceps muscle attaches to the infraglenoid tubercle, which is a triangular surface where the inferior glenoid rim joins the lateral scapular border (3).

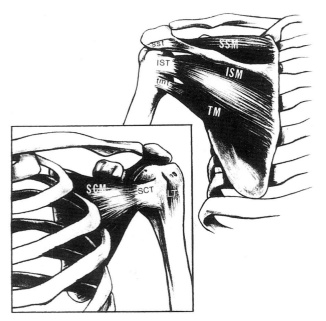

FIGURE 5.1. Rotator cuff muscles and tendons. The supraspinatus tendon inserts more superiorly and anteriorly on the greater tuberosity, the infraspinatus and teres minor more posteriorly and inferiorly. The subscapularis is a broader band and is anterior. It inserts in a fanlike fashion on the lesser tuberosity. ISM, infraspinatus muscle; IST, infraspinatus tendon; LT, lesser tuberosity; SSM, supraspinatus muscle; SST, supraspinatus tendon; SCM, subscapularis muscle; SCT, subscapularis tendon; TM, teres minor muscle; TMT, teres minor tendon.

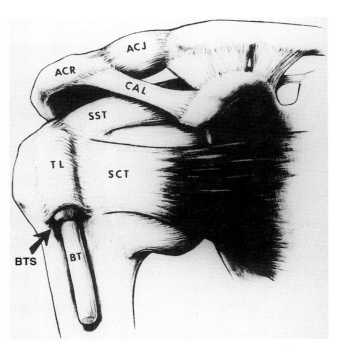

FIGURE 5.3. The coracoacromial arch and surrounding structures. Note the relationship of the supraspinatus tendon to the anterior acromion, acromioclavicular joint, and coracoacromial ligament. The long head of biceps tendon also courses through this region, surrounded by its own synovial sheath. ACJ, acromioclavicular joint; ACR, acromion; BT, biceps tendon; BTS, biceps tendon sheath; CAL, coracoacromial ligament; CN, conoid ligament; CP, coracoid process; SCT subscapularis tendon; SST, supraspinatus tendon; TL, transverse humeral ligament.

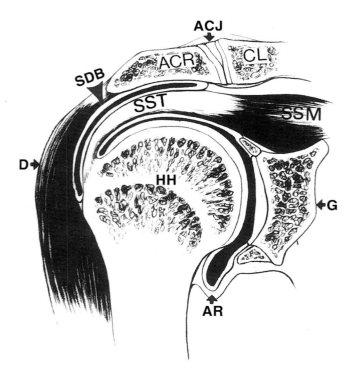

FIGURE 5.2. Cross sectional diagram illustrating several important structures and relations of the shoulder. ACJ, acromioclavicular joint; ACR, acromion; AR, axillary recess; CL, clavicle; D, deltoid muscle; G, glenoid; HH, humeral head; SDB, subdeltoid bursa; SSM, supraspinatus muscle; SST, supraspinatus tendon.

Hyaline articular cartilage lines the surfaces of the humeral head. The cartilage on the humeral head is thickest at its center. The blood supply to the humeral head is via the anterior humeral circumflex artery. There is a normal "sulcus" located posteriorly on the humeral head (5). This represents an area of "bare bone" between the insertion of the posterior capsule and overlying synovial membrane and the edge of the articular surface of the humeral head. The sulcus results from the expected aging process, commencing in the third decade, where the capsule and synovium retract and expose a sulcus of bare bone. The appearance of this sulcus on cross sectional images has sometimes been confused with a Hill-Sachs lesion.

The glenoid fossa is situated on the superolateral aspect of the scapula (Fig. 5.6). The superior portion of the fossa is narrow, the inferior portion is broad. In man there is greater anterior tilt to the glenoid fossa and therefore greater anterior instability (6,7). The glenoid fossa is lined by articular cartilage, thinner in the center than at the outer edges. The glenoid labrum rims the glenoid cavity, and provides inherent stability to the glenohumeral joint, restricting anterior and posterior excursion of the humerus (2) (Fig. 5.6). The labrum consists of hyaline cartilage, fibrocartilage, and fibrous tissue.

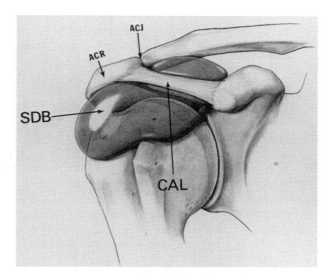

FIGURE 5.4. Diagram illustrating the extent of a fully distended subacromial-subdeltoid bursa (SDB). CAL, coracoaromial ligament; ACJ, acromioclavicular joint; ACR, anterior acromion.

Mosely (8) has shown that unlike the meniscus of the knee, which is mainly fibrocartilage, fibrocartilage is present in the labrum only in a small transition zone, at the attachment to the osseous glenoid rim. The blood supply of the labrum is through small periosteal and capsular vessels. The vessels supply the outermost portion of the labrum. The inner portion is without vessels, similar to the knee meniscus.

The glenoid labrum is variable in size and thickness. In young patients, the labrum is closely attached at its base to the glenoid, blending with the fibrils of hyaline articular cartilage. In later years, especially the superior portion of the

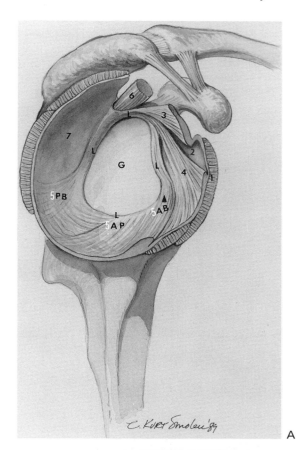

A

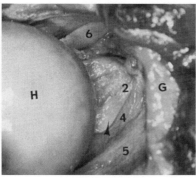

B

FIGURE 5.6. A: Diagram of capsular mechanism and surrounding structures. B: Corresponding cadaver specimen dissected from posterior. The capsule and glenohumeral ligaments are seen. The opening into the subscapularis bursa, located above the middle glenohumeral ligament, is identified. The anterior band of the inferior glenohumeral ligament is prominent in the specimen in B, in keeping with its role in anterior inferior stability. Also note its close relationship and attachment to the labrum. The long head of biceps tendon arises in the supraglenoid region, with the superior labrum, forming the biceps-labral anchor. 1, subscapularis muscle; 2, anterior capsule; 3, superior glenohumeral ligament; 4, middle glenohumeral ligament; 5, inferior glenohumeral ligament; AB, anterior band; AP, axillary pouch; PB, posterior band; 6, biceps tendon, long head; 7, posterior capsule; 8, posterior rotator cuff; L, glenoid labrum; G, glenoid; H, humeral head. Black arrowhead indicates opening into subscapularis bursa. (From Zlatkin MB, Bjorkengren AG, Gylys-Morin V, et al. Cross-sectional imaging of the capsular mechanism of the glenohumeral joint. *Am J Roentgenol* 1988;150:151–158, with permission.)

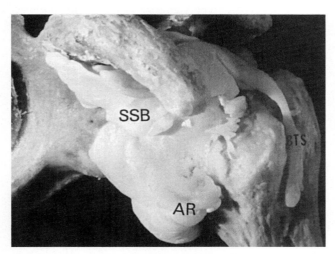

FIGURE 5.5. Shoulder specimen injected with methyl methacrylate illustrates the appearance of a distended joint capsule. Note the axillary recess (AR) and the subscapularis bursa (SSB). The tendon sheath of the long head of the biceps tendon communicates with the joint and can also be identified (BTS). (From Donald Resnick, M.D., San Diego, CA, with permission.)

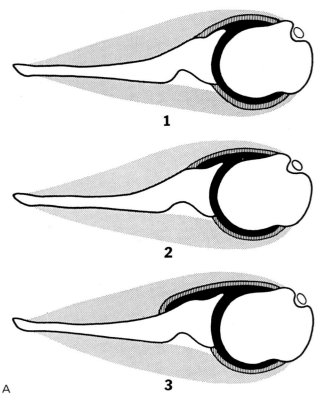

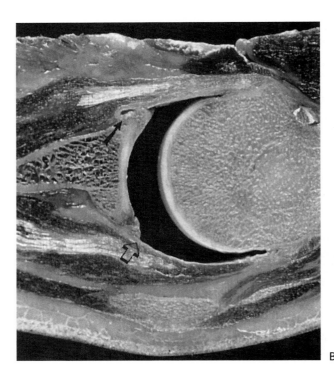

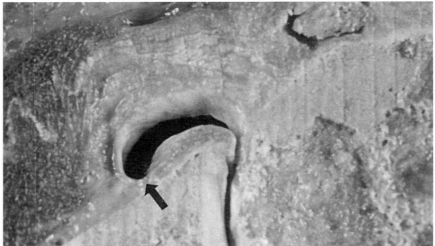

FIGURE 5.7. A: Diagram illustrating the three types (1–3) of anterior capsular insertions. **B:** Cadaver section depicting a type 1 anterior capsular insertion (*black arrow*). The posterior capsule most commonly inserts directly into the labrum (*open black arrow*). **C:** Cadaver section illustrating a more medial anterior capsule insertion, type 2 (*black arrow*). (From Zlatkin MB, Bjorkengren AG, Gylys-Morin V, et al. Cross-sectional imaging of the capsular mechanism of the glenohumeral joint. *Am J Roentgenol* 1988;150:151–158, with permission.)

labrum may rest free on the edge of the glenoid (9), such that a probe may be placed between the labrum and the glenoid articular surface. This may arise as a result of pull by the superior glenohumeral ligament and biceps tendon (9). When the labrum has this appearance, it may be distinguished from a labral tear by its smooth borders. In young athletes, superior quadrant labral tears may result from traction by these same two structures in overhead throwing (10).

The fibrous glenoid labrum deepens and enlarges the shallow glenoid fossa. The glenoid is also deepened by the thin cartilaginous lining in the center of this structure. Al-

though this was felt to increase the stability of the joint, some investigators believe this is not as significant as once believed. Recently, the importance of the labrum as a site for ligamentous attachment has been stressed (Fig. 5.6) (11). It is believed that the strong intertwining between the collagen fibers of the glenohumeral ligaments and the labrum is more resistant to injury than the glenolabral junction/union. There appears to be a strong pathophysiological relationship between the locations of labral lesions and the attachment sites of the glenohumeral ligaments and proximal biceps tendon (Fig. 5.6) (12). The inferior portion of the labral-ligamentous complex is more important than the superior portion in stabilizing the glenohumeral joint. It is this portion of the labrum that is more commonly injured in patients with anterior glenohumeral instability. Nonetheless, the superior labrum does play some role in the stability of the glenohumeral joint where it functions in conjunction with the biceps tendon, through the biceps labral complex (Fig. 5.6). If tension is placed on the biceps tendon, it does stabilize the humeral head. It is the superior and anterior superior portions of the labrum that are more variable in terms of their attachment to the glenoid, as is discussed in more detail later, while the more inferior portion of the labrum is typically fixed.

A loose, redundant fibrous capsule envelops the joint. It is lined by a synovial membrane and has a surface area that is approximately twice that of the humeral head (3) (Figs. 5.2, 5.5). It encompasses all the intracapsular soft-tissue structures, including the biceps tendon, glenohumeral ligaments, labrum, and synovial recesses. In the bursal recesses, this membrane may be redundant. Superiorly, the capsule encroaches on the root of the coracoid process and inserts in the supraglenoid region. Laterally, the capsule inserts into the anatomic neck of the humerus and inferiorly into the periosteum of the humeral shaft. With the arm at the side, the lower part of the capsule is lax, forming the axillary recess (Figs. 5.2, 5.5). Posteriorly and inferiorly, the capsule is continuous with the capsular border of the labrum and the adjacent bone. Medially, the anterior capsular insertion may be variable (13) based on its relationship to the glenoid labrum (Fig. 5.7). It may insert directly into the labrum, type 1, which is considered the most stable and most common (14). In 23% of cases (14), it inserts progressively more medially along the scapular neck, Types 2 and 3, which have been considered to be less stable. Type 2 capsules insert more medially, but less than 1 cm from the labrum on the glenoid, whereas Type 3 capsules insert greater than 1 cm along the scapular neck (15,16). In Types 2 and 3, the capsule is not directly continuous with the anterior portion of the labrum. More medial capsular insertions have been thought to contribute to, be predisposed to, or be associated with anterior shoulder instability. A type 3 capsule may potentially be difficult to distinguish from healed anterior capsular stripping on cross sectional imaging, but in anatomic location, it is more superior on the glenoid than the typical site of a capsular lesion associated with instability. More recent study with MRI and MR arthography has called into question the correlation between the type of capsular insertion and glenohumeral instability (17).

The fibrous capsule is strengthened in several areas. The coracohumeral ligament is a strong fibrous band extending from the coracoid process over the humerus, to attach to the greater tuberosity. It has a more important function in shoulder stability than previously thought (18,19). It also supports the long head of biceps tendon in the intertubercular groove. Anteriorly the capsule may thicken to form the

superior (SGHL), middle (MGHL), and inferior glenohumeral ligaments (IGHL) (9) (Fig. 5.6). These ligaments reinforce the anterior portion of the capsule and act as a check to external rotation of the humeral head (9). They extend from adjacent to the lesser tuberosity to the anterior border of the glenoid fossa.

The superior glenohumeral ligament, together with the coracohumeral ligament, stabilizes the shoulder joint when the arm is in the adducted dependent position. The ligament consists of two proximal attachments: one to the superoanterior aspect of the labrum conjoined with the biceps tendon, and the other to the base of the coracoid process (Figs. 5.6, 5.8). This ligament projects in a lateral fashion to insert along the anterior aspect of the anatomic neck of the humerus, superior and medial to the lesser tuberosity (2,5), and is present in 90% to 97% of cadaveric dissections (11) and approximately 85% of cases with MR arthrography (20).

The middle and inferior glenohumeral ligaments blend with the labrum at a level lower than that of the superior ligament although fibers from the MGHL extend to the upper half of the labrum as well (Figs. 5.6, 5.8). These ligaments and the recesses between them have been shown to be quite variable (9). The greatest variation is seen in relation to the middle glenohumeral ligament, which is absent in approximately 27% of cadaveric dissections (11). The recesses may be quite large. When large, they may be associated with a small or absent middle glenohumeral ligament, a medial capsular insertion on the scapular neck, and a prominent subscapularis bursa. This may form a large anterior pouch, which may then offer no passive restraint to anterior dislocation. The middle glenohumeral ligament provides stabilization to the glenohumeral joint when the shoulder is abducted 45°, and it has been identified in 85% of cases with MR arthrography (11). It originates from just beneath the superior glenohumeral ligament along the anterior border of the glenoid to the junctions of the middle and inferior third of the glenoid rim. It blends with the anteroinferior aspect of the capsule and inserts along the anterior aspect of the surgical neck of the humerus, anterior and inferior to the lesser tuberosity (2,5).

The inferior glenohumeral ligament has a complex configuration (21) (Figs. 5.6, 5.8, 5.9). It may be identified as a distinct structure or as just a diffuse thickening of the capsule. It is the thickest portion of the capsule. It consists of three portions: the anterior band, posterior band, and axillary pouch/recess of the capsule. It stabilizes the glenohumeral joint when the arm is abducted to approximately 90° and has been identified in 91% of cases with MR arthrography (Figs. 5.8, 5.9) (11). The ligament has a triangular configuration, with its origin from the anteroinferior and posterior margin of the glenoid rim below its epiphyseal line. As opposed to the other glenohumeral ligaments, its origin is inseparable from the base of the labrum. Turkel et al. (22) found that the inferior glenohumeral ligament consistently attaches to the anterior and anteroinferior aspects of

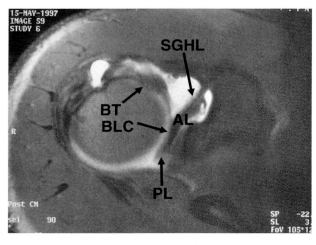

A

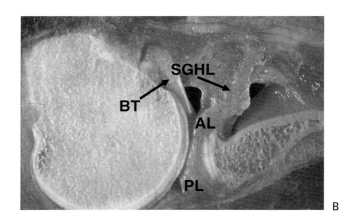

B

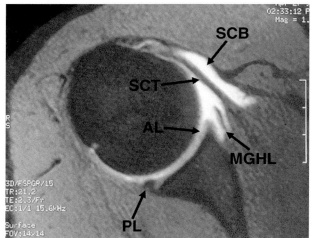

C

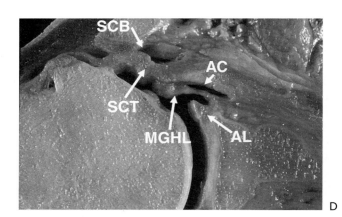

D

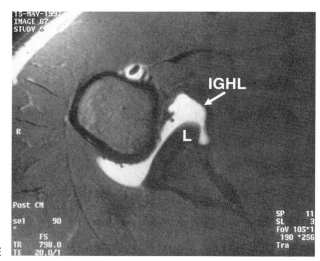

E

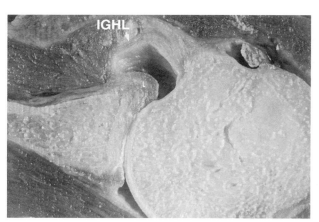

F

FIGURE 5.8. Cross sectional anatomy of the glenohumeral ligaments and surrounding structures (axial plane). MR images obtained after intraarticular gadolinium injection, TR/TE (800/20) images, with fat saturation, and corresponding cadaver sections **(A, B)**. The superior attachments of the superior glenohumeral ligament are seen, with the biceps tendon into the superior glenoid with the superior labrum and more anteriorly along the coracoid. The confluence of the biceps tendon long head and superior labrum form the biceps-labral anchor. AL, anterior superior labrum; BLC, biceps-labral complex; BT, biceps tendon long head; PL, posterior superior labrum; SGHL, superior glenohumeral ligament. **C, D:** Midglenoid level shows the relationship of the anterior labrum (*AL*) to the middle glenohumeral ligament (*MGHL*), anterior capsule (*AC*), and subscapularis tendon (*SCT*). The subscapularis bursa is continuous with the joint and extends anterior to the subscapularis tendon (*SCB*). **E, F:** Anterior inferior glenoid level. Here the anterior band of the inferior glenohumeral (*IGHL, white arrow*) ligament and subjacent capsule is thick and forms a complex with the labrum (*L*), which is usually also round and thick at this level.

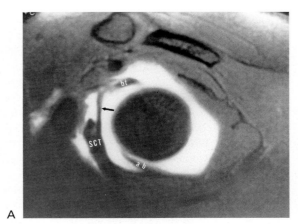 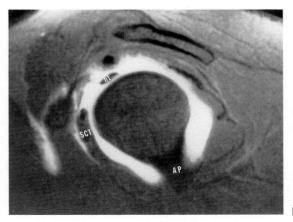

FIGURE 5.9. A, B: Glenohumeral ligaments. Sagittal oblique MR images obtained after intra-articular gadolinium injection, TR/TE (800/20) images, with fat saturation. The anterior band (*AB*) and axillary pouch portions (*AP*) of the inferior glenohumeral ligament can be well seen in this plane when contrast is present. BT, biceps tendon; SCT, subscapularis tendon. Small arrow in A, middle glenohumeral ligament coursing obliquely and superiorly.

the labrum, and, as such, these structures should be conceptually regarded as one and the same (5). The inferior glenohumeral ligament inserts along the inferior aspect of the surgical neck of the humerus. The thickest aspect of the IGHL is along its superior edge, further defined as the *superior band* of the inferior glenohumeral ligament, which functions in association with the subscapularis muscle and middle glenohumeral ligament in the middle ranges of abduction (22).

Glenohumeral joint stability is primarily achieved through soft-tissue restraint, as articular surface conformity offers little inherent stability, and the joint capsule and ligaments have been shown to provide static limitation to translations of the glenohumeral joint. The ligamentous support structures/capsule, however, are lax throughout most of glenohumeral rotation; therefore, large excursions of the humeral head on the glenoid are possible in the absence of active muscle contractions across the joint (23).

On all sides of the capsule except the inferior portion, it is reinforced by the tendons of the rotator cuff muscles: the supraspinatus, infraspinatus, teres minor, and subscapularis muscles. These tendons all blend with the fibrous capsule over varying lengths, averaging approximately 2.5 cm to form the musculotendinous cuff, also known as the *fibrotendinous* or *capsulotendinous cuff* (Figs. 5.1, 5.6). Of the rotator cuff tendons the supraspinatus tendon is the one that is most often injured. The primary function of the supraspinatus muscle and tendon complex is to abduct the humerus, but it also has a role in humeral rotation. The abductor function is carried out by the fibers of the supraspinatus tendon enveloping the superior surface of the humerus, whereby tension on these fibers tends to depress the humeral head, counteracting the uplifting force of the deltoid muscle (3). The innervation of the supraspinatus muscle is provided by the suprascapular nerve (C5 and C6 roots), which passes through the suprascapular notch. The suprapinatus tendon

has been traditionally described as being identified and arising primarily on the anterior margin of the muscle belly. It then extends over the top of the humeral head to insert on the greater tuberosity superiorly. Recent study, however, indicates that the supraspinatus may in fact consist of two distinct portions. The ventral portion originates from the anterior supraspinatus fossa inserting anteriorly onto the greater tuberosity. In addition, less well known is that this ventral portion of the supraspinatus tendon may additionally have a site of insertion onto the lesser tuberosity. This portion of the supraspinatus may also function as an internal rotator of the arm. The second portion of the supraspinatus is located more posteriorly, with muscle fibers originating from the posterior aspect of the supraspinatus fossa and spine of the scapula with a "straplike" configuration. It has several small tendon slips that coalesce into a broad fibrous attachment inserting more posteriorly onto the greater tuberosity. This is the portion that acts primarily as a shoulder abductor (24). In addition medially originating fibers from both muscle portions merge in a bipennate fashion to form a strong tendon eccentrically located within the muscle with a mean obliquity to the coronal plane of 50°.

The main function of the infraspinatus muscle–tendon unit is external rotation of the humerus. It also functions to depress the humeral head and, as a static stabilizer of the glenohumeral joint, resists posterior subluxation of the humeral head in internal rotation (3). The infraspinatus muscle is innervated by the distal fibers of the suprascapular nerve. The infraspinatus tendon is posterior to the supraspinatus tendon and inserts on the middle facet of the greater tuberosity, inferior and posterior to the supraspinatus tendon. It courses more obliquely than the supraspinatus tendon. In addition to the infraspinatus muscle's function as an external rotator, it also helps keep the humeral head centered (25).

The teres minor is posteroinferior to the infraspinatus (Fig. 5.1). It inserts more inferiorly on the lowermost facet of the greater tuberosity. The least commonly injured, it is a powerful external rotator of the humerus. It also helps resist subluxation of the humeral head (3). The teres minor muscle is innervated by branches of the axillary nerve. The teres minor also forms part of the border of the quadrilateral space as well as the triangular space. The quadrilateral space is bounded by the teres minor muscle superiorly, the long head of the triceps muscle medially, the teres major muscle inferiorly, and the surgical neck of the humerus laterally. It is important as the posterior humeral circumflex artery and vein and axillary nerve course through the space. With compression or entrapment of the axillary nerve, patients can present with shoulder pain, nondermatomal paresthesia, and deltoid weakness, referred to clinically as *quadrilateral space syndrome* (26). Medial to the triceps muscle is the triangular space, bordered superiorly by the teres minor muscle and inferiorly by the teres major muscle. This space contains the circumflex scapular artery.

The subscapularis is the largest and most powerful muscle of the rotator cuff with a broad-based belly that takes origin from much of the anterior scapula (Fig. 5.1). It has four to six strong tendon slips that arise medially deep within the muscle. These slips converge to form a main tendon that inserts along the superior aspect of the lesser tuberosity (27). Additional tendon fibers from the subscapularis merge with the transverse humeral ligament and extend across the floor of the bicipital groove, fusing with those of the supraspinatus tendon into a sheath that encompasses the biceps tendon (28). The subscapularis muscle is supplied by the upper and lower subscapular nerve (3). In addition to the subscapularis's primary role in active internal rotation, it also functions in adduction, depression, flexion, and extension. The subscapularis tendon also reinforces the anterior joint capsule and becomes continuous with it. The subscapularis tendon is separated from the rest of the rotator cuff tendons by the rotator cuff interval, discussed later.

The rotator cuff tendons fuse along their distal attachments to the greater and lesser tuberosities to provide a continuous water-tight unit (29). Prior to their fusion, the anatomic space between the supraspinatus and subscapularis along the anterosuperior aspect of the shoulder is the rotator interval (Fig. 5.10). It is a complex region and can be conceptualized in layers (30,31). The outermost layer consists of fibrofatty tissue; beneath this fibrofatty tissue is the coracohumeral ligament, the rotator interval capsule, and then the superior glenohumeral ligament. The coracohumeral ligament courses from the coracoid process into the interval, fusing with the interval capsule. This capsule–ligament complex extends superiorly, merging and fusing with the anterior margin and superficial/deep fascial fibers of the supraspinatus anteriorly. The interval capsule and ligament also extend inferiorly to the superior margin of the subscapularis and project laterally to insert on the greater and lesser tuberosities. The superior glenohumeral ligament also is a contributor to this complex of structures, originating from the

supraglenoid tubercle contiguous to the attachment of the long head of the biceps tendon, and then coursing laterally to insert at the lesser tuberosity, where it fuses with the coracohumeral ligament (29). This fused rotator interval capsule and coracohumeral ligament are important stabilizers and anterosuperior supporting structures for shoulder function, and they can be conceptualized as a roof over the intraarticular course of the biceps tendon, which is the deepest structure in the interval. When the interval capsule and coracohumeral ligament are disrupted, the shoulder may be susceptible to posterior inferior subluxation and instability (29).

The biceps brachii functions primarily as a supinator of the forearm and a flexor of the elbow joint. There are two tendinous origins of the biceps muscle. Recent biomechanical and clinical studies have clarified its role in stabilizing the humeral head in the glenoid during abduction of the shoulder (32). The intraarticular portion of the LHB arises from the supraglenoid tubercle (Figs. 5.6, 5.8, 5.9, 5.11) and the posterosuperior glenoid labrum. It runs across the superomedial aspect of the humeral head and enters the intertubercular sulcus, which is formed by the greater tuberosity, the lesser tuberosity, and soft tissue, including the insertion of the subscapularis tendon and coracohumeral ligament (32). It penetrates the rotator cuff between the supraspinatus and subscapularis at the rotator interval. The biceps tendon is surrounded by a synovial sheath, which is continuous with the synovial sheath of the shoulder joint (Fig. 5.3). Therefore, any disorder that involves the capsule may also involve the biceps tendon sheath. The anterior relationships of the proximal long head of the biceps include the coracohumeral ligament, the superior glenohumeral ligament, the anterior supraspinatus tendon, and the subscapularis tendon. These are the stabilizers of this portion of the tendon. The tendon is secured within the groove by the transverse humeral ligament, which passes between the tuberosities, over the synovial sheath of the tendon. The transverse humeral ligament is formed by a few fibers of the capsule, or as a continuation of the subscapularis tendon.

The LHB does not slide; rather, the humeral head moves on the fixed tendon during motion at the shoulder joint, the bicipital gliding mechanism (32). The biceps tendon mainly functions through its distal insertion at the elbow, but it also has some function at the shoulder, where it acts as a stabilizer, as well as a humeral head depressor. In external rotation, the humeral head and bicipital groove may act as an osseous fulcrum for the tendon's function as a depressor. With internal rotation, the biceps relies on a ligamentous/capsular pulley, over which the biceps tendon curves from the bicipital groove into the rotator interval. This sling also receives contributions from the coracohumeral ligament and superior glenohumeral ligament, which fuse together onto their common insertion on the lesser tuberosity. The proximal transverse humeral ligament, which forms the roof over the bicipital groove, also associates intimately with the ligamentous pulley (29). Its action as a depressor of the humeral

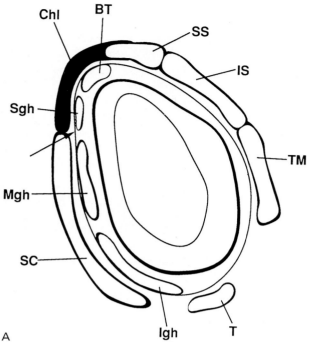

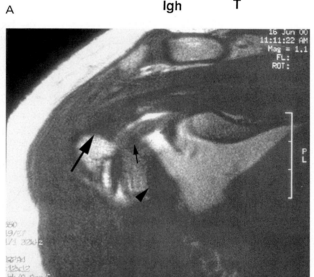

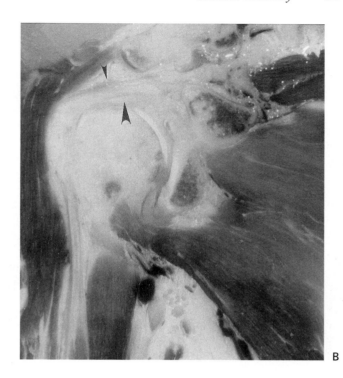

FIGURE 5.10. Rotator interval structures. **A:** Sagittal diagram through the left shoulder; structures of the anterior interval. The first layer of the interval includes the subscapularis (*SC*) and supraspinatus (*SS*) tendons and the coracohumeral ligament (*Chl*). Deep to this is the articular capsule (*black arrow*), followed by the superior glenohumeral ligament (*Sgh*) and the biceps tendon (*BT*) and its sheath. Also shown is the infraspinatus (*IS*), teres minor (*TM*), middle glenohumeral ligament (*Mgh*), inferior glenohumeral ligament (*Igh*), and triceps long head (*T*). **B:** Anatomic section reveals the anterior supraspinatus tendon (*small arrowhead*) and biceps tendon (*large arrowhead*). **C:** Coronal oblique MRI arthrogram, TR/TE (550/19), demonstrates the anterior supraspinatus tendon (*large arrow*), the biceps tendon (*small arrow*), and the distal subscapularis tendon (*arrowhead*).

head is thought to be increased in patients with impingement lesions. It is closely associated functionally with the rotator cuff. The short head arises from the tip of the coracoid process. The conjoined tendon of the coracobrachialis muscle and the short head of the biceps brachii muscle join on the tip of the coracoid process.

In addition to the principal muscles that act on the glenohumeral joint, which are the deltoid and the rotator cuff muscles, and the biceps mechanism, other important muscles that act on this joint include the teres major, the coracobrachialis, triceps, pectoralis major, and latissimus dorsi.

There are a number of bursae about the glenohumeral joint. The subdeltoid bursa is the largest bursa in the human body (Figs. 5.2, 5.4). It is composed primarily of a subacromial and subdeltoid portion. The size and configuration of the subdeltoid bursa vary considerably, extending between the complex of the acromion and coracoacromial arch of which it is a part, and the rotator cuff. The bursa is firmly adherent to the periosteum of the undersurface of the acromion, coracoacromial ligament, and superior surface of the rotator cuff. Its lateral extent projects deep to the deltoid muscle approximately 3 cm along the outer margin of the greater tuberosity. Medially, the bursa exhibits considerable variability extending as far as 2 cm medial to the acromioclavicular joint. Anteriorly, the bursa covers the superior aspect of the bicipital groove; posteriorly, the bursa extends

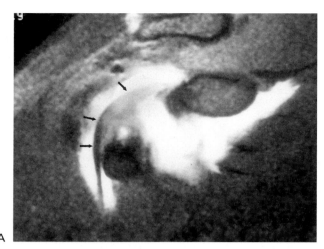
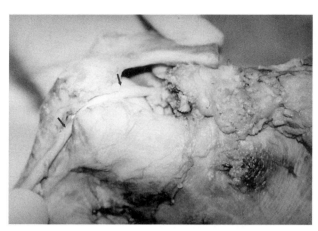

FIGURE 5.11. Biceps tendon. **A:** Coronal oblique MR images obtained after intraarticular gadolinium injection, TR/TE (600/20) images, with fat saturation. **B:** Dissected anatomic specimen. The long head of biceps tendon is seen extending from the supraglenoid region, into the intertubercular groove (*black arrows*).

between the deltoid muscle and rotator cuff musculature. In a recent study, the subdeltoid bursa demonstrated continuity between the subdeltoid and subacromial components in all specimens (33). The bursa on histological analysis demonstrates a synovial-lined potential space within a fine layer of mature areolar-adipose tissue that lubricates motion between the rotator cuff and the acromion and acromioclavicular joint; hence, it is often inflamed in patients with impingement and rotator cuff disease. It communicates with the joint cavity only if a full-thickness tear of the rotator cuff opens through the joint capsule into the floor of the bursa.

The subcoracoid bursa resides between the subscapularis tendon and the combined tendon of the coracobrachialis and the short head of the biceps tendon. It is identified in nearly 97% of gross specimens and communicates with the subdeltoid bursa in 11% of anatomic specimens (34). The subcoracoid bursa should not communicate with the glenohumeral joint under normal circumstances. Subcoracoid bursitis may rarely be implicated as the sole cause of shoulder pain typically presenting as nonspecific anterior shoulder discomfort.

The subcoracoid bursa should not be confused with the subscapularis bursa which is found in up to 90% of the population (Figs. 5.5, 5.6, 5.8). The subscapularis bursa is not truly a separate bursa but rather an outpouching of the glenohumeral joint protruding between the superior and middle glenohumeral ligaments and residing between the posterior aspect of the subscapularis muscle-tendon and the anterior surface of the scapula. The opening into the bursa between these two ligaments is known as the *foramen of Weitbrecht*. Another less common opening into this bursa between the middle and inferior glenohumeral ligament is known as the *foramen of Rouviere*. The subscapularis bursa communicates with the joint cavity and protects the subscapularis tendon as it passes under the coracoid, or over the

neck of the scapula. The subscapularis recess may extend over the subscapularis tendon and therefore acts as a gliding mechanism for this structure (Fig. 5.8). Synovitis and loose bodies are often found here. In patients with anterior instability, the recess may be particularly large.

The *infraspinatus bursa* is a small infrequent bursa between the infraspinatus tendon and the scapula that does not communicate with the joint space (3).

The *acromioclavicular joint* is a small, relatively immobile synovial articulation between the medial aspect of the acromion and the lateral portion of the clavicle (Fig. 5.2). Its range of motion between the extremes of shoulder position is approximately 20° (35). The articular surfaces of the acromion and clavicle are covered with fibrocartilage. In the central portion of the joint is an articular disk that is fibrocartilaginous in nature and usually incomplete. A synovium-lined articular capsule surrounds the joint. It is reinforced by the superior and inferior acromioclavicular ligaments. The inferior portion of the joint is also reinforced by fibers of the coracoacromial ligament, which blends with the undersurface of the capsule (3). The coracoclavicular ligament complex is the major source of stability of the acromioclavicular joint. The coracoclavicular ligament forms a fan-shaped ligament complex that connects the base of the coracoid process to the overlying clavicle. This ligament has two components, the posteromedial conoid and anterolateral trapezoid ligaments, and is identified on oblique coronal and oblique sagittal images (27). The main function of these ligaments is to prevent upward dislocation of the clavicle (Fig. 5.3).

The coracoacromial arch (Figs. 5.3, 5.4) is a strong, bony, and ligamentous arch that protects the humeral head and rotator cuff tendons from direct trauma (13). It consists of the acromion, acromioclavicular joint, coracoid process, and the coracoacromial ligament. Portions of the rotator cuff tendons, including the supraspinatus tendon and the superior

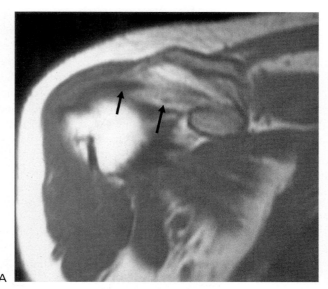
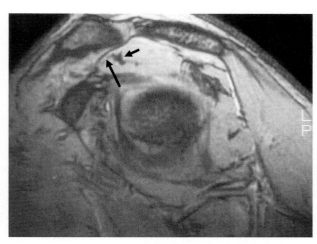

FIGURE 5.12. Coracoacromial ligament. **A:** Coronal Oblique MR image TR/TE (800/20). **B:** Sagittal oblique Gradient echo image. TR/TE (600/15), flip angle 30°. Note the close relationship of the coracoacromial ligament (*larger arrows*) to the supraspinatus tendon (*smaller arrows*).

20% of the infraspinatus and subscapularis tendons, pass under this arch as they extend to their insertion on the humerus (Fig. 5.11) (3). The coracoacromial ligament is unyielding in nature and is close to the humeral head during abduction (Fig. 5.12). It limits the space available to the rotator cuff, subdeltoid bursa, and biceps during this motion. The ligament can be variable in its appearance, which is important with regard to surgical planning (36). In approximately two-thirds of subjects, the ligament morphology follows the classical description: a strong, fibrous, triangular-shaped structure composed of two conjoined or closely adjacent bands. The ligament is attached at its base to the anterior two-thirds of the coracoid. Superiorly, the two bands blend into an apex that inserts onto the tip of the acromion. This superior attachment site usually continues along the lateral margin of the acromion for a variable distance posteriorly. In the other third of cases, the base of the ligamentous triangle is broadened and extends posteriorly all the way to the base of the coracoid. There is often a gap (0.5–1.5 cm) between the two bands that persists as they converge toward the acromial insertion. This results in a broad acromial insertion site, with the ligament carpeting the entire undersurface of the anterior medial acromion and underlying a substantial portion, if not all, of the acromioclavicular joint (37). This broad acromial insertion site is thought to be worsened with certain acromial shapes, thickening of the coracoacromial ligament, and bony osteophytes on the anterior acromion or acromioclavicular joint. This may then contribute to the process of chronic impingement and attrition of the rotator cuff and associated tendons beneath this arch, particularly when the arm is moved into overhead motion.

Acromial morphology has been categorized utilizing plain radiographic analysis by Morrison and Bigliani: Type I, flat; Type II, curved; Type III, hooked (Fig. 5.13) (38). This configuration can be assessed with MR imaging utilizing the sagittal images, although this approach has met with variability and poor reliability among investigators (39,40). Some observers believe that the J- or hook-shaped Type III morphology, with its abrupt downward-facing leading edge anteriorly, has the highest association with impingement syndrome and rotator cuff abnormalities (3).

The coracohumeral ligament originates from the lateral margin of the base of the coracoid process, blends with the supraspinatus tendon, and attaches to both the greater and lesser tuberosities, creating a tunnel for the biceps tendon. This ligament stabilizes the long head of the biceps tendon and also projects within the rotator interval (Fig. 5.10) (41). The ligament also is believed to restrain external rotation of

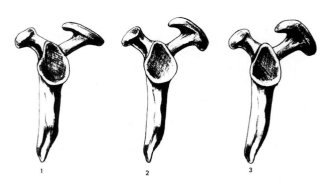

FIGURE 5.13. Acromion shape. The three types of anterior acromion: Type I, flat; Type II, curved; Type III, hook shaped.

the humerus and, in conjunction with the supraspinatus muscle, supports the dependent arm (3).

The suprascapular notch lies just lateral to the base of the coracoid process. The superior transverse scapular ligament converts the notch to a foramen through which the suprascapular nerve passes through. The suprascapular vessels project superior to this ligament (3). The inferior transverse scapular ligament is present inconsistently and extends from the scapular spine to the glenoid rim lateral to the spinoglenoid notch. The subscapular nerve passes between this ligament and notch (3).

MRI AND MRI ARTHROGRAPHIC ANATOMY

MRI Anatomy

The shoulder is typically imaged with the patient in a supine position with the arm at the side in a position of neutral or mild external rotation (Figs. 5.14–5.17). Progressive improvements in surface coil developments and design with

newer and faster pulse sequences have resulted in higher-quality MR images. For example, the newer phased array and quadrature shoulder coil configurations have proved to be of great value in imaging of the shoulder. Typical planes obtained in shoulder imaging include the following; axial, extending from the level of the acromion through the glenoid; oblique coronal obtained parallel to the scapula and supraspinatus, and extending through the subscapularis tendon anteriorly and the infraspinatus tendon posteriorly; and oblique sagittal, from the level of the scapula neck through the lateral border of the greater tuberosity, perpendicular to the coronal plane (38).

The pulse sequences utilized are variable, but typically they will include oblique coronal dual echo fast spin echo (DE-FSE) with the second echo of the sequence with fat saturation, axial DE-FSE with fat saturation, axial gradient echo, and sagittal T2-weighted FSE sequences with or without fat saturation. Fast short TI inversion recovery (STIR) sequences can also be used instead of the T2-FSE with fat saturation sequence. More recently, many have begun to use

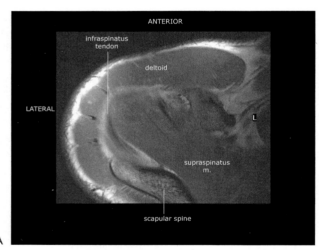

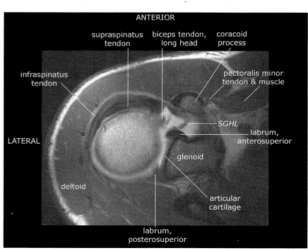

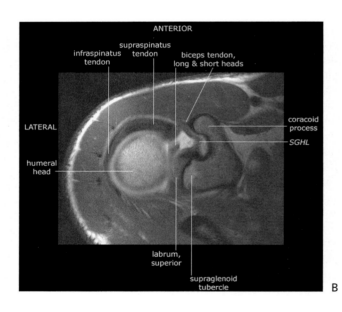

FIGURE 5.14. A–G: Axial MRI and MR arthrographic anatomy. Superior to inferior; short TR/TE images (800/20). IGHL, inferior glenohumeral ligament; MGHL, middle glenohumeral ligament; SGHL, superior glenohumeral ligament; subscap, subscapularis; pect., pectoralis; m, muscle.

FSE sequences with intermediate weighting and fat suppression in place of the dual echo sequences along with higher imaging matrices.

In the normal state, subcutaneous fat, intermuscular fat planes, and bone marrow have the highest signal on short TR/TE or long TR short TE images, due to their relatively short T1. On long TR/TE images, they are of intermediate signal intensity. Muscles and hyaline cartilage have an intermediate to high signal intensity on all spin echo pulse sequences, and on gradient echo sequences articular cartilage tends to have high signal intensity. Due to a relative lack of mobile protons, a long T1, and a short T2, certain structures should have essentially a very low or no MR signal. These structures include cortical bone, the glenoid labrum, the fi-

brous capsule, the glenohumeral, and other ligaments and tendons, such as the tendinous insertions of the rotator cuff musculature, and the long head of biceps tendon, as it courses in the bicipital groove (42,43). Numerous studies have shown that signal may be present in the ligaments, tendons, and fibrocartilage of asymptomatic people due to age-related degeneration, subclinical pathology, partial volume averaging of normal tissues, or artifacts including magic angle effects (44–51).

Axial images (Fig. 5.14) demonstrate the relationship between the humeral head and glenoid fossa. Articular cartilage and the glenoid labrum are well depicted. The superior and middle portions of the anterior glenoid labrum are usually triangular in this plane, whereas the more anterior inferior

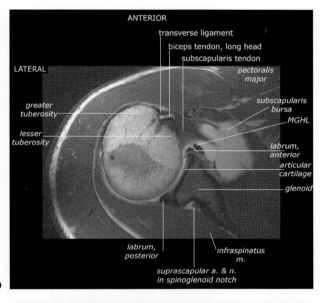

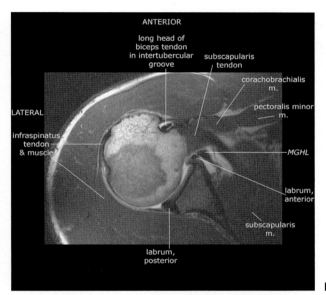

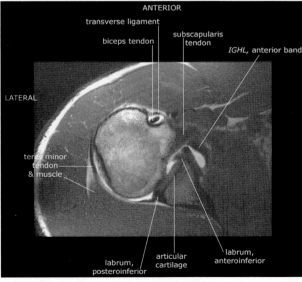

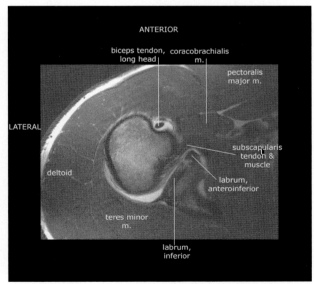

FIGURE 5.14. *(continued)*

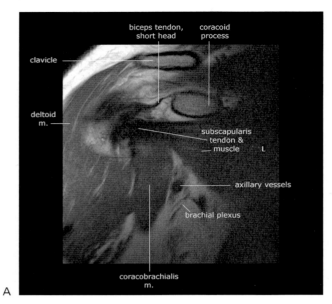

A

- clavicle
- biceps tendon, short head
- coracoid process
- deltoid m.
- subscapularis tendon & muscle
- L
- axillary vessels
- brachial plexus
- coracobrachialis m.

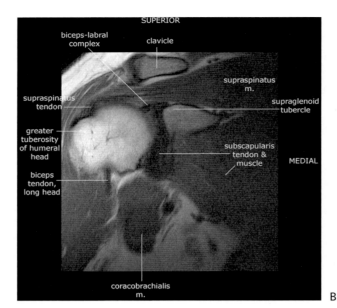

B

SUPERIOR

- biceps-labral complex
- clavicle
- supraspinatus tendon
- supraspinatus m.
- supraglenoid tubercle
- greater tuberosity of humeral head
- biceps tendon, long head
- subscapularis tendon & muscle
- MEDIAL
- coracobrachialis m.

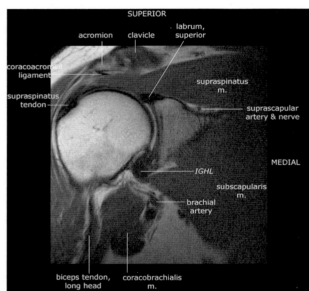

C

SUPERIOR

- acromion
- clavicle
- labrum, superior
- coracoacromial ligament
- supraspinatus m.
- supraspinatus tendon
- suprascapular artery & nerve
- MEDIAL
- IGHL
- subscapularis m.
- brachial artery
- biceps tendon, long head
- coracobrachialis m.

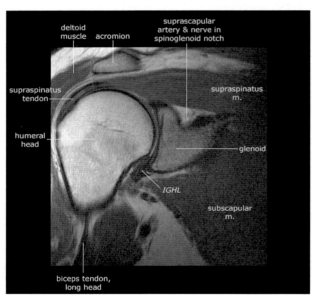

D

- deltoid muscle
- acromion
- suprascapular artery & nerve in spinoglenoid notch
- supraspinatus tendon
- supraspinatus m.
- humeral head
- glenoid
- IGHL
- subscapular m.
- biceps tendon, long head

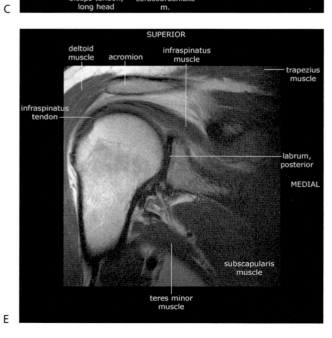

E

SUPERIOR

- deltoid muscle
- acromion
- infraspinatus muscle
- trapezius muscle
- infraspinatus tendon
- labrum, posterior
- MEDIAL
- subscapularis muscle
- teres minor muscle

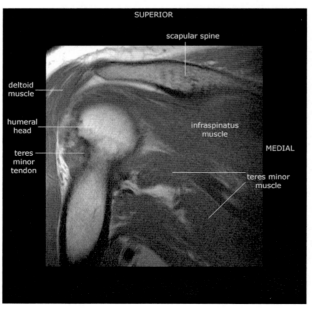

F

SUPERIOR

- scapular spine
- deltoid muscle
- humeral head
- infraspinatus muscle
- MEDIAL
- teres minor tendon
- teres minor muscle

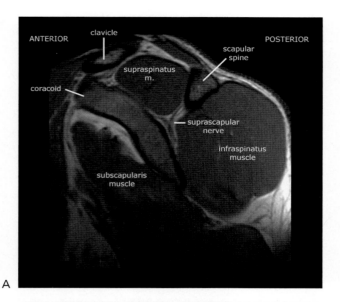

A

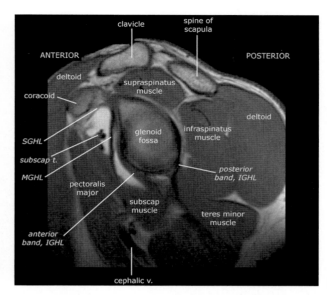

B

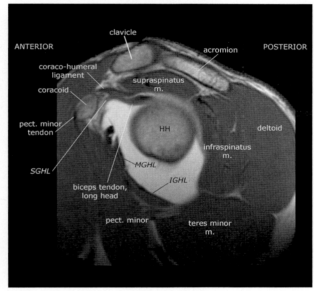

C

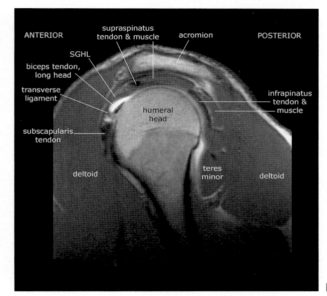

D

FIGURE 5.16. A–E: Sagittal oblique MRI and MR arthrographic anatomy. Medial to lateral; short TR/TE images (800/20). IGHL, inferior glenohumeral ligament; MGHL, middle glenohumeral ligament; SGHL, superior glenohumeral ligament; subscap, subscapularis; pect., pectoralis; m, muscle; t, tendon.

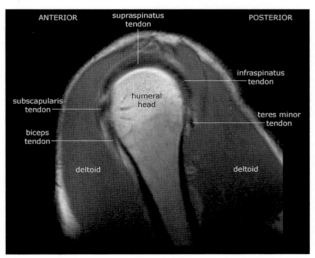

E

FIGURE 5.15. A–F: Coronal oblique MRI and MR arthrographic anatomy. Anterior to posterior; short TR/TE images (800/20). IGHL, inferior glenohumeral ligament; MGHL, middle glenohumeral ligament; SGHL, superior glenohumeral ligament; subscap, subscapularis; pect., pectoralis; m, muscle.

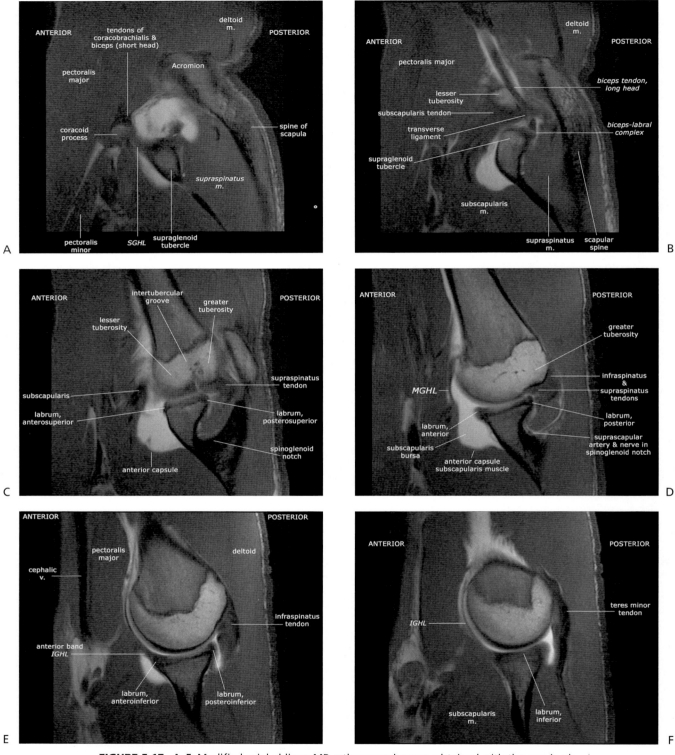

FIGURE 5.17. A–F: Modified axial oblique MR arthrogram images, obtained with the arm in abduction and external rotation (*ABER*). Superior to inferior; short TR/TE images (800/20). IGHL, inferior glenohumeral ligament; MGHL, middle glenohumeral ligament; SGHL, superior glenohumeral ligament; subscap, subscapularis; pect, pectoralis; m, muscle.

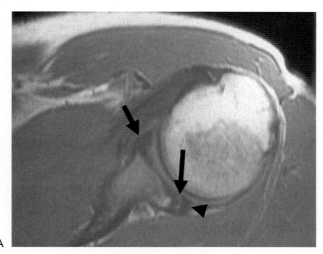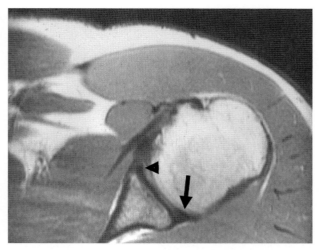

FIGURE 5.18. Labral shape and variation. Axial short TR/TE images (800/20). **A:** The triangular appearance of the anterior labrum (*small arrow*) and the smaller more round appearance of the posterior labrum (*arrowhead*). Longer arrow outline hyaline articular cartilage undercutting the posterior labrum. **B:** Image reveals the small near absent anterior labrum (*arrowhead*), and the posterior labrum to be larger and more triangular (*longer arrow*).

labrum may be round. The anterior labrum can be variable in appearance and size (Fig. 5.18) and may be rounded or cleaved or even, rarely, absent (52). The posterior labrum is also said to typically be triangular, but it may rounded, flat, or absent (53). The normal bright signal of hyaline cartilage at the base of the labrum should not be mistaken for a tear or detachment (Fig. 5.18) (54). Linear or globular foci of increased signal can be observed near the base of the labrum in normal subjects (15). The magic angle phenomenon can cause areas of increased signal in the posterosuperior/ anteroinferior labrum on proton density– and T1-weighted images. This signal should not approach fluid on T2-weighted images (15,55). On MRI, labral shape may vary with humeral rotation. Cleaved or notched (53) configurations are normal variants and should not be mistaken for tears. Labral size, shape, and appearance are also not necessarily bilateral and symmetrical. Partial imaging of the glenohumeral ligaments (16) (Figs. 5.6, 5.8, 5.9, 5.14) may also simulate cleavage planes or notches in the labrum or even tears or avulsed fragments. A similar problem may also occur with partial imaging of the subscapularis tendon. This may be most notable in the absence of an effusion when the glenohumeral ligaments and subscapularis tendons are closely applied to the anterior labrum. Superiorly, fluid may be seen in a sublabral recess or foramen (41). Fluid or contrast beneath the labrum at the level of the coracoid or below (below the equator or epiphyseal line) is considered pathologic and indicative of a tear or detachment. The *vacuum phenomenon* (56) occurs where low signal intensity gas is seen intraarticularly on GRE images, and it should not be mistaken for a labral tear or cartilage lesion. It is accentuated with the arm in external rotation and is located superiorly.

The subscapularis muscle and tendon are also well visualized in the axial plane (Figs. 5.8, 5.14). The subscapularis recess or bursa is identified in the presence of synovial fluid. This bursa can extend anterior to the subscapularis tendon, as well as between the capsule and posterior surface of the tendon (Fig. 5.8). The anterior capsule and its insertion into the glenoid margin can be identified on axial images. It is best seen on long TR/TE images in the presence of joint fluid, with gradient echo imaging, or with MR arthrography. The glenohumeral ligaments may not be easily separated from the subscapularis tendon on routine spin echo axial images but are more easily identified when an effusion is present. They may also be better seen with MRI arthrography (Figs. 5.8, 5.9, 5.14–5.17). On superior sections, the superior glenohumeral ligament and superior capsule may be seen inserting in the supraglenoid region, where the superior labrum and biceps tendon may be identified. At the midglenoid level, the middle glenohumeral ligament is best identified posterior to the subscapularis tendon and the capsule. At the inferior portion of the glenoid cavity, the inferior glenohumeral ligament inserts as a thick complex with the inferior capsule into the labrum. When an effusion is present or with MR arthrography, the three bands of the inferior glenohumeral ligament may be identified separately. Of particular importance in the setting of anterior instability is visualization of the anterior band as it forms part of the anterior inferior labral-ligmentous complex (Figs. 5.8, 5.9, 5.14–5.17).

The biceps brachii functions as a supinator of the forearm and a flexor of the elbow joint. It also is believed to be a flexor of the shoulder joint. The long head of the biceps tendon is seen arising from the supraglenoid region (Fig. 5.11).

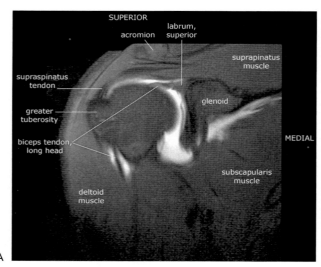
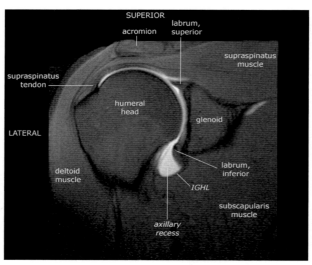

FIGURE 5.19. A, B: Anterior coronal oblique MRI arthrogram images. Short TR/TE images (800/20), with fat suppression. The addition of fat suppression helps separate contrast in the subdeltoid bursa from the higher signal of the peribursal fat, and it outlines the high signal intraarticular contrast, against the low signal of the supraspinatus tendon undersurface. It distends the axillary recess, as well as highlighting the biceps tendon in the tendon sheath and the confluence of the biceps tendon with the superior labrum at the biceps labral anchor region.

At the level of the superior pole of the glenoid, four separate attachments of the biceps tendon may be observed. These include the supraglenoid tubercle, the posterior superior labrum, the anterior superior labrum, and an extraarticular attachment to the lateral edge of the base of the coracoid process. The biceps labral complex corresponds to the superior one-third of the glenoid. Stoller has described variability in the pattern of insertion of the long head into the supraglenoid region as it forms part of the biceps labral anchor complex (57). As it exits the supraglenoid region, the tendon courses obliquely and anteriorly over the humeral head. Proximally it may be best seen on coronal and sagittal oblique images (Figs. 5.11, 5.15, 5.16). It then courses inferiorly into the intertubercular groove, where it is well seen on axial sections and appears as a round signal void (Fig. 5.14). Its synovial sheath is seen as a ring of moderate signal intensity (57), which may often contain a small amount of fluid as a normal finding (58).

The tendons of the rotator cuff complex are well seen on serial coronal oblique images, since this plane courses parallel to the supraspinatus muscle and tendon (Fig. 5.15). The infraspinatus and teres minor tendons are also well delineated in this orientation. The subscapularis tendon is identified on more anterior coronal oblique images but is better evaluated on axial images (Figs. 5.14, 5.19). It may also be delineated on sagittal oblique images (Fig. 5.16). The subdeltoid bursa is a potential space and therefore is not visualized as a separate structure, unless filled with fluid, although on occasion a thin rim of fluid signal may be seen on fat-suppressed images in this region (59,27). The subdeltoid peribursal fat plane (60,61) is seen on short TR-/

TE- and proton density–weighted sequences, as a high signal intensity line separating the rotator cuff tendons from the acromioclavicular joint, acromion, and overlying deltoid muscle.

On anterior coronal oblique images, the coracoclavicular (conoid and trapezoid) and acromioclavicular ligaments, as well as the acromioclavicular joint, may be identified. The anterior acromion can be seen. The coracoacromial ligament may also be delineated, although less constantly identified (Fig. 5.12). The anterior edge of the supraspinatus tendon can be depicted, along with the long head of biceps tendon and the subscapularis muscle and tendon (Fig. 5.10). The space and tissues between these two tendons, the rotator interval, may be seen on these sections as well (Fig. 5.10). The superior and inferior labrum can be identified in this plane, as can the axillary recess.

The sagittal oblique plane demonstrates the rotator cuff muscles and tendons in cross section (Fig. 5.16). The anteroposterior extent of the rotator cuff tendons can be visualized. In this plane the relationship of the acromion process, the acromioclavicular joint and the coracoacromial ligament to the supraspinatus and other cuff tendons are best depicted (Figs. 5.12, 5.16). The shape of the anterior acromion can be discerned on sagittal oblique images (Fig. 5.16). With fluid in the joint or with MRI arthrography (see later discussion) (Figs. 5.9, 5.16), the labrum, capsule, and the glenohumeral ligaments can be depicted; in particular, the three limbs of the inferior glenohumeral ligament are best seen in this plane.

The rotator interval may be well evaluated on oblique sagittal images taken parallel to the plane of the glenoid fossa and orthogonal to the long axis of the rotator cuff (Figs.

5.10A, 5.16). The coracohumeral ligament is an important landmark on the sagittal images, coursing from the coracoid process into the interval to blend with the interval capsule. The most proximal portion of the biceps can be found immediately inferior and deep to the posterior aspect of the coracohumeral ligament and interval capsule at the level of the superior biceps labral anchor complex. The fused coracohumeral ligament and capsule may be followed posterosuperiorly to the level of the anterior margin and leading edge of the supraspinatus (29). The long head of the biceps tendon should be demonstrated as a smooth low signal intensity structure that on sequential sagittal images (Fig. 5.16) can be followed within the rotator interval from medial to lateral to the bicipital groove, after which axial images are best for following the tendon from the proximal bicipital groove (Fig. 5.14) more distally along the humeral shaft (29).

MR Arthrographic Anatomy

Conventional MR imaging, as discussed earlier, affords direct visualization of major anatomic structures. MR arthrography can improve the anatomic delineation of smaller intraarticular structures, including the glenoid labrum, glenohumeral ligaments, capsule, and articular surface of the rotator cuff tendon complex. Two standard techniques have been described: one uses dilute gadolinium chelate with T1-weighted fat-suppressed images; the other uses normal saline as the contrast agent supplemented with T2-weighted fat-suppressed sequences (62). The latter are more typically done with fast spin echo acquisitions. A combined approach may also be utilized, with T1-weighted fat–suppressed images, followed by T2-weighted fast spin echo acquisitions with fat suppression.

The standard intraarticular gadolinium examination utilizes a 0.5% (1:200) gadolinium concentration, which can be easily titrated administering 0.1 ml of Gd-DTPA with a tuberculin syringe into 20 ml of bacteriostatic saline. Approximately 12 to 15 ml of the solution is administered into the glenohumeral joint utilizing an anterior approach under fluoroscopic guidance with a 20-gauge spinal needle. The patient returns to the MRI unit, where postinjection images are obtained.

The sequences utilized for an MR arthrography examination are varied. If preinjection images are obtained (oblique coronal PD-FSE, T2-FSE fat-suppressed; axial DE-FSE fat-suppressed images), a typical postinjection sequence would include oblique coronal, oblique sagittal, and axial T1-weighted fat-saturated, and oblique coronal T2-weighted FSE fat-suppressed images. For further investigation of the labral-capsular anatomy or undersurface rotator cuff tears, many investigators perform axial images with the arm placed in the position of abduction-external rotation (ABER) (Fig. 5.17). This position places traction on the inferior glenohumeral ligament and causes separation and distraction of an otherwise unrecognized anterior labral tear (62).

Intravenous gadolinium arthrography may also be utilized to visualize the labrum and capsule. After the intravenous administration of 15 ml Gd-DTPA, the patient is exercised for 10 minutes, which encourages the development of a joint effusion with subsequent diffusion of gadolinium into the joint. The patient usually is imaged within 15 minutes after injection, with a similar three-plane T1-weighted pulse sequence protocol with fat suppression.

The glenoid labrum, the fibrous capsule, the glenohumeral ligaments, the rotator cuff tendons, and the long head of the biceps tendon should have low or absent signal, outlined against the high signal gadolinium contrast, or fluid on T2-weighted sequences with saline-enhanced studies (Figs. 5.8, 5.9, 5.14–5.17).

Normal variations in labral morphology, especially the anterior labrum, can be challenging even on MR arthrographic images. An example would include the differentiation between a blunted, degenerated labrum and a small, rounded normal labrum. Also, sublabral sulci can be a source of diagnostic confusion. As discussed later, sulci are located at the labral-articular cartilage interface and are usually located at the region of the biceps labral anchor/complex, or between the origins of the middle and inferior glenohumeral ligaments (62). Sublabral foramina, also discussed in more detail later, are often identified anterior to the biceps labral complex in the anterior superior labral quadrant.

The anterior capsule and its insertion along the bony glenoid margin can be best identified with MR arthrography. The capsular insertion onto the scapula on MR imaging has proven to be unreliable as the medial insertion of the capsule may often be variable and may be related to variability in the size of the subscapularis recess with which it is continuous and not necessarily be related to capsular stripping (62). A stripped capsule may, however, heal back and be continuous with a large subscapularis recess and therefore be difficult to distinguish from a variant insertion, unless the morphological changes and the more inferior extent are recognized. This is more easily accomplished with MR arthrography. Studies have been conflicting in determining whether types of capsular insertions are statistically different in stable and unstable shoulders; therefore, the use of the type of capsular insertion in the assessment of anterior instability is dubious (62,63).

The glenohumeral ligaments are also more easily identified with MRI arthrography (Figs. 5.8, 5.9, 5.14–5.17). The glenohumeral ligaments reinforce the joint capsule by attaching to the labrum and anchoring the humerus to the glenoid rim (64,20). The complex of the glenohumeral ligaments and labrum is known as the labral-ligamentous complex (65). They function together as a unit to reinforce the joint capsule. On superior sections, as noted earlier, the superior glenohumeral ligament and superior capsule may be seen inserting in the supraglenoid region, where the superior labrum and biceps tendon may be identified (16). The confluence of labrum and biceps long head in this region is known as the *biceps-labral anchor* or *complex*, and it is better depicted at MR arthrography (Figs. 5.14–5.17) (66). The superior glenohumeral ligament courses anteriorly, merging with the coracohumeral ligament in the rotator interval. The middle glenohumeral ligament may also arise in the supraglenoid region; hence, it courses obliquely and often may only be visualized in partial section in axial MR arthrographic images (16). At the midglenoid level, the middle glenohumeral ligament may be better separated with joint distension and is best identified as it courses posterior to the subscapularis tendon and the joint capsule (16). It then merges with the subscapularis tendon as it inserts on the lesser tuberosity. Its thickness varies from threadlike to cordlike (67,68). At the inferior portion of the glenoid cavity, the inferior glenohumeral ligament is identified as a thick complex posterior to the inferior capsule and attaching firmly in conjunction with the labrum. The inferior sling formed by the inferior glenohumeral ligament is considered to be the most important ligament in stabilizing the shoulder. As already noted, it has three components: the anterior band, axillary pouch, and posterior band (69), which are only reliably identified in their respective portions with MR arthrography (Figs. 5.9, 5.14–5.17). With the arm in the ABER position (Fig. 5.17), the anterior band of the inferior glenohumeral ligament becomes taut and can be optimally characterized throughout its entire extension on MR arthrograms obtained with the arm in this position (11). Occasionally, increased signal can be observed at the insertion site of the anterior band of the inferior glenohumeral ligament on MR arthrograms in asymptomatic subjects. This likely represents partial volume averaging of the ligament with subjacent contrast medium (15).

The long head of the biceps tendon is seen arising from the supraglenoid region. Contrast will normally extend into the biceps tendon sheath since it communicates with the joint. Proximally, the biceps tendon is outlined by contrast on the coronal and sagittal oblique images, and then as it courses inferiorly into the intertubercular groove, it is seen on axial sections as a round signal void outlined against the high signal contrast. Its synovial sheath is seen as a ring of moderate signal intensity, against the high signal of contrast (58).

On serial coronal oblique images, the rotator cuff tendons are outlined between the peribursal fat and contrast solution on the articular surface. The articular surface of the tendon should be linear in contour, smooth, and of low signal. Fat suppression helps separate the high signal of the peribursal fat from contrast extravasating through a cuff defect into the subdeltoid bursa (Fig. 5.19) (70).

On anterior coronal oblique images (Fig. 5.19), contrast outlines the anterior edge of the supraspinatus tendon, which can be depicted along with the long head of biceps tendon, subscapularis muscle and tendon, and the rotator interval. The superior and inferior labrum can be outlined in this plane, as can the axillary recess, which may be redundant and filled with contrast in neutral rotation.

On the sagittal oblique plane images, the undersurface of the anteroposterior aspect of the rotator cuff tendons can be outlined against the high signal of the distending contrast. The structures of the anterior interval, including the anterior supraspinatus, the biceps tendon, and the subscapularis may also be best depicted when contrast outlines the joint cavity and distends it (Fig. 5.16). With contrast in the joint, the labrum, capsule and the glenohumeral ligaments, and in particular the three limbs of the inferior glenohumeral ligament are well depicted, especially with respect to their superior inferior course and extent (Fig. 5.9).

NORMAL VARIATIONS AND DIAGNOSTIC PITFALLS

This difficult topic is discussed in detail elsewhere in the text, particularly in Chapter 3, but some of these topics are reviewed here as well, because of their importance and for emphasis.

Rotator Cuff

Most early descriptions on MRI of the rotator cuff describe its appearance as a homogeneous signal void. More recently, most observers have agreed that it is common to observe increased intratendinous signal on short TR-/TE- and proton density–weighted images even in asymptomatic individuals. The uncertainty regarding the etiology and significance of this increased signal in the rotator cuff has led to a number of investigations to try to explain these findings (59,45–50,71,72). Some investigators have attributed this signal to partial volume averaging of adjacent normal tissue such as muscle, fat, or other soft tissue (59,44,47,50,54,71). Others have attributed this signal to technical factors or artifacts, including internal rotation of the arm (50) or T2 prolongation associated with tendons oriented 55° to the main magnetic field, the "magic angle" phenomenon (51). Others have attributed this signal to subclinical pathology. One study (44) with cadaveric correlation indicated that this increased signal could be secondary to ongoing rotator cuff impingement, occurring with daily life and activities that have not or may never cause the patient any difficulty. Similar MR findings in cadaveric shoulders (49) showed histological evidence of scarring and eosinophilic and mucoid degeneration. Supporting the prevalence of subclinical rotator cuff pathology, one study (48) indicated that asymptomatic MR evident cuff abnormalities including partial and complete rotator cuff tears are common and increase in prevalence with age. In the majority of cases, these causes of increased intratendinous signal can be distinguished from a rotator cuff tear by the absence of fluid signal on images with T2 contrast. MR arthrography can help distinguish increased intratendinous signal from a cuff tear that communicates with the articular

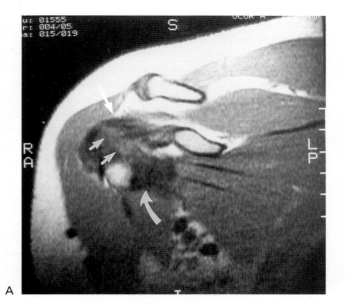

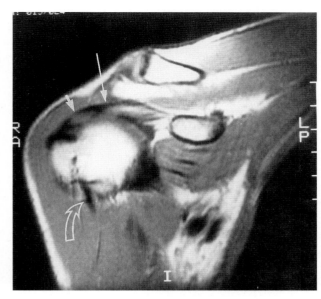

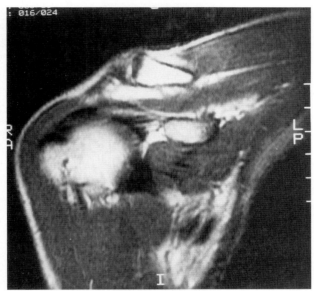

FIGURE 5.20. Anterior interval pitfall. **A, B:** Anterior interval increased signal. Anterior coronal oblique short TR/TE image (1,000/20). Intermediate signal is demonstrated at and beneath the anterior supraspinatus tendon (*short white arrows*) at the interval between the supraspinatus (*long white arrow*) and subscapularis tendons (*curved white arrow*). Also note the biceps tendon (*curved open arrow*). **C:** The signal fades on the anterior coronal oblique long TR/TE image (2,200/70), thus differentiating it from a cuff tear.

surface, as contrast will not extend into a tear/defect on an MR arthrographic exam.

The anatomy of the rotator interval may also contribute to the appearance of intratendinous signal anteriorly (Fig. 5.20). As previously noted, the anterior rotator interval is the space between the superior border of the subscapularis muscle and tendon below and the supraspinatus muscle and tendon (73,54,74) above. Increased signal seen in the anterior supraspinatus tendon in this region may reflect averaging of normal tissues anterior to the tendon from the rotator interval, including the superficial fibrofatty or membranous tissues (54,75), but other structures may contribute, such as the biceps tendon sheath (54,76). This "interval pitfall" is usually only seen on only one or two anterior images,

whereas true pathology in the tendon should typically be identified on serial images. This area of signal increase may be particularly problematic at lower field where thicker imaging sections may often be necessary due to signal-to-noise considerations, including extremity-type magnets. This pitfall may also be avoided by using thinner imaging sections whenever possible.

Others (59,6) have referred to a similar appearing area of increased signal in the anterior supraspinatus tendon approximately 1 cm from the greater tuberosity (62) as due to the critical zone. The size of the critical zone may increase with age. The supraspinatus tendon lacks special nutritional vessels and the main vascular supply derives from (a) the vessels of the osteotendinous attachment, the ascending branches of the anterior circumflex humeral artery projecting along the intertubercular groove and ramifying over the greater tubercle of the humerus and distal end of the supraspinatus; and (b) vessels from the middle of the muscles—specifically, branches of the suprascapular artery within the muscles, nurturing the proximal end of the tendon. The critical zone is said to lie between the vessels of the osteotendinous attachment and the muscular branches (77). Presumably, the differing vascularity in this area leads to the change in signal, or that degeneration is more apt to be present here (59,46).

Another potential cause of intermediate signal on coronal short TR/TE and proton density images mimicking intratendinous pathology is a prominent or thickened region of humeral head articular cartilage beneath the midsupraspinatus tendon (Fig. 5.21). Histological examination reveals that the transitional zone of hyaline articular accounts for the majority of this increase in thickness. The transitional zone is responsible for the highest signal from cartilage on MR imaging (44). Careful review of the images, including review of accompanying sagittal oblique images, will reveal that this increased signal is beneath and separate from the supraspinatus tendon. Three distinct lines can be identified, from inferior to superior. First is the signal void of cortical bone, then the intermediate signal of cartilage, and then the signal void of the tendon itself.

Signal isointense to muscle on all pulse sequences on more posterior coronal oblique sections in place of the expected signal void of tendons is another type of intermediate signal on short TR/TE and proton density images (Fig. 5.22). One proposed explanation is that in these cases, muscle bundles extend more laterally over the humeral head in the space between the supraspinatus and infraspinatus tendons, as they diverge toward their insertions on the humeral head (78). Vahlensieck and coworkers (72) have described a posterior straplike portion of the supraspinatus tendon, with several shorter tendinous slips arising from muscle fibers separate from those forming the anterior dominant tendon. Imaging of this seemingly different posterior portion of the tendon is another possible explanation for this appearance of interposed muscle tissue, which would occur between the supraspinatus and infraspinatus tendons. Changes in humeral rotation may further exacerbate this problem.

Labrum and Capsule

Similar to the rotator cuff, increased signal on short TR/TE and proton density sequences has also been observed within the labrum, in some asymptomatic volunteers (79,45). This may reflect degeneration as has been observed in cadaver sections (49).

Other difficulties in interpretation related to the labrum and capsule include fronds or folds of capsular tissue or partial imaging of glenohumeral ligaments within the subscapularis bursa that can be mistaken for loose bodies or labral fragments (Fig. 5.23). Variations in insertions of the medial anterior capsule can be mistaken for capsular stripping or detachment. Difficulties in interpretation of labral pathology may arise owing to the articular cartilage beneath the labrum and normal variation in its morphology. Hyperintense hyaline articular cartilage at the base of the labrum can be problematic on axial images and on anterior coronal oblique images (Figs. 5.18, 5.24). This *hyaline cartilage undercutting*

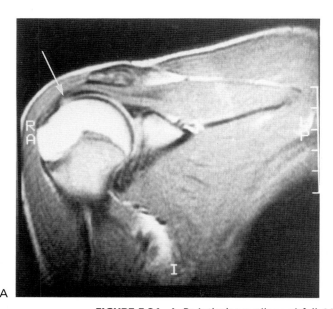
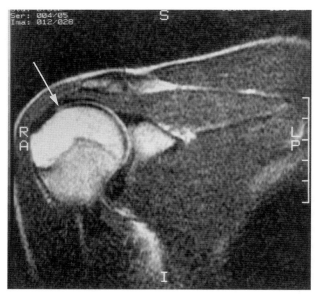

A   B

FIGURE 5.21. A, B: Articular cartilage pitfall. Midcoronal oblique images TR/TE (2,200/20/70). Intermediate signal is identified just beneath the middistal supraspinatus tendon (*arrow*) on the proton density image in A. This signal is continuous with the articular cartilage but can mistakenly appear to be within the tendon. This signal fades on the long TR/TE image in B (*arrow*).

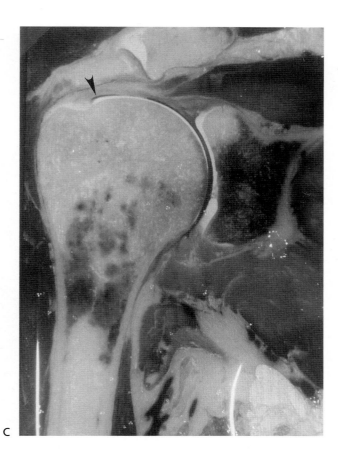

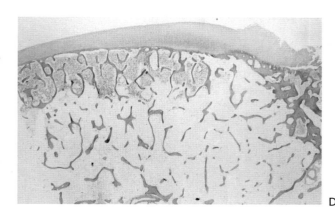

FIGURE 5.21 *(continued).* **C:** Cryomacrocut section. The articular cartilage appears to be thicker (*black arrowhead*) in a similar region to the focus of increased signal on the MR image. **D:** Low power (9×) photomicrograph of this thicker portion of articular cartilage stained with safranin O and fast green. The red stained area is located at the region shown in A and B, and it corresponds to the transitional layer.

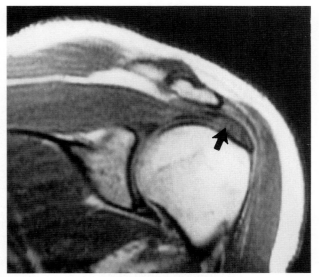

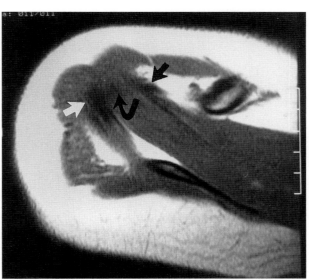

FIGURE 5.22. Interposed "muscle" pitfall. **A:** Mid coronal oblique short TR/TE image (550/20). Signal isointense to muscle is seen continuing from the supraspinatus muscle to its insertion on the greater tuberosity (*arrow*). **B:** Superior axial short TR/TE images (550/20). Axial images demonstrate the low signal intensity dominant anterior supraspinatus tendon (*black arrow*) extending anteriorly to its distal insertion. Posteriorly to this is the posterior straplike portion of the supraspinatus tendon, with several shorter tendinous slips arising from muscle fibers separate from those forming the anterior dominant tendon (*curved black arrow*) extending distally. Imaging of this seemingly different posterior portion of the tendon is a possible explanation for this appearance of interposed "muscle" signal, as seen in A, which would occur between the supraspinatus and infraspinatus tendon (*white arrow*).

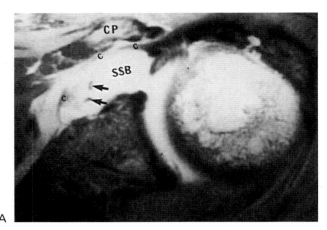

A

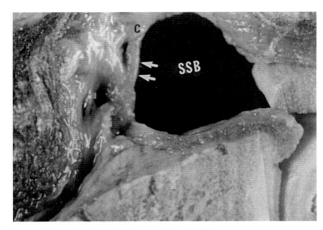

B

FIGURE 5.23. MRI scan of cadaver injected with saline **(A)**, TR/TE 2,500/70, corresponding cadaver section **(B)**. The superior aspect of the subscapularis bursa *(SSB)* is prominent. Folds or fronds of capsular tissue *(black arrows in A and white arrrows in B)* may often be seen in this region and are identified as structures of decreased signal on the MR images. They should not be mistaken for loose bodies. C, joint capsule; CP, coracoid process.

may represent a transitional zone of fibrocartilage or fibrovascular tissue, beneath the labrum. MR arthrography can help resolve the problem of cartilage undercutting as contrast should not imbibe into these regions, and if it does, the high signal of contrast should be easily distinguished from the intermediate signal of hyaline cartilage.

Partial imaging of the glenohumeral ligaments or subscapularis tendon adjacent to the labrum may also simulate

loose bodies, labral tears, or avulsed labral fragments (Fig. 5.25). MR arthrography may help resolve by separating the glenohumeral ligaments from the labrum when the joint is distended with contrast (Figs. 5.8, 5.9, 5.14–5.17) (74). With MR arthrography, these structures can be followed from their origins to their insertions and viewed in multiple planes (Figs. 5.14–5.17). The middle glenohumeral ligament may also attach directly to the labrum, which can

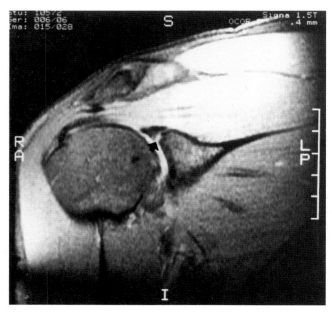

FIGURE 5.24. Coronal oblique long TR short TE image (2,500/20), with fat saturation. High signal at the base of the superior labrum *(arrow)* represents articular cartilage and should not be interpreted as a superior labral tear or detachment. This normal finding is sometimes referred to as *cartilage undercutting.*

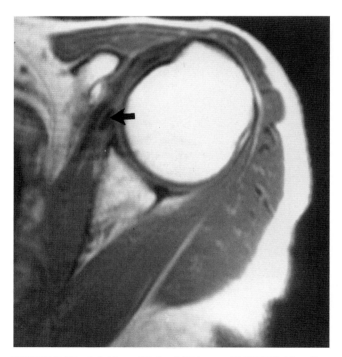

FIGURE 5.25. Axial long TR short TE image (2,500/20): Visualization of a prominent middle glenohumeral ligament *(arrow)* adjacent to the anterior labrum should not be mistaken for a labral tear, detachment, or loose body.

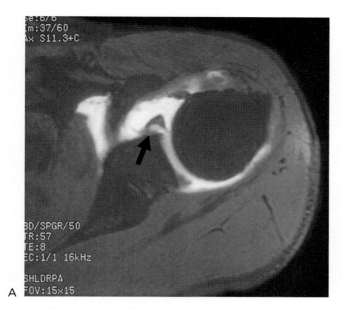

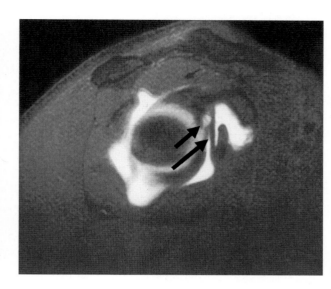

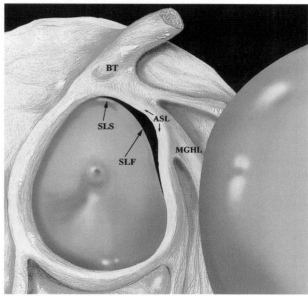

FIGURE 5.26. Sublabral foramen. Axial **(A)** and sagittal oblique MR arthrogram. Spoiled gradient echo image **(A)**, short TR/TE images (800/20) **(B)**, with fat suppression. High signal contrast outlines a smooth appearing sublabral foramen (*short arrows in A and B*). A thick middle glenohumeral attaches anterosuperiorly in B (*longer arrow*). Note there is no sublabral sulcus more superiorly. **C:** Diagram in lateral view illustrates the sublabral foramen. It is anterior and inferior to the sublabral sulcus. BT, long head of the biceps tendon; MGHL, middle glenohumeral ligament; ASL, anterior superior labrum; SLS, sublabral sulcus; SLF, sublabral foramen.

result in the appearance of an elongated and redundant labrum (80).

The anterosuperior labrum is the most common site of normal anatomic labral-ligamentous variations, with specific variations described in up to 13.5% of the population in investigational studies (81,67). These variations in labral attachment occur above the equator of the glenoid, which occurs at the 3 o'clock position on the glenoid margin. Below the equator the labrum should be firmly attached (Fig. 5.8). The anterosuperior labrum is not attached to the bony glenoid in 8% to 12% of the population, referred to as a *sublabral foramen* or a *sublabral hole* (82,15) (Fig. 5.26). This finding is located anterior to the biceps-labral complex (83). A *sublabral recess*, also referred to as a *sublabral sulcus*, is

a recess/synovial reflection between the biceps-labral complex and the superior margin of the glenoid (82). On occasion, a sublabral recess can be continuous with a sublabral foramen (83). In cadaver studies, a sublabral recess has been demonstrated in up to 73% of shoulders (84). The anterosuperior labrum can also be focally absent, usually associated with a thickened, cordlike middle glenohumeral ligament, which approaches the thickness of the proximal biceps tendon. This entity is referred to as the *Buford complex*, believed to be present in approximately 1.5% of the population (83,15) (Fig. 5.27). Pathologic lesions occurring or originating in, or extending into, the anterosuperior labral quadrant can also be distinguished from normal anatomic variations if they extend below the level of the coracoid process tip

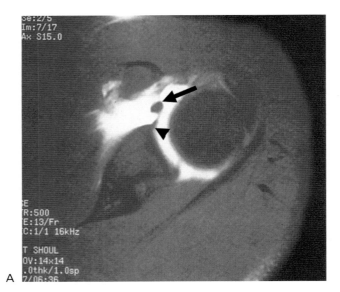

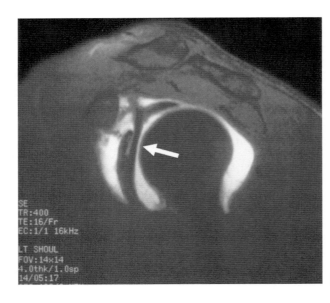

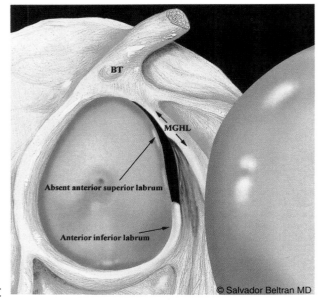

FIGURE 5.27. Buford complex. Axial **(A)** and sagittal oblique MR arthrogram. Short TR/TE images (800/20), with fat suppression. The labrum is nearly absent anterosuperiorly (*arrowhead*). The thick cordlike middle glenohumeral ligament is identified partially in A (*black arrow*) and continuously in B (*whole arrow*), attaching to the superior labrum directly. (*arrow*) **C:** Diagram in lateral view of the Buford complex. Note the absent anterior superior labrum and the thick, cordlike middle glenohumeral ligament that is attaching anterosuperiorly. BT, long head of the biceps tendon; MGHL, middle glenohumeral ligament.

(which helps mark the equator) toward or into the anteroinferior labrum or posteriorly into the posterosuperior quadrant (beyond the biceps labral anchor) (15). Therefore, a Buford complex should be suspected if the contiguous anteroinferior and superior labrum appear normal (67). Morphological alterations help distinguish pathologic lesions as well. MR arthrography will delineate this anatomy to better advantage and help distinguish the variant anatomy from pathologic lesions.

Bone Marrow

Although the majority of the appendicular skeleton undergoes conversion of hematopoetic to fatty marrow, the proximal humerus is a site of residual hematopoietic marrow in adults. On T1-weighted images, foci of decreased signal are therefore routinely observed within the proximal humeral metaphysis. Patients with anemia or marrow replacement disorders may have an increased amount of hematopoetic marrow, due to reconversion of fatty to hematopoetic marrow. Residual or reconverted marrow can be distinguished from marrow replacement by the lack of expansion, soft tissue mass, cortical destruction or significant increased signal on T2-weighted images. One study of patients presenting for shoulder MRI demonstrated residual hematopoetic marrow within the proximal humerus in 99% of patients, with some patchy extension to the epiphysis in 62%. This epiphyseal extension of hematopoetic marrow was more com-

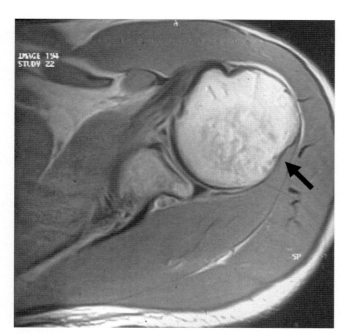

FIGURE 5.28. Axial image at the level of the mid glenoid, TR/TE 500/20, normal appearance of the posterior humeral notch (*arrow*). This should be distinguished from a Hill-Sachs lesion, which occurs more superiorly and is more wedge shaped.

mon among females and in those with more extensive hematopoetic marrow present within the proximal humeral metaphysis. The most characteristic pattern was a curvilinear distribution of red marrow involving the subcortical bone of the medial aspect of the humeral head, indicating that not all instances of nonfatty epiphyseal marrow are pathologic (90).

Occasionally, ossification centers may persist, such as the superior apophysis of the glenoid or an os acromiale. An os acromiale should be reported as it may be unstable, as discussed in more detail elsewhere in the text, and may contribute rotator cuff impingement (15). It may be hypermobile and tilt anteriorly at its attachment site to the coracoacromial ligament, resulting in impingement (91).

There is a region of normal flattening/groove along the posterolateral aspect of the humerus, just proximal to the insertion site of the teres minor (Fig. 5.28). This occurs 20 mm or more inferior to the proximal humeral head. This should not be confused with a Hill-Sachs lesion, which occurs more superiorly, at or above the level of the coracoid process tip (15).

Pseudospurs along the undersurface of the acromion can be caused by prominence/hypertrophy at the insertion site of the coracoacromial ligament or from tendon slips of the deltoid musculature (15).

Subcoracoid impingement, resulting in degeneration/ tearing of the subscapularis tendon, can be associated with developmental enlargement of the coracoid process and close proximity of the coracoid to the lesser tubercle (38,84).

Joint Space and Biceps Tendon

In a study of asymptomatic volunteers (58), some fluid was found within the glenohumeral joint and/or biceps tendon sheath in nearly all subjects. Most of the fluid was minimal in quantity, thin in character, and reported in the range of 1 to 2 ml (15), with only a sliver in the axillary and subscapularis recess (85). Any fluid distending the subscapularis or axillary recess, or biceps tendon sheath, should be considered a joint effusion. The majority of shoulders in this study with a significant effusion also had an abnormal tendon, most of which were complete tears. Significant isolated effusions of the biceps tendon sheath were identified in only a small number of volunteers in this study (3%).

Increased signal has been found to occur along the lateral aspect of the bicipital groove, thought to be due to branches of the anterior circumflex humeral artery and vein. This may be prominent on gradient echo sequences due to flow related enhancement and may simulate a small fluid collection (46). Increased signal in the biceps tendon may also be observed as a result of magic angle effects and may simulate tendonitis (57).

With respect to the long head of the biceps tendon (LHBT), the most widely known variations relate to its relationship with the superior glenoid labrum. In about 50% of cadavers, the tendon arises directly from the superoposterior portion of the labrum or, less commonly, both the superoanterior and superoposterior portions of the labrum. In the remaining 50% of cadavers, it arises from the supraglenoid tubercle (86). A recent case report by Yeh et al. described a patient with an apparent intracapsular origin of the LHBT, where it merged into the superior joint capsule about 2 cm distal to its usual attachment to the superior labrum (86). In other reports, the tendon may be absent; it may be extrasynovial, lying within the fibrous capsule. Other anomalies that have been described include a double biceps tendon and the presence of a mesentery of the tendon (86).

The biceps labral anchor complex has been shown to have three types of attachment to the glenoid fossa (89,82). The attachments are superior to that of the anterosuperior labral quadrant, but the variability in attachment of this complex is related to that of this portion of the labrum. A type 1 complex adheres firmly to the superior aspect of the glenoid rim (Fig. 5.29). There is no sublabral foramen in the anterior superior labral quadrant. In a type 2 classification, the complex is attached several millimeters medial to the glenoid rim with an associated small sublabral sulcus, which may be continuous with a sublabral foramen and may also communicate with the subscapularis bursa. A type 3 biceps-labral complex has a labrum that is shaped like a meniscus with a large sublabral sulcus that projects under the labrum and over the cartilaginous pole of the glenoid (Fig. 5.30). The presence of these sublabral sulci, in conjunction with a sublabral foramen, should not be mistaken for a superior labral anterior to posterior (SLAP) lesion.

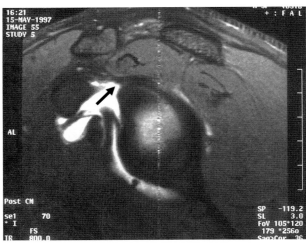
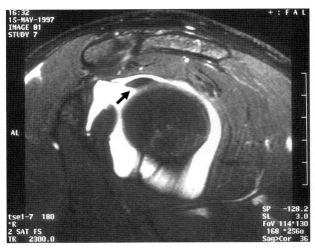

FIGURE 5.29. Type 1 biceps labral complex. Sagittal oblique MR arthrograms; CSE, TR/TE images (800/20) (**A**), TSE 2300/45 (**B**), with fat suppression. The biceps labral complex attaches directly to the glenoid (*arrows*).

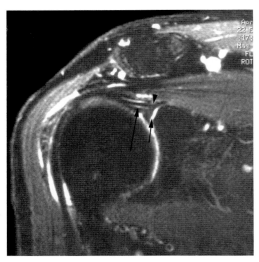
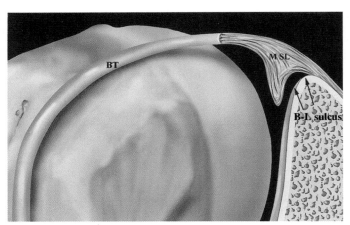

FIGURE 5.30. Type 3 Biceps labral complex. **A.** FSE TR/TE 2400/65, with fat suppression. There is a large fluid filled sulcus between the labrum and glenoid (*arrow*). The superior labrum has a meniscoid shape (*arrowhead*). Note is made of a small split like defect in the proximal biceps tendon (*longer arrow*). **B.** Diagram of Type 3 Biceps labral complex. BT, biceps tendon. MSL, meniscoid superior labrum. B-L, Biceps-Labral sulcus.

REFERENCES

1. Warwick R, Williams PL. Arthrology. In: *Gray's Anatomy*, 35th ed. London: Longman Group, 1973:424–429.
2. Carson WG. Arthroscopy of the shoulder: anatomy and technique. *Orthop Rev* 1992;21(Feb):143–153.
3. Petersilge CA, Witte DH, Sewell BO, et al. Normal regional anatomy of the shoulder. *MRI Clin North Am* 1997;5(Nov):667–681.
4. Davidson PA, Elattrache NS, Jobe CM, Jobe FW. Rotator cuff and posterior-superior glenoid labrum injury associated with increased glenohumeral motion: a new site of impingement. *J Shoulder Elbow Surg* 1995;4:384–390.
5. Matthews LS, Terry G, Vetter WL. Shoulder anatomy for the arthroscopist. *Arthroscopy* 1985;1(2):83–91.
6. Saha AK. Dynamic stability of the glenohumeral joint. *Acta Orthop Scand* 1972;42:491–505.
7. Hill JA, Tkach L, Hendrix RW. A study of glenohumeral orientation in patients with anterior recurrent shoulder dislocations using computerized axial tomography. *Orthop Rev* 1989;18:84–91.
8. Mosely HF, Overgaard B. The anterior capsular mechanism in recurrent anterior dislocation of the shoulder. *J Bone Joint Surg* 1962;44B:913–927.
9. Depalma AF. *Surgery of the shoulder*. 3rd ed. Philadelphia: Lippincott, 1983:47–64.
10. Andrews JR, Carson WG, McLeod WD. Glenoid labrum tears related to the long head of the biceps. *Am J Sports Med* 1985;13:337–341.
11. Beltran J, Rosenberg ZS, Chandnani VP, et al. Glenohumeral in-

stability: evaluation with MR arthrography. *Radiographics* 1997; 17:657–673.

12. Palmer WE, Brown JH, Rosenthal DI. Labral-ligamentous complex of the shoulder: evaluation with MR arthrography. *Radiology* 1994;190:645–651.

13. Rothman RH, Marvel JP, Heppenstall RB. Anatomic considerations in the glenohumeral joint. *Orthop Clin North Am* 1975;6: 341–352.

14. Uhthoff HK, Piscopo M. Anterior capsular redundancy of the shoulder: congenital or traumatic? *J Bone Joint Surg* 1985;67B: 363–366.

15. Tsao LY, Mirowitz SA. MR imaging of the shoulder: imaging techniques, diagnostic pitfalls, and normal variants. *MRI Clin North Am* 1997;5:683–704.

16. Zlatkin MB, Bjorkengren AG, Gylys-Morin V, et al. Cross-sectional imaging of the capsular mechanism of the glenohumeral joint. *Am J Roentgenol* 1988;150:151–158.

17. Palmer WE, Caslowitz PL. Anterior shoulder instability: diagnostic criteria determined from prospective analysis of 121 MR arthrograms. *Radiology* 1995;197:819–825.

18. Neer II CS, Saterlee CC, Dalsey RM, et al. The anatomy and potential effects of contracture of the coracohumeral ligament. *Clin Orthop* 1992;280:182–185.

19. Ferrari D. Capsular ligaments of the shoulder: anatomical and functional study of the anterior superior capsule. *Am J Sports Med* 1990;18:20–24.

20. Palmer WE, Caslowitz PL, Chew FS. MR arthrography of the shoulder: normal intraarticular structures and common abnormalities. *AJR* 1995;164:141–146.

21. Obrien SJ, Neves MC, Arnoczky SP, et al. The anatomy and histology of the inferior glenohumeral ligament complex of the shoulder. *Am J Sports Med* 1990;18:449–456.

22. Turkel SJ, Panio MW, Marshall JL, et al. Stabilizing mechanism preventing anterior dislocation of the glenohumeral joint. *J Bone Joint Surg Am* 1981;63:1208–1217.

23. McMahon PJ, Debski RE, Thompson WO, et al. Shoulder muscle forces and tendon excursions during glenohumeral abduction in the scapular plane. *J Shoulder Elbow Surg* 1995;4:199–208.

24. Vahlensieck M, an Haack K, Schmidt HM. Two portions of the supraspinatus muscle: a new finding about the muscles macroscopy by dissection and magnetic resonance imaging. *Surg Radiol Anat* 1994;16:101–104.

25. Celli L, Rovesta C, Marangiu MC, et al. Transplantation of teres major muscle for infraspinatus muscle in irreparable rotator cuff tears. *J Shoulder Elbow Surg* 1998;7:485–490.

26. Mochizuki T, Isoda H, Masui T, et al. Occlusion of the posterior humeral circumflex artery: detection with MR angiography in healthy volunteers and in a patient with quadrilateral space syndrome. *Am J Radiol* 1994;163:625–627.

27. Totterman SM, Miller RJ, Meyers SP. Basic anatomy of the shoulder by magnetic resonance imaging. *Top Magn Reson Imaging* 1994; 6:86–93.

28. Patten RM. Tears of the anterior portion of the rotator cuff (the subscapularis tendon): MR imaging findings. *AJR* 1994;162: 351–354.

29. Ho CP. MR imaging of rotator interval, long biceps, and associated injuries in the overhead-throwing athlete. *MRI Clin North Am* 1999;7:23–37.

30. Clark JM, Sidles JA, Matsen FA. The relationship of the glenohumeral joint capsule to the rotator cuff. *Clin Orthop* 1990;254:29–34.

31. Clark JM, Harryman DT. Tendons, ligaments and capsule of the rotator cuff: gross and microscopic anatomy. *J Bone Joint Surg* 1992;74A(5):713–725.

32. Sakurai G, Ozaki J, Tomita Y, et al. Morphologic changes in long head of biceps brachii in rotator cuff dysfunction. *J Orthop Sci* 1998;3:137–142.

33. Mitchell MJ, Causey G, Berthoty DP, et al. Peribursal fat plane of the shoulder: anatomic study and clinical experience. *Radiology* 1988;168:699–704.

34. Schraner AB, Major NM. MR imaging of the subcoracoid bursa. *AJR* 1999;172:1567–1571.

35. Inman VT, Saunders JB, Abbott LC. Observations on the function of the shoulder joint. *J Bone Joint Surg* 1994;26:1–30.

36. Holt EM, Allibone RO. Anatomic variants of the coracocromial ligament. *J Shoulder Elbow Surg* 1995;4:370–375.

37. Edelson JG, Luchs J. Aspects of coracoacromial ligament anatomy of interest to the arthroscopic surgeon. *Arthroscopy* 1995;11:715–719.

38. Fritz RC, Stoller DW. MR imaging of the rotator cuff. *MRI Clin North Am* 1997;5:735–754.

39. Haywood TM, Langlotz CP, Kneeland JB, et al. Categorization of acromial shape: interobserver variability with MR imaging and conventional radiography. *AJR* 1994;162:1377–1382.

40. Peh WCG, Farmer THR, Totty WG. Acromial arch shape: assessment with MR imaging. *Radiology* 1995;195:501–505.

41. Erickson SJ, Fitzgerald SW, Quinn S, et al. Long bicipital tendon of the shoulder: normal anatomy and pathologic findings on MR imaging. *AJR* 1992;158:1091–1096.

42. Kieft GJ, Bloem JL, Obermann WR, Verbout AJ, Rosing PM, Doornbos J. Normal shoulder: MR imaging. *Radiology* 1986;159: 741–745.

43. Seeger LL, Ruszkowski JT, Bassett LW, Kay SP, Kahmann RD, Ellman H. MR imaging of the normal shoulder: anatomic correlation. *AJR* 1987;148:83–91.

44. Rafii M, Firooznia H, Sherman O, et al. Rotator cuff lesions: signal patterns at MR imaging. *Radiology* 1990;177:817–823.

45. Chandnani VP, Ho C, Gerharter J, et al. MR findings in asymptomatic shoulders: a blind analysis using symptomatic shoulders as controls. *Clin Imag* 1992;16:25–30.

46. Kaplan PA, Bryans KC, Davick JP, Otte M, Stinson WW. MR imaging of the normal shoulder: variants and pitfalls. *Radiology* 1992;184:519–524.

47. Neumann CH, Holt RG, Steinbach LS, et al. MR imaging of the shoulder: appearance of the supraspinatus tendon in asymptomatic volunteers. *AJR* 1992;158:1281–1287.

48. Sher J, Uribe J, Posada A, Murphy BJ, Zlatkin MB. Abnormal shoulder MRI exams in asymptomatic volunteers. *J Bone Joint Surg* 1994;77A:10–16.

49. Kjellin J, Ho CP, Cervilla, et al. Alteration of the supraspinatus tendon at MR imaging: correlation with histopathologic findings in cadavers. *Radiology* 1991;181:837–841.

50. Davis SJ, Teresi LM, Bradley WG, Ressler JA, Eto RT. Effect of arm rotation on MR imaging of the rotator cuff. Radiology 1991;181:265-268.

51. Erickson SJ, Cox IH, Hyde JS, Carrera GF, Strandt JA, Estkowski LD. Effect of tendon orientation on MR imaging signal intensity: a manifestation of the magic angle phenomenon. *Radiology* 1991; 181:389–392.

52. McNiesh LM, Callaghan JJ. CT arthrography of the shoulder; variations of the glenoid labrum. *AJR* 1987;149:963–966.

53. Neumann CH, Petersen SA, Jahnke AH. MR imaging of the labral-capsular complex: normal variations. *AJR* 1991;157: 1015–1021.

54. Tsai JC, Zlatkin MB. Magnetic resonance imaging of the shoulder. *Radiol Clin North Am* 1990;28:279–291.

55. Loredo R, Longo C, Salonen D, et al. Glenoid labrum: MR imaging with histologic correlation. *Radiology* 1995;196:33–41.

56. Patten RM. Vacuum phenomenon: a potential pitfall in the interpretation of gradient recalled echo MR images of the shoulder. *AJR* 1994;162:1383.

57. Stoller DW, Wolf EM. The shoulder. In: Stoller DW, ed. *Magnetic resonance imaging in orthopedics and sports medicine.* 2nd ed. Philadelphia: Lippincott Williams & Wilkins, 1997:511–633.

58. Needel S, Zlatkin MB, Sher J, Uribe J, Murphy B. MR imaging of the rotator cuff: peritendinous and bony abnormalities in an asymptomatic population. *AJR* 1996;166:863–867.
59. Mirowitz SA. Normal rotator cuff: MR imaging with conventional and fat-suppression techniques. *Radiology* 1991;180:735–740.
60. Mitchell MJ, Causey G, Berthoty DP, et al. Peribursal fat plane of the shoulder: anatomic study and clinical experience. *Radiology* 1988;168;699–704.
61. Zlatkin MB, Reicher MA, Kellerhouse LE, McDade W, Vetter L, Resnick D. The painful shoulder: MR imaging of the glenohumeral joint. *J Comput Assist Tomogr* 1988;12:995–1001.
62. Tirman PF, Palmer WE, Feller JF. MR arthrography of the shoulder. *MRI Clin North Am* 1997;4:811–839.
63. Iannotti JP, Zlatkin MB, Esterhai JL, Kressel HY, Dalinka MK, Spindler KP. Magnetic resonance imaging of the shoulder. *J Bone Joint Surg Am* 1991;73:17–29.
64. Chandnani VP, Gagliardi JA, Murnane TG, Bradley YC, DeBerardino TA, Spaeth J, Hansen MF. Glenohumeral ligaments and shoulder capsular mechanism: evaluation with MR arthrography. *Radiology* 1995;196:27–32.
65. Coumas JM, Waite RJ, Goss TP, et al. CT and MR evaluation of the labral capsular ligamentous complex of the shoulder. *AJR* 1992;158:591–597.
66. Snyder SJ, Karzel RP, Delpizzo W, Ferkel RD, Friedman MJ. SLAP lesions of the shoulder. *Arthroscopy* 1990;6:274–279.
67. Tirman PFJ, Feller JF, Palmer WE, Carroll KW, Steinbach LS, Cox I. The Buford complex—a variation of normal shoulder anatomy: MR arthrographic imaging features. *AJR* 1996;166:869–873.
68. Tuite MJ, Orwin JF. Anterosuperior labral variants of the shoulder: appearance on gradient-recalled-echo and fast spin-echo MR images. *Radiology* 1996;199:537–540.
69. Obrien SJ, Warren RF, Schwartz E. Anterior shoulder instability. *Orthop Clin North Am* 1987;18:395–408.
70. Fritz RC, Stoller DW. Fat-suppression MR arthrography of the shoulder. *Radiology* 1992;185:614–615.
71. Liou JTS, Wilson AJ, Totty WG, Brown JJ. The normal shoulder: common variations that simulate pathologic conditions at MR imaging. *Radiology* 1993;186:435–441.
72. Vahlensieck M, Pollack M, Lang P, Grampp S, Genant HK. Two segments of the supraspinatus muscle: cause of high signal at MR imaging? *Radiology* 1993;186:449–454.
73. Nobuhara K, Ikeda H. Rotator interval lesion. *Clin Orthop* 1987;223:44–50.
74. Post M. Surgical and non surgical treatment. In: Post M, ed. *The shoulder*. Philadelphia: Lea & Febiger, 1978.
75. Zlatkin MB. Anatomy of the shoulder. In Zlatkin, MB, ed. *MRI of the shoulder*. New York: Raven Press, 1991:21–40.
76. Gurley AM, Roth SI. Bone. In: Sternberg SS, ed. *Histology for pathologists*. New York: Raven Press,1992:66–67.
77. Ling SC, Chen CF, Wan RX. A study on the vascular supply of the supraspinatus tendon. *Surg Radiol Anat* 1990;12:161–165.
78. Falchook FS, Zlatkin MB, Buck BE. Pitfalls in imaging of the rotator cuff. Anatomic and surgical correlation. *Radiology* 1992;185(P)240.
79. McCauley TR, Pope CF, Jokl P. Normal and abnormal glenoid labrum: assessment with multiplanar gradient-echo MR imaging. *Radiology* 1992;183:35–37.
80. Rafii M, Firooznia H, Golimbu C, Minkoff J, Bonomo J. CT arthrography of the capsular structures of the shoulder. *AJR* 1986;146:361–367.
81. Williams MM, Snyder SJ, Buford D. The Buford complex—the cordlike middle glenohumeral ligament and absent anterosuperior labrum complex: a normal anatomic capsulolabral variant. *Arthroscopy* 1994;10:241–247.
82. Kwak SM, Brown RR, Resnick D, et al. Anatomy, anatomic variations, and pathology of the 11- to 3-o'clock position of the glenoid labrum: findings on MR arthrography and anatomic sections. *AJR* 1998;171:235–238.
83. Stoller DW. MR arthrography of the glenohumeral joint. *Radiol Clin North Am* 1997;35:97–115.
84. Smith DK, Chopp TM, Aufdemorte TB. Sublabral recess of the superior glenoid labrum: study of cadavers with conventional nonenhanced MR imaging, MR arthrography, anatomic dissection, and limited histologic examination. *Radiology* 1996;201:251–256.
85. Schweitzer ME, Magbalon MJ, Fenlin JM. Effusion criteria and clinical importance of glenohumeral joint fluid: MR imaging evaluation. *Radiology* 1995;194:821–824.
86. Yeh L, Pedowitz R, Kwak S. Intracapsular origin of the long head of the biceps tendon. *Skeletal Radiol* 1999;28:178–181.
87. Bowen MK, Warren RF. Ligamentous control of shoulder stability based on selective cutting and static translation experiments. *Clin Sports Med* 1991;10(Oct,4):757–782.
88. Rodosky MW, Harner CD, Fu FH. The role of the long head of the biceps muscle and superior glenoid labrum in anterior stability of the shoulder. *Am J Sports Med* 1994;22:121–130.
89. Stoller DW. *MRI, arthroscopy, and surgical anatomy of the joints*. Philadelphia: Lippincott–Raven, 1999:1–132.
90. Mirowitz, SA. Hematopoietic bone marrow within the proximal humeral epiphysis in normal adults: investigation with MR imaging. *Radiology* 1993;188(3):689–693.
91. Bigliani LU, Levine WN. Current concepts review: subacromial impingement syndrome. *J Bone Joint Surg* 1997;79-A:1854–1868.

ROTATOR CUFF DISEASE

MICHAEL B. ZLATKIN

The rotator cuff mechanism is very important to shoulder function. Disease of this mechanism is a very common clinical problem facing the physician who sees patients with shoulder pain. Disease of the rotator cuff is commonly related by many orthopedists and other clinicians to chronic impingement, which may eventually result in a cuff tear, although there are other causes that may be causative or considered in the development of pathology to the rotator cuff. This chapter will review the pathophysiology of rotator cuff disease, discussing these various causes and theories in its development. It will review the classification and incidence of this disease process. Although some of the clinical features and therapy of this disease process will be reviewed here, these features will be discussed in more detail elsewhere in this text. The MRI features of the spectrum of rotator cuff pathology will be described, including problems in diagnosis, such as differentiating tendinosis from artifact or partial tear, partial tears from scarring and surface degeneration, as well as accurately delineating partial tears and small complete tears. The use of some of the more current techniques, such as fast (turbo) spin echo imaging, fat suppression, and MRI arthrography, will also be addressed.

ROTATOR CUFF FUNCTION

The rotator cuff is the complex of muscles that arise from the scapula, blend in with the capsule, and attach to the greater and lesser tuberosities. The tendons of four muscles contribute to the rotator cuff of the shoulder and include the supraspinatus, the infraspinatus, the teres minor, and the subscapularis muscles. The first three muscles insert on the greater tuberosity, and the subscapularis tendon attaches anteriorly to the lesser tuberosity. The space between the supraspinatus and subscapularis tendons is known as the *rotator interval*.

Electromyographic studies have indicated that all four muscles of the rotator cuff are active during movement of the joint but with varying force (1). Biomechanical analysis has revealed that the rotator cuff contributes between one-third and one-half of the power of the shoulder in abduction predominantly carried out by the infraspinatus tendon and 80% to 90% in external rotation (2–5), primarily undertaken by the infraspinatus and teres minor. In that regard, these muscles are involved in the initial phases of abduction of the arm (6). They counteract the superior translational force produced by the deltoid. In contrast, the subscapularis tendon functions in internal rotation.

The rotator cuff also functions as a dynamic stabilizer of the glenohumeral joint in normal as well as abnormal motion (7,8). In that respect, it may act by reinforcing or creating tension in the glenohumeral joint in the midrange of motion. The function of dynamic stabilization may occur by compressing the humeral head into the glenoid fossa (9,10). This may be referred to as *concavity compression* (10). The cuff musculature may directly reinforce the superior (supraspinatus and infraspinatus), anterior (subscapularis), and posterior (infraspinatus and teres minor) portions of the glenohumeral joint capsule.

The rotator cuff also functions in providing muscular balance to the glenohumeral joint; thus, its absence or weakness can potentially result in abnormal kinematics and abnormal humeral head excursion (8,10).

The function of the rotator cuff in maintaining a watertight joint space and allowing continuation of normal synovial fluid mechanics has also been described, suggesting that it may play a role in cartilage nutrition with prevention of secondary osteoarthritis (11).

PATHOPHYSIOLOGY

Controversy continues concerning the pathogenesis of rotator cuff disease. A variety of different factors are felt to be important in the etiology of rotator cuff disease and ultimately rotator cuff tears. There are two more extensively described and studied mechanisms: rotator cuff impingement beneath the coracoacromial arch (extrinsic impingement) and primary degeneration of the cuff, which may or may not be vascular (ischemic) in origin (12–15) and shows progressive worsening with age. Trauma, overuse related to occupational and athletic activities, and glenohumeral joint instability also play a role. Acute and chronic inflammation such as that seen in rheumatoid arthritis is a less common cause.

IMPINGEMENT (EXTRINSIC CAUSES)

Rotator cuff impingement may be divided into primary extrinsic impingement, secondary extrinsic impingement (secondary to instability), internal impingement (posterosubglenoid), and subscoracoid impingement.

Primary Extrinsic Impingement

Meyer (16), in 1937, was the first to propose that attrition of the aponeurosis against the undersurface of the acromion was the main cause of rupture of the supraspinatus tendon and to dispute Codman's theory of degenerative tendinopathy (12–14). Neer, although not the first to describe this pathophysiologic mechanism (17,18), is most responsible for popularizing this concept of cuff impingement and using this as an aid in guiding and planning the clinical management of these patients. Neer (17,18) showed that the functional arc of shoulder elevation is in a forward direction. When the shoulder elevates in this functional arc, the rotator cuff and surrounding soft-tissue structures impinge in the space beneath the coracoacromial arch. Neer (17,18) stated that 95% of rotator cuff tears occur as a result of chronic impingement beneath this arch. The space below this arch is defined by the acromion superiorly, the coracoacromial ligament superomedially, and the coracoid process anteriorly (19). Known sites of impingement in this arch include the anteroinferior edge of the acromion, the coracoacromial ligament, and occasionally the undersurface of the acromioclavicular joint (17–20).

Variation in anterior acromion shape is also correlated with cuff tears (Fig. 6.1). This has been described by Bigliani

and colleagues (21). They described three types of acromion based on their shape (Fig. 6.1). They correlated the shape of the acromion in cadavers as seen on supraspinatus outlet radiographs with the occurrence of rotator cuff pathology. A Type I acromion has a flat surface, Type II has a curved undersurface, and Type II has a hooked undersurface.

A fourth type of acromion shape (Type IV) has also been recently described (Fig. 6.1). This has a convex inferior surface (22). It was found in 7% of the patient population studied by MR imaging in 30 patients. It can potentially cause narrowing of the subacromial space near the midposterior portion of the distal acromion, rather than at its anterior tip. This is a relatively uncommon configuration (23). As yet no statistical correlation has been found between this type of acromion and impingement.

Type I acromions have the least association with impingement syndrome. Only 3% of Type I acromions are associated with a rotator cuff tear (24). The hook-shaped acromion (Type III) has been shown to have the most significance (24) (Fig. 6.1) and may be the most common cause of anterior acromial impingement (24–26). It has the highest correlation with rotator cuff pathology, particularly rotator cuff tears. Correlation with surgical and arthrographic results revealed a 70% to 80% association of rotator cuff tears with Type III acromions (24,26).

The Type III acromion may be a congenital variant or possibly be related to an acquired osteophyte due to traction on the coracoacromial ligament or calcification of the acromial attachment of the coracoacromial ligament. These spurs or osteophytes may develop on the anterior and inferior aspect of the acromion and at the origin of the coracoacromial ligament. The presence of a Type III anterior acromion may increase in frequency with age (27). In the study by Tuite et al. (28), the presence of a Type III acromion was felt to be useful in separating patients with primarily shoulder impingement from those with shoulder instability.

Bigliani and Morrison (26) in their study of 140 cadaver shoulders found Type I acromions in 18.6% of cases, Type II

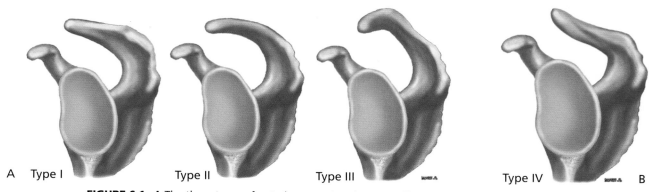

FIGURE 6.1. A: The three types of anterior acromion shape are illustrated, as described by Morrison and Bigliani (26): Type I, flat; Type II, curved; Type III, hooked. Type III is most clearly associated with impingement. **B:** Type IV acromion. This is more recently described. It has not been associated with impingement.

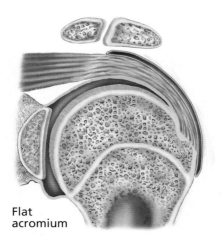 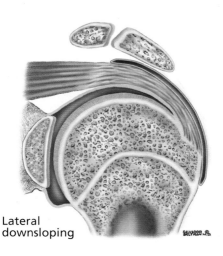

Flat
acromium

Lateral
downsloping

FIGURE 6.2. Diagram depicting lateral down-sloping of the anterior acromion as seen on coronal section.

acromions in 42% of cases, and Type III acromions in 38.6% of cases. The relative frequency of each type of acromion was studied in 394 cadaver scapular specimens by Getz and colleagues (29). Type I acromions were found in 22.8%, Type II in 68.5%, and Type III in 8.6% of cadavers (29). In this study, there was a symmetry between left and right shoulders in 70% of shoulders, and subacromial enthesophytes were most common when a Type III acromion was present. Type III acromions were more common in males in this study. With respect to origin of the different types of acromion shape, this study of scapular specimens (29) suggested that the variability of these acromion shapes was related to the presence of these enthesophytes and that these enthesophytes were more likely to be developmental, rather than acquired.

The importance of the slope of the acromion, as distinct from a hooked undersurface in the pathogenesis of the shoulder impingement syndrome, has been described in the literature (30). The lateral aspect of the normal acromion is nearly horizontal or upward sloping from posterior to anterior. Lateral or anterior downward sloping of the acromion, relative to the distal clavicle may also contribute to impingement and narrowing of the supraspinatus outlet (Fig. 6.2). The importance of the lateral edge of the acromion has been downplayed, however, by some (31,32). Farley and coworkers (33) did not find an association between this type of acromion on coronal oblique MR imaging sequences and the presence of a rotator cuff tear. At least in one of the studies, however (32), lack of association between lateral downsloping and impingement may relate to the inclusion of less severe cases of lateral tilting (34).

A low-lying acromial position, relative to the distal clavicle, may decrease the space between the acromion and the humerus and may predispose certain individuals to shoulder impingement. Edelson and coworkers (30) in a study of dry scapula specimens found an association between a low-lying acromion and degenerative changes of the acromion. Instability of the acromioclavicular joint may also contribute to impingement if it results in a low-lying acromion (35).

Osteophytes arising from the acromioclavicular joint and extending inferiorly may play some role in the impingement process as well. When the arm is abducted, the suprasapinatus component of the rotator cuff slides under the acromion and reaches a position under the acromioclavicular (AC) joint. Here distally pointing degenerative osteophytes of the acromioclavicular joint cause injury to the cuff due to their close proximity to the supraspinatus tendon in this position. They tend to compress the supraspinatus tendon when the arm is moved in this direction. A study by Peterson and coworkers (20) revealed an association of the AC joint osteophytes and supraspinatus tendon pathology. This study revealed that 51% of patients with supraspinatus ruptures had these osteophytes, as compared to 14% of patients with no tear. Kessel and Watson (36) found these changes in one-third of their patients with a "painful arc syndrome" and lesions of the supraspinatus tendon. In this study, these osteophytes were found to be more common than anterior subacromial spurs, although they frequently occur together. Osteoarthritis of the AC joint is not, however, specific for patients with impingement and may be identified on MRI exam in a large percentage of asymptomatic individuals (37).

Spurs on the anterior and inferior aspect of the acromion are also important (17,18). These spurs extend from the anteroinferior surface of the acromion in a medial and slightly inferior direction toward the coracoid process. They arise at the acromial attachment of the coracoacromial ligament. The presence of these spurs is considered presumptive evidence of shoulder impingement. Spur size may be strongly associated with the incidence of a rotator cuff tear (38). As discussed, these spurs may occur as a result of traction caused by repetitive impingement of the greater tuberosity on the coracoacromial ligament in this region. A recent study (37) found a significant incidence of acromioclavicular joint osteophytes in asymptomatic volunteers, especially with increasing age. Subacromial spurs were also present in this study. Subacromial spurs are felt to be the more correlative marker of impingement changes and rotator cuff disease (37,40) than acromioclavicular joint osteophytes. In this study (37), these spurs were present in 79% of patients with full-thickness defects on MRI exam, 68% with partial-thickness defects, 33% with tendinopathy, and 11% of patients with normal tendons. Although in this study these spurs were increased in patients of older age, they were also more closely associated with tendon pathology than with patient age.

Variation in size and thickness of the coracoacromial ligament, especially the wide portion inferior to the acromion, may be an additional factor in narrowing the subacromial space, thus causing attritional changes of the rotator cuff (41). Posttraumatic calcification or ossification of the coracoacromial ligament is another rare cause of impingement (42). The coracoacromial ligament has a trapezoid shape and attaches to the undersurface of the acromion in a broad or wide insertion. The average measurement of the coracoacromial ligament thickness has been studied anatomically and at arthroscopy (43). Its average thickness is 3.9 mm, with a range of 2 to 5.6 mm. Others have stated however that the thickening of the ligament may occur secondary to the impingement process (44), although certainly, once present, it may exacerbate the process.

An unfused apophysis of the anterior acromion, known as the *os acromiale*, may contribute to shoulder impingement (45–51). The acromion is formed by the fusion of three separate ossification centers. These normally fuse by 25 years of age. Fusion failure may occur in 8% of the population and thus form an os acomiale (49). They may be bilateral in 60% of shoulders (51). It is not known what proportion of these patients may be symptomatic. The unfused segment of the acromion can be united to the remaining portion of the acromion via an articulation. This articulation may be composed of fibrous tissue, cartilage, periosteum, or synovium (45). The os acromiale is classified as a pre-, meso-, meta-, or basiacromion based on the regions of articulation with the acromion, with the basi most proximal and the preaacromial most distal (45) (Fig. 6.3). The most common are the meso or metaacromial type (50).

The os acromiale may cause impingement because if it is unstable, it may be pulled inferiorly during abduction by the deltoid, which attaches here. In addition, hypertrophy and spurring may develop at the junction of the os acromiale and the more posterior aspect of the acromion, along its undersurface, and may contribute to impingement and subsequent rotator cuff tears in this manner (45,49,50). An unstable os acromiale is also associated with acromioclavicular joint degeneration. When recognized, a small unstable os acromiale may be excised, whereas a large unstable fragment may require fusion.

The clinical syndrome of impingement was outlined in the studies by Neer (17,18). He described the technique of anterior acromioplasty to relieve the symptoms of impingement. In the original description three progressive stages of impingement lesions were described (17,18). This was based on the age of the patient, the type of activity that presum-

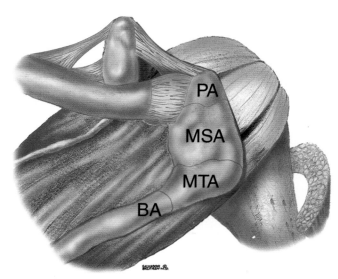

FIGURE 6.3. Axial diagram depicting the four different types of os acromiale. The mesoacromion (MSA) and metaacromion (MTA) are more common. PA, preacromion; BA, basiacromion.

ably led to the injury and the pathologic findings. Stage 1 typically results from excessive overhead use such as in sports. It generally occurs in young patients, usually less than 25 years of age, but may occur at any age. Histologically, edema and hemorrhage are said to be present in the rotator cuff tendons at this stage. If treated conservatively, this phase of the disease is usually reversible, and these patients may return to normal function. Neer (17,18) believes that patients seen in this state who get better with conservative management may account for some of the confusion regarding the prognosis and treatment of rotator cuff tears, as patients at this stage may present a similar clinical picture as those with fully developed rotator cuff tears (stage 3).

Stage 2 disease consisted of fibrosis and thickening of the rotator cuff tendons as well as the subacromial-subdeltoid bursa. It occurs in patients between 25 to 50 years of age and is less common than stage 1. The shoulder will usually become symptomatic after vigorous overhead use, such as in throwing sports. Traditionally surgery is considered in these patients when they have failed a conservative approach to therapy. The procedure at this stage of is removal of the thickened subacromial bursa and dividing the coracoacromial ligament. According to Neer (17,18), anterior acromioplasty in this group of patients who are less than 40 years old should not be performed unless overhang and prominence of the undersurface of the anterior acromion are present.

Stage 3 results from further impingement wear. At this stage, incomplete (3A) or complete tears (3B) of the rotator cuff are present. These lesions are most common in patients over 40 years of age. Lesions of the biceps tendon consisting of mechanical inflammation are usually present, although true tears of the biceps tendon are much less common than the associated cuff tears. This may be mediated by a laterally placed or shallow bicipital groove. Secondary bone changes are very common, particularly those related to the anterior acromion, greater tuberosity, and acromioclavicular joint. Acromioplasty and cuff repair are often required due to pain and/or weakness.

Secondary Extrinsic Impingement (Impingement Associated with Instability)

Fu and associates (52) subdivided impingement syndromes into two major categories: primary extrinsic impingement (discussed earlier), which occurs in nonathletic persons and is related to alterations in the coracoacromial arch, and secondary impingement, which occurs mainly in athletes involved in sports requiring overhead motion of the arm and which has a relationship to glenohumeral joint instability (52,53).

This distinction has been known for some time as Hawkins et al. described the (54) situation of the high-profile competitive athlete who may present with a rotator cuff tear that develops over a shorter period of time and at a younger age because of repetitive use of the shoulder. These patients may develop symptoms without any abnormality of the bony anatomy of the coracoacromial arch. Jobe (55,56) believed that in the athlete, particularly the throwing athlete, rotator cuff disease resulted from a continuum that involves not only impingement, but instability as well. This continuum progresses from instability, to subluxation, to impingement, and finally to rotator cuff tear. Anterior instability, he believed, was the primary lesion, with microtrauma from repetitive overhead use leading to breakdown or stretching of the static stabilizers of the shoulder. Tears of the anterior labrum and abnormalities of the inferior glenohumeral ligament were the most common pathologic lesions found in these patients. The resultant anterior instability also results in fatigue and overload of the dynamic stabilizers, the rotator cuff. These factors allow anterior and superior subluxation (translation) of the humeral head; when the arm is abducted and externally rotated, the anterior subluxation causes "dynamic" impingement of the rotator cuff against the acromion and the coracoacromial ligament. Subluxation of the humeral head may then cause impingement by anterior and superior compression of the rotator cuff between the humeral head and coracoacromial ligament and anterior acromion.

These patients usually have less advanced rotator cuff pathology, including tendinosis or partial or very small rotator cuff tears (54). This distinction is important, since therapy should be directed to the underlying instability. Conservative treatment is aimed at strengthening the rotator cuff and scapular rotators. Throwing athletes with glenohumeral instability and secondary impingement who do not respond to conservative treatment may be treated with an anterior capsular labral reconstruction. In the less common

situation where alterations of the bony coracoacromial arch may also be identified (mixed pathology), then subacromial decompression may be necessary, in addition to anterior stabilization.

Scapulothoracic instability may also cause a similar type of secondary extrinsic impingement. The scapulothoracic muscles include the trapezium, serratus anterior, rhomboids, and lattisimus dorsi. Abnormal scapulothoracic motion and alteration of the scapulohumeral rhythm may also lead to impingement via functional narrowing of the subacromial space during overhead throwing (54).

Posterosubglenoid (Internal) Impingement

Another type of impingement recognized recently is impingement of the rotator cuff on the posterosuperior portion of the glenoid in throwing athletes (58–64). This is also known as *internal impingement* (65). This particular type of impingement occurs during the late cocking phase of throwing with abnormal contact between the posterosuperior portion of the glenoid rim and the undersurface of the rotator cuff, and it is thought to occur at the extremes of abduction and external rotation. It has also been recognized in nonathletes who frequently rotate the shoulder into the extremes of abduction and external rotation (60). It is not clear whether actual instability is necessary to develop this clinical problem.

A triad of findings will be present including injury to the rotator cuff undersurface at the junction of the infraspinatus and supraspinatus tendons, degenerative tearing of the posterosuperior glenoid labrum, as well as subcortical cysts and chondral lesions in the posterosuperior glenoid and humerus due to repetitive impaction. The lesion on the humerus may at times simulate a Hill-Sachs lesion. There may in addition be an injury to the inferior glenohumeral ligament and anterior inferior labrum. The inferior glenohumeral ligament may be injured because it limits abduction and external rotation of the glenohumeral joint and is therefore under tension in this position.

Edelson and Teitz (65) recently examined a large number of skeletal shoulder specimens (1,232 shoulders) and found the characteristic telltale patterns of internal impingement impressed into the bones on both sides of the joint in many of these specimens. Based on these findings, these authors believe that internal impingement between the glenoid and the humeral head may be a significant mechanism in the development of rotator cuff pathology. On the basis of these findings, they called into question the rationale for some acromioplasty operations.

Subcoracoid Impingement

Impingement beneath the coracoid process relates to encroachment of the subscapularis tendon insertion on the lesser tuberosity (66,67), secondary to narrowing of this space between the coracoid process and the humeral head. This may often go unrecognized, and patients may undergo subacromial decompression before this diagnosis is considered. Subcoracoid impingement is most prominent with the humeral head in forward flexion and medial rotation where the coracohumeral distance is least. Developmental enlargement of the coracoid process that projects more laterally may be the underlying cause. This can be exacerbated by acquired conditions including fractures of the coracoid or lesser tuberosity, calcification of the subscapularis tendon, glenoid osteotomy, or procedures in which the coracoid process is transferred, such as the Bristow procedure for treatment of instability (see Chapters 4 and 9).

Subcoracoid impingement may occur when the distance between the coracoid and lesser tuberosity measures below 11 mm, with the arm positioned in maximal internal rotation (68). CT has been used as a method of obtaining a measurement of the lateral extent of the coracoid process and can be used to assess the degree of subcoracoid impingement, but similar measurement may be undertaken with MRI.

Other Causes of Impingement

Other causes may include such entities as supraspinatus muscle hypertrophy in athletes who perform repetitive overhead activity, such as swimmers. In patients with supraspinatus muscle hypertrophy, impingement may occur in the presence of a normal coracoacromial arch. They may have symptoms of impingement with shoulder adduction as the enlarged muscle is shifted into the supraspinatus outlet. In these patients, the enlarged supraspinatus muscle belly may seem to be deformed beneath the AC joint on coronal oblique MR images (34).

Impingement may also occur related to prominent healed callus from a greater tuberosity fracture. Patients with extra bone about the greater tuberosity, related to the fracture deformity, may undergo impingement of this more prominent area beneath the lateral aspect of the acromion. Displaced greater tuberosity fractures that heal with deformity may also cause impingement or block normal motion during abduction.

Primary Rotator Cuff Degeneration (Intrinsic Causes)

There are other theories on the etiology of rotator cuff tears and many who disagree with the predominant or exclusive role of impingement in the development of cuff tears. Codman (12–14) suggested that degenerative changes within the cuff itself lead to tears. According to Codman (12–14), this may have a vascular or ischemic basis. He described a critical portion in the rotator cuff at the distal supraspinatus tendon approximately 1 cm medial to its insertion into the greater tuberosity. He referred to the pattern of degenerative cuff failure as a "rim rent" in which the deep surface of the cuff is torn at its attachment to the tuberosity. He stated that these tears tended to begin on the deep surface and then extend outward until they become full-thickness defects. He pointed out that it would be hard to explain this on the basis of erosion from contact from the acromion process.

This area of decreased vascularity in the supraspinatus tendon has been documented by other cadaver studies of the microcirculation (69). Lindblom (70) and Rothman (71) found this area to be hypovascular or avascular. It may therefore be prone to ischemia and be more susceptible to the development of degenerative changes (71). This region of the tendon may be most avascular in the resting position of adduction and neutral rotation. According to these studies, the position of the rotator cuff tendons predisposes them to constant pressure from the humeral head, which tends to drain blood from the vessels (69).

In another study based on findings in cadavers that also drew the conclusion that tears are degenerative, related to intrinsic factors and not due to extrinsic impingement, Uthoff and coworkers (72) found that most rotator cuff tears begin from the articular side. They indicated that if rotator cuff tears arose primarily from extrinsic impingement, then the majority of rotator cuff tears should begin from the bursal side. On that basis, they felt that rotator cuff tears are therefore degenerative in origin and nature and that extrinsic causes therefore play a secondary role. Ozaki and coworkers (73) have shown in cadavers that the majority of pathologic changes of the undersurface of the acromion occurred in specimens in which the cuff tear was incomplete and on the bursal side of the cuff. All specimens that had a complete tear also had pathologic changes on the undersurface of the acromion. In contrast in specimens that had an incomplete tear that involved the humeral head side of the cuff (the articular side), which was the most common pathologic state in their study, the undersurface of the acromion was always intact. These authors felt that these findings indicated that the lesion of the undersurface of the anterior one-third of the acromion is a secondary change that follows a tear of the cuff on the bursal side. They indicated that a vicious cycle then develops, so that the irregularity of the acromion abrades the cuff, and vice versa. Their conclusion, then, was that the majority of cuff tears are caused by intrinsic degenerative changes due to age and that cuff tearing that occurs from impingement and documented by lesions present on the undersurface of the acromion are secondary phenomena.

In another study, Lohr and Uthoff (74) revealed differential vascularity between the bursal and articular surfaces of the rotator cuff. The bursal surface was observed to be well vascularized, whereas the articular surface demonstrated a sparse arteriolar pattern. The results of this study were thought to indicate that this differential vascularity predisposed the articular surface of the rotator cuff to degenerative changes and failure.

Mosley and Goldie (75) in a microinjection study of 72 cadaver shoulders renamed this critical portion in the rotator cuff "the critical zone." In their research, however, they found this region to be a watershed area, occurring between osseous and tendinous vessels supplying the rotator cuff tendons.

Pettersson (76) has described the histological pattern of age-related degeneration in the tendon. He demonstrated changes in cell arrangement, calcium deposition, fibrinoid thickening, fatty degeneration, necrosis, and rents. Although this pattern of degeneration may not be symptomatic, it may impair the tensile and elastic strength of the tendon. Kumagai and coworkers (77) revealed an alteration in the pattern of collagen fibers in such patients, in which there was a transformation from Type II to fibrovascular containing Type III collagen.

Intraoperative laser Doppler flowmetry has also been used to assess the rotator cuff tendon vascularity in symptomatic patients. The study by Swiontowski et al. (78) was undertaken to clarify the discrepancy between surgical findings of increased vascularity in patients with "impingement syndrome" and the cadaveric reports discussed earlier demonstrating a hypovascular zone in the rotator cuff. The conclusions of these studies were felt to support impingement as a mechanism of rotator cuff pathology. Particularly in patients with intact tendons and tendinosis but also in patients with partial and complete tears, increased vascularity was found in the region of the critical zone. The authors concluded that impingement of the tendon in this region generates a hypervascular response that results in the resorption of injured tendon fibers by neovascular tissue and mediates the progression of rotator cuff disease. These findings also corroborated an earlier cadaveric study in an increase in the number of blood vessels was found in degenerated tendon regions. The vessels invaded degenerative tendons through ingrowth of granulation tissue from the bursal and synovial surfaces. This was not observed in normal tendons, where in fact the number of arterioles decreased with age (79,80). Brooks and coworkers (81) also carried out perfusion studies that they felt did not support an ischemic zone in the distal anterior supraspinatus tendon. They identified the critical zone in their study and found that it was not relatively more hypovascular and that the vascular portions of the supraspinatus and infraspinatus tendons are similar. Both tendons were hypovascular in their distal 15 mm. No significant difference was demonstrated between the vascularity of supraspinatus and infraspinatus. They concluded that factors other than vascularity are important in the pathogenesis of supraspinatus rupture.

In a study in support of intrinsic degeneration as the underlying cause of rotator cuff failure, Nirschl (82) found acromial spurs in only 10% of patients referred for surgery for rotator cuff "tendonitis." Rotator cuff degeneration has also been observed in the absence of subacromial spurs (86).

Rotator cuff tendinitis/tendinosis and subsequent failure has been attributed to repeated eccentric tensile overload of the rotator cuff tendons. Expanding on these concepts, a more recent article by Budoff, Nirschl, and Guidi (84) argues that most patients with rotator cuff abnormalities have as their primary underlying etiology, intrinsic degeneration, rather than extrinsic impingement, which they believe occurs secondary to rotator cuff failure. These authors state that the supraspinatus, since it is a small and relatively weak muscle, is in a key position and is therefore susceptible to overuse and injury. When eccentric tensile overload occurs at a rate that is greater than the ability of the cuff to repair itself, injury occurs, resulting in weakness of the musculotendinous rotator cuff unit. Trauma to the shoulder may initiate the process as well, and a weak, fatigued, or injured rotator cuff is unable to oppose the superior pull of the deltoid effectively, which is then unable to keep the humeral head centered on the glenoid during elevation of the arm, causing it to elevate, which then functionally narrows the subacromial space. Continued dysfunction of the rotator cuff and further superior migration of the humeral head cause the greater tuberosity and the rotator cuff to abut against the undersurface of the acromion and the coracoacromial ligament, leading to signs of secondary extrinsic impingement.

The secondary impingement between the greater tuberosity and the acromion may lead to reactive and degenerative osseous changes, such as ostephytic spurring of these structures. The already injured and weakened rotator cuff is then damaged further by this process of secondary impingement, especially by osteophytes on the undersurface of the acromion. Trauma superimposed on this may then cause the weakened cuff to rupture. These authors believe that although subacromial impingement does occur, it is a secondary process, rather than a primary one. They indicate that it is a dynamic process, secondary to intrinsic failure of the tendon, that in time results in reactive osseous changes, causing the classic radiographic changes seen with the impingement syndrome, including erosions or exostosis of the greater tuberosity. In this process, the coracoacromial ligament may undergo degeneration or a traction spur at its insertion into the anteromedial corner of the acromion, which may mimic the Type III acromion. These authors believe that since changes to the CA ligament and the undersurface of the anterior acromion are secondary processes and since they do not occur in many patients, these structures should be preserved if their anatomy is not altered. They believe that these structures play an important role as passive stabilizers against superior migration of the humeral head and therefore should not be sacrificed. They believe that removal of the structures with a subacromial decompression/acromioplasty does not address the primary problem in most symptomatic cuffs, which is intratendinous degeneration or tendinosis. In other words, they do not believe that impingement is the primary cause of rotator cuff pathology and tears. They state the results of Burkhead and coworkers (85), who found that an injection into the subacromial space does not relieve pain caused by resisted abduction in patients who have a partial-thickness tear, corroborate their findings. These authors therefore recommend debridement of the degenerated cuff tissue arthroscopically and only resecting of clearly identified excrescences. This approach, they feel, is direct treatment of the primary pathoanatomy. They do not perform a complete acromioplasty and do not remove the coracoacromial ligament.

There is thus considerable debate as to the origin of rotator cuff disease. It is not clear whether the cuff degenerates from within as a process of aging and overuse, which may be related to vascular and ischemic factors and then may undergo secondary impingement after it is further weakened due to overload, or whether injury occurs primarily from extrinsic factors due to chronic attrition underneath the coracoacromial arch (primary impingement). It is likely that many of these factors coexist and each contribute to the development of a cuff tear or that they may contribute to different degrees in individual patients, depending on age, activity, pathoanatomy, and so forth. Whether or not an avascular region exists, the supraspinatus tendon does undergo age-related degeneration. In addition, because of its particular location and surrounding bony anatomy, it is also vulnerable to the process of mechanical impingement and thus to the development of cuff tears in this region. Neer (17,18), in fact, noted that elevation of the arm, particularly in internal rotation, causes the "critical area" of the cuff to pass under the coracoacromial arch, thus reflective of the contribution of both of these etiologies to rotator cuff disease. The combination of these stresses may then lead to cumulative injury to the collagen fibers of the tendon, which may eventually lead to tears.

Trauma

Trauma is felt to play a secondary role in the etiology of rotator cuff tears (17,18). While a history of recent trauma may often be elicited, the injury may not be of significant force, as little force may be needed to tear a tendon that is already degenerated by long-standing impingement wear, perhaps related to underlying tendinosis and repeated episodes of peritendinous inflammation. Fifty percent of patients with cuff tears may have no recollection of any episode of trauma, according to Neer (17,18). He indicates that a history of preexistent, often long-standing shoulder pain, is often elicited upon the questioning of patients. The trauma from a fall or dislocation may therefore complete or enlarge a preexistent small or incomplete tear or tear an already degenerated tendon. Norwood and coworkers (86), on the other hand, found that in patients with larger tears of more than one tendon, more frequently a history of acute trauma was elicited (80%). These patients however were generally older and nonathletic. In this series of patients, it was felt

that the acute trauma, superimposed on chronic degenerative changes, caused the cuff rupture. In distinction, patients with tears of only a single tendon were less likely to have a history of trauma and were younger, more commonly athletic, and more likely to have had episodes of shoulder pain requiring treatment, and chronic mechanical impingement was felt to play the most significant role in the etiology of their tears.

Notwithstanding these points, a tear may occur following an anterior dislocation of the shoulder, usually in an older patient in whom a cuff rupture occurs rather than an injury to the glenoid labrum and/or shoulder capsule (87–89). Studies show that a cuff tear may occur in 14% to 63% of patients with acute anterior dislocations (76,90,91). The incidence will be higher with older patients. In Pevny's study of 52 patients over the age of 40 with dislocations after skiing injury (92), 18 (35%) rotator cuff tears were identified. The supraspinatus tendon may tear with variable degrees of infraspinatus involvement.

Deutsch (93) studied traumatic tears of the subscapularis tendon in 13 surgically confirmed patients. In all but three patients, the mechanism of injury was traumatic hyperextension or external rotation of the abducted arm. Six shoulders had full-thickness tears of the subscapularis tendon, and seven shoulders had full-thickness tears associated with concomitant biceps tendon pathologic conditions, including subluxation, dislocation, or rupture. Isolated ruptures of the subscapularis may also occur with anterior dislocations, again predominantly in patients older than 40 and in men (88,94). Avulsive fractures of the lesser tuberosity at the site of insertion of the subscapularis may occur in elderly women and men (95). With a posterior dislocation, there may be disruption of the infraspinatus or teres minor tendons (88–90,96). Superior dislocations of the humeral head may also result in cuff rupture as the humeral head is driven upward acutely through the cuff. As noted earlier, however, many of these lesions may occur superimposed on preexistent rotator cuff disease. Minor tendinous avulsive injuries are said to occur in the "normal" tendons of athletes (97).

A cuff tear may also arise following a dislocation when the greater tuberosity is fractured. It may also develop following an avulsion fracture of the greater tuberosity. Neer reported that a displaced greater tuberosity fracture results in an obligate longitudinal cuff tear at the region of the rotator interval (98). Posterior dislocations may also result in a fracture of the lesser tuberosity, in which case a tear of the subscapularis tendon may result (8). Although a nondisplaced greater tuberosity fracture may result in injury to the cuff (87), recent evidence with MRI (99,100) indicates that this may more often result in a tendon contusion, or intact cuff, rather than a tear, and the pain may more commonly be related to the bony injury.

In a study by Mason and coworkers (100), one-part greater tuberosity fractures referred for MR revealed no associated cuff abnormalities that required early surgery. Reinus and coworkers (99) reported on six patients with subtle greater tuberosity fractures who were sent for MRI because of possible rotator cuff tear. MRI exam revealed findings consistent with a nondisplaced greater tuberosity fracture in all cases. Plain shoulder radiographs before MRI were interpreted as normal in all cases. Full-thickness rotator cuff tears were not present in any of the cases.

Impingement and the Biceps Tendon

The biceps tendon is also an integral part of the impingement syndrome, and bicipital problems are usually a manifestation of a more significant underlying impingement process. The progression of involvement in the biceps tendon is similar to that in the supraspinatus tendon, although often less rapid or advanced. A similar zone of hypovascularity is thought to be present in the biceps tendon. This is important given the increasing understanding of the critical role the biceps tendon plays as a stabilizer of the humeral head during abduction of the shoulder in the scapular plane. As noted earlier, a shallow or laterally placed bicipital groove may predispose the biceps tendon to impingement by the anterior one-third of the acromion (17,101). In Murthi's study (102) of the biceps tendon in patients who underwent arthroscopic subacromial decompression for impingement syndrome, a high incidence of chronic inflammation of the long head of the biceps tendon was found in patients with coincident rotator cuff disease. Disease of the biceps tendon is more fully discussed in Chapter 8.

The subdeltoid bursa is involved in the impingement process as well, often resulting in subdeltoid bursitis and eventually fibrosis. The subacromial bursa tends to undergo proliferative or degenerative changes in patients with impingement syndrome. Kronberg and Saric (103) studied 21 patients with impingement syndrome who underwent acromioplasty, and in each case biopsies from the subacromial bursa were taken. Ten patients had severe fibrosis, eight had moderate fibrosis, and one patient had no fibrosis at all. All normal controls had no fibrosis.

Other factors (10,104) that may be operative in the development of rotator cuff pathology include a frozen shoulder, or weakness of the rotator cuff muscles. With a frozen shoulder, stiffness of the posterior capsule may aggravate the impingement process by forcing the humeral head up against the anteroinferior acromion as the shoulder is flexed. Rotator cuff muscle weakness due to a number of different factors may cause loss of the normal humeral head depressor mechanism. Contraction of the deltoid then results in upward displacement of the humeral head, compressing the cuff against the arch.

In summary, tears of the rotator cuff most likely occur in tendons that are weakened by some combination of age, repeated small episodes of trauma, impingement, hypovascularity of the tendon, major injuries, and previous partial tearing (10,104).

CLASSIFICATION, LOCATION, AND INCIDENCE OF ROTATOR CUFF TEARS

A *full-thickness rotator cuff tear* is defined as one that extends from the articular surface to the bursal surface of the cuff. Codman (108) defined a *complete tear* as one in which the whole thickness of the rotator cuff and capsule are torn, resulting in direct communication between the subdeltoid bursa and the joint cavity. In contrast, partial-thickness tears are tears that do not involve the entire thickness of the cuff (Fig. 6.4). They will involve only one surface of the cuff, either the inferior or the superficial surface. A special type of partial tear is one that involves only the midsubstance of the cuff. Tears of the inferior surface are also referred to as *deep* or *articular surface tears,* those of the midsubstance as *intrasubstance tears*, and those of the superficial surface as *superior* or *bursal surface tears*. Retraction of tendinous fibers from the greater tuberosity may also be considered a partial tear (106).

Rotator cuff tears may be classified according to age. *Acute tears* are those that occur suddenly, usually secondary to an injury and are less common. An acute tear is one that has been present for less than 6 weeks. A *subacute tear* is defined as 6 weeks to 6 months old (105). *Chronic tears* are much more common (92%) and are those that have existed for a longer period of time and are insidious in onset of their symptoms (104). Ellman et al. (108) define chronic tears as those that are 6 months to 1 year old, and he considers tears older than a year to be old tears. A chronic tear may also undergo acute extension, with the sudden failure of additional fibers, and the onset of new clinical manifestations (108).

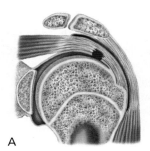

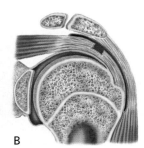

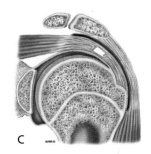

FIGURE 6.4. Classification of partial tears by location. **A:** Articular surface partial tear; **B:** bursal surface partial tear; **C:** intrasubstance partial tear.

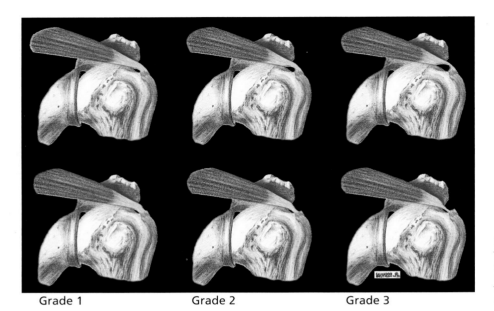

Grade 1   Grade 2   Grade 3

FIGURE 6.5. Classification of partial tears by depth. Grade 1, up to 3 mm; grade 2, 3–6 mm; grade 3, more than 6 mm. Articular side partial tears are on the upper level; bursal side partial tears are on the lower level.

The shape of rotator cuff tears can be classified according to the pattern they assume. Small tears tend to be transverse in nature. As these tears enlarge, they assume a triangular or crescentic configuration. Massive tears result from an enlargement of one of these two patterns, either over time or through superimposed trauma (109,110). Ellman (107) describes a more elaborate classification scheme based on the size and location of a tear, which he describes as transverse linear, crescent-shaped, L-shaped, reverse L-shaped, trapezoidal, and massive.

Partial tears have been classified by Ellman (111) as follows (Fig. 6.5): grade 1 (low grade) are less than 3 mm deep and only the capsule or superficial fibers are involved; grade 2 (intermediate) are 3 to 6 mm deep and less than 50% of the cuff thickness is involved; and grade 3 (high grade or deep) is greater than 6 mm, in which more than 50% of the cuff thickness is involved.

Complete cuff tears can be classified by size. The size is measured at the widest point of retraction after minimal debridement of 1 to 2 mm. Small tears as those less than 1 cm, medium size tears as those less than 3 cm, and large tears as those 3 to 5 cm. Massive tears are those greater than 5 cm (105). Other authors consider small tears as those less than 2 cm and massive tears those greater than 4 cm (112). Ellman has pointed out that the length of a tear does not always correspond to the difficulty of repair and proposes that the area of a tear be measured in square centimeters (112). He calculates this using the base of the tear along the former insertion site times the depth of the muscle retraction. On MRI exam, the size of tears should be determined with regard to the length of detachment from the humerus both in a medial to lateral extent and an anterior to posterior extent. The size of the rotator cuff tear in both anterior posterior and mediolateral dimensions is a very important prognostic factor in de-

termining surgical outcome (113). Other important prognostic factors to be discussed later in this chapter include the quality of the tissues, the presence of a chronic rupture of the long head of the biceps tendon, and the degree of preoperative shoulder weakness (113,114).

Another classification uses the number of tendons involved to size tears (115). If the supraspinatus tendon alone is involved, the tear is classified as small (stage 1B). If the supraspinatus is involved and at least a portion of the infraspinatus, it is stage 2 and is considered moderate in size. With the involvement of the supraspinatus infraspinatus and subscapularis, the tears are stage 3 and are considered large or massive. Stage 4 is rotator cuff arthropathy.

Patte (116) has provided an extensive classification system based on the extent of tears and their topography in the sagittal and coronal planes (Fig. 6.6) and the quality of the involved muscle, particularly with respect to the presence of atrophy and the status of the long head of the biceps tendon (intact, torn, or dislocated). His classification scheme was designed to provide prognostic and diagnostic data for both operative and nonoperative patients. While the various components of this system are all important and should be addressed on imaging exams, it is not apparent how these components correlate with each other (105). One important factor that is addressed in Patte's scheme (116) that is not dealt with in other schemes is the degree of muscle atrophy (trophicity). This is important in prognosis and the ultimate postoperative result with respect to the ability to rehabilitate the shoulder toward recovery of muscle strength (105).

Neer (101) classified rotator cuff tears according to etiology and divided them into impingement tears; traumatic tears due to single injury, or repetitive microtrauma; tears due to supreme violence; and "rotator interval tears due to multidirectional dislocation" and acute dislocations after the

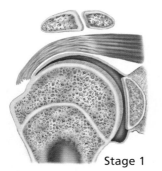 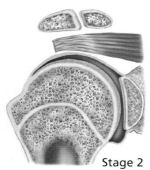 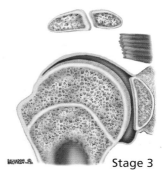

Stage 1 Stage 2 Stage 3

FIGURE 6.6. Different stages of tendon retraction as seen in the coronal plane. Stage 1, near the tendon insertion; stage 2, at the level of the humeral head; stage 3 at the glenoid margin.

age of 40. Impingement tears were the majority of cuff tears in his classification scheme (95%). In this group, patients are older than 40, and the tears involve the supraspinatus. They may be suddenly enlarged by a trivial injury (acute extension). Traumatic tears occur in younger patients, are often incomplete, and involve the supraspinatus. Supreme violence results in massive cuff avulsion often with nerve injury. Rotator interval tears result in enlargement of the rotator interval. Tears in acute glenohumeral dislocations occur after age 40, resulting in injuries of the rotator interval and subscapularis tendon.

With regard to the site of a tear, most partial- and small full-thickness rotator cuff tears are centered in the anterior half of the supraspinatus (117). Supraspinatus tears begin on the deep surface anteriorly and distally at the greater tuberosity insertion, near the biceps tendon, and then extend outward until they become full-thickness defects. In supraspinatus tears occurring just proximal to the greater tuberosity, a small remnant of tendon may still be attached to the greater tuberosity in smaller defects. Once in the supraspinatus, the defects then propagate posteriorly and medially through the remaining portions of the supraspinatus and then into the infraspinatus. This then puts progressive stress on the biceps tendon. Changes in the biceps tendon may initially be of less severe degree and may only consist of tendinosis, but it may eventually rupture, especially in chronic defects. The defect may then propagate across the bicipital groove to involve the subscapularis tendon starting at the top of the lesser tuberosity and extending inferiorly. Involvement of the subscapularis tendon, may occur with larger tears, and anterior tears. In this case it may often involve the superior articular surface fibers and the rotator interval capsule. It may also be involved in subcoracoid impingement. Acute ruptures of the subscapularis can occur with severe trauma (118), especially with abduction and external rotation (119,120), or in elderly patients with recurrent anterior dislocations. As the lesions propagate anteriorly into the subscapularis they may be associated with disruption of the stabilizers of the biceps, such as the transverse humeral ligament and then result in medial dislocation of the biceps tendon.

Isolated infraspinatus full-thickness tears are uncommon. They can occur in the spectrum of posterior superior (inter-

nal) subglenoid impingement or with severe trauma with posterior dislocation. Partial tears occurring at the junction of the posterior supraspinatus and anterior infraspinatus can occur in overhead-throwing athletes in association with posterior superior (internal) subglenoid impingement (63). In some situations, these partial tears may be seen even more posteriorly, primarily in the infraspinatus tendon. Tears of the teres minor tendon are distinctly rare, even in the setting of massive tears, although partial tears of the superior aspect of the teres minor have been reported in a series of massive, irreparable, rotator cuff tears (121). These may occur with trauma, in association with posterior capsular rupture as well as infraspinatus tendon tears, in the setting of a posterior dislocation. In this situation, teres minor muscle and capsular injuries may occur without the typical reverse Bankart lesion (122). In Ovesen's cadaver study (123), a posterior subspinous dislocation of the humeral head was provoked. All ten of the specimens in this study showed total rupture of the posterior capsule and teres minor, in most cases together with a partial lesion of the infraspinatus. In the majority of the specimens, lesions were also seen in the lower part of the subscapularis muscle and in the proximal part of the anterior capsule (123). A rare association of chronic massive rotator cuff defects is spontaneous detachment of the deltoid origin. It is associated with an acute, sudden onset of shoulder weakness. This was recently reported in three patients with four affected shoulders (124).

With progressive disruption of the rotator cuff tendons, the humeral head can then rise under pull of the deltoid muscle. This then leads to abrasion of the humeral head articular cartilage against the coracoacromial arch, causing subacromial impingement that in time erodes the anterior portion of the acromion and the acromioclavicular joint. There are also nutritional factors related to the rotator cuff tear that cause atrophy of the glenohumeral articular cartilage and osteoporosis of the subchondral bone of the humeral head. Eventually the soft, atrophic head collapses, producing the complete syndrome of cuff-tear arthropathy (17). The incongruous head may eventually erode the glenoid so deeply that the coracoid becomes eroded as well.

One other factor that is important when evaluating rotator cuff tears is the assessment of the status of the torn rotator cuff tendon edges. On imaging exams as well as at surgery, the appearance of the torn edges may be classified as good, fair, or poor (125,126). The status of the rotator cuff musculature as emphasized by Patte (116), with regard to the degree of atrophy, can also be quantified in a relative manner, as mild, moderate, or severe (125,126). It is best determined on imaging exam (125,126), but it can be correlated with clinical strength-testing systems.

Ciepela and Burkhead (105) have emphasized the need of achieving a unified classification system that takes into account the factors discussed in the above classification schemes. He proposes an equation for comparing complete rotator cuff tears: duration of tear in weeks × anterior posterior extent of the tear × degree of retraction × degree of atrophy divided by the humeral head diameter. The last factor is added to take into account the relative size of patients' humeral heads, as a 2-cm tear in a patient with a large diameter humeral head would be different than in one with a small diameter humeral head.

The incidence of rotator cuff tears has also been evaluated. According to Ellman (127), rotator cuff tendinopathy, regardless of its etiology, will lead to rupture in more than 20% of patients. Much of the data on the incidence of rotator cuff tears has been derived from cadaver studies. In these studies, full-thickness cuff tears range in incidence from less than 5% (17) to 20% to 27% (128,129). Partial tears may also be common. Fukuda has reported an incidence of partial-thickness tears of 13% (130). Intratendinous partial tears were the most common (7.2%), followed by articular surface tears (3.6%) and bursal side tears (2.4%). Depalma found an even higher incidence of partial tears (131). In his study of 96 specimens aged 18 to 74, 37% were found to have partial tears.

Data on the incidence of rotator cuff tears in living patients are more difficult to obtain. The incidence of rotator cuff tears also increase with increasing age as the strength of human tendons decreases with older individuals. The general consensus is that partial-thickness tears are more common than full-thickness tears and that those of the articular side of the rotator cuff are slightly more common than those of the bursal side (42). In the study by Sher and coworkers (132) of 100 asymptomatic volunteers who underwent MRI examination, 22% of patients had partial tears and 14% had complete tears. The incidence of rotator cuff tears increased with age. Partial tears were rare in those less than 40 (4%), and complete tears rarely occurred in individuals less than 60 years old; however, in asymptomatic individuals older than 60 years old, 54% had a tear of the rotator cuff. Ellman (111) studied a series of 130 patients who underwent arthroscopic subacromial decompression and in whom the cuff was inspected from both the bursal and articular surfaces. Twenty-two patients (17%) had full-thickness tears of the rotator cuff, and 20 (15%) had partial-thickness tears. Of the partial-thickness tears, 40% involved the bursal surface and 60% the articular surface.

CLINICAL FEATURES

The clinical manifestations of patients with shoulder pain due to the impingement syndrome and rotator cuff tears has been discussed in more detail in Chapter 4. The development of shoulder impingement is more common in certain occupations such as fruit picking, tree pruning, carpentry, or painting. It is more common in certain athletic activities such as overhead throwing, swimming, and tennis (108). Patients complain of chronic shoulder pain, stiffness, and weakness, and the findings may be accentuated when the arm is flexed or internally rotated. There may be a limited range of motion. Pain may be provoked by elevation of the shoulder. There may be a painful arc, between 60° and 120° of abduction. The clinical manifestations often worsen with more advanced stages of the disease process. Injection of local anesthetic into the subacromial space may lead to relief of pain in patients with an impingement process. Patients with rotator cuff tears that communicate with the articular surface may also obtain relief with intraarticular injection of anesthetic, but other intraarticular pathology may be relieved by this method as well.

The earlier stages of tendon pathology such as tendinitis/tendinosis predominate among younger patients. Rotator cuff tears, as noted earlier, are more common in older patients and predominate in patients over the age of 40, in men, and in the dominant arm. Shoulder pain, stiffness, and weakening are the most common clinical manifestations of patients with rotator cuff tears. In patients with rotator cuff tears, night pain may be present. On physical exam, shoulder crepitus may be elicited when the arm is internally rotated, abducted, and flexed. Weakness of flexion, abduction, and external rotation of the arm may be apparent.

An accurate diagnosis of a rotator cuff tear may be evident from the clinical findings; however, they may be simulated by other shoulder disorders such as adhesive capsulitis and calcific tendinitis, or less advanced stages of rotator cuff disease and impingement. The presence of clinical features of impingement at clinical exam may also not be predictive of the presence and extent of rotator cuff pathology, which may be more correlative with the age of the patient (133). As such, imaging studies such as MRI and, in selected situations, MR arthrography can be useful in establishing the correct diagnosis and determining the extent and nature of the pathologic process involved.

MRI IMAGING
Technique

Imaging of the shoulder has been reported at field strengths as low as 0.2 T (134) and more recently with dedicated extremity systems (Shellock F, 2000, unpublished data). Images with the highest resolution can be obtained with higher field strength systems. The surface coils utilized in the evaluation of the shoulder have been described in greater detail in Chapter 2. Most of our studies carried out at high field are done with a dedicated shoulder coil, using a four-channel phased array system (MRI Devices Corporation, Waukeshah, WI).

We position patients in a supine position in the magnet. The arm is usually placed in a position that is most comfortable for the patient—generally with the entire arm by the side and the wrist in neutral rotation. External rotation of the humeral head should be avoided, as this is usually an uncomfortable position and therefore may also result in an increase in motion artifact, as does placing the arm over the abdomen. In addition, placing the arm in external rotation may project the long head of the biceps tendon close to the critical zone of the supraspinatus tendon, and fluid within the biceps tendon sheath may simulate the appearance of a rotator cuff tear (134,135).

After the appropriate localizing sequences are obtained, axial images are obtained from below the level of the acromion to the inferior glenoid margin. They are undertaken with a dual echo fast spin echo sequence. The axial images are used as a localizing image to determine the correct plane for the oblique coronal and oblique sagittal images. They are also used as a screening series for any glenoid labral or capsular pathology that may be present in these patients. Anterior rotator cuff tears related to the supraspinatus tendon may be visualized in this plane, as is pathology related to the subscapularis tendon and long head of the biceps tendon.

The oblique coronal images are oriented perpendicular to the glenoid margin, parallel to the supraspinatus muscle and tendon. This plane is best for assessing the continuity of the supraspinatus muscle and tendon and in visualizing any cuff pathology. The relationship of the anteroinferior acromion and acromioclavicular joint to the supraspinatus muscle and tendon can also be discerned in this plane. These images can be obtained as a combined a fast spin echo (FSE) proton density and T2-weighted sequence, with fat saturation on the second echo. Other alternatives to obtain similar contrast are to acquire a short TR/TE (T1-) weighted sequence, followed by an FSE inversion recovery sequence (FSE IR), or a dual echo FSE sequence without fat saturation, followed by either an FSE inversion recovery sequence or FSE T2-weighted sequence with fat saturation. The use of fat suppression aids in conspicuity for rotator cuff pathology (136) as well as depicting occult bone marrow injuries in the greater tuberosity (140) and elsewhere.

Sagittal oblique images, which are obtained parallel to the glenoid margin and perpendicular to the supraspinatus muscle and tendon, are helpful in determining the relationship of the anterior acromion and the acromioclavicular joint to the rotator cuff, the shape of the anterior acromion, and the presence of spurs. They give the best impression of the volume of the space beneath the anterior acromion and AC joint, the "subacromial space." Utilizing this dual echo gradient echo series, the sagittal oblique images are also useful as a "second look" for cuff pathology. When a cuff tear is present, they are also very helpful in assessing the anterior to posterior dimensions of the tear. These images can be obtained as an FSE sequence, usually with an intermediate echo (40–50 microseconds) with fat saturation.

The technique of MR arthrography is discussed elsewhere in this text but is reviewed here. Patients are prepped and draped in the usual sterile fashion. A 20-gauge spinal needle is used to enter the glenohumeral joint. A traditional anterior or anterosuperior approach may be used (138). Next 0.1 ccs of gadolinium from a tuberculin syringe is injected into a mixture of 20 ccs of saline and nonionic iodinated contrast (isovue 300), to achieve a 1/200 gadolinium dilution (139). Twelve to 15 ml of contrast are injected into the joint. A digitally subtracted rapid sequence conventional arthrogram is obtained (143), followed by conventional overhead images. If a conventional arthrogram is not desired, then the gadolinium can be mixed into a 20-cc syringe filled with saline. The patient is then taken to the MRI suite. T1-weighted images with fat saturation in the axial, coronal oblique, and sagittal oblique planes are obtained next (Fig. 6.7A). Coronal oblique FSE sequences with fat saturation may be obtained as well and are particularly useful if a noncontrast MRI has not been obtained prior to the MR arthrogram (Fig. 6.7B). These will help detect any non-joint-communicating defects, such as bursal-sided partial rotator cuff tears.

In addition to traditional guidance of glenohumeral injection with fluoroscopy with conventional or C arm technique, other methods of entering the glenohumeral joint for MR arthrography include nonfluoroscopically guided injections using anatomic guidelines (141), ultrasound guidance (142), and MR guidance with MR guidance (143).

Some authors choose to do saline MR arthrography (141, 144,145). For saline MR arthrography, the gadolinium is omitted from the solution, and postcontrast imaging is done with fast spin echo T2-weighted sequences with fat saturation, in all three planes. Using T2-weighted fast spin echo techniques, good-quality images can be obtained in a reasonable scan time.

Although exercise is traditionally done with conventional arthrography, a recent study (146) revealed that using exercise with direct shoulder MR arthrography has no beneficial or detrimental effect on image quality or on the depiction of rotator cuff tears.

Indirect (intravenous) gadolinium MR arthrography is a relatively new MR technique improving articular and periarticular contrast (147), and it may also be helpful to image the rotator cuff, labrum, and capsule (148) (Fig. 6.7C). It is achieved by injection of paramagnetic MR contrast media intravenously instead of intraarticular injection as in direct MR arthrography. In this approach, 0.1 mmol/kg body

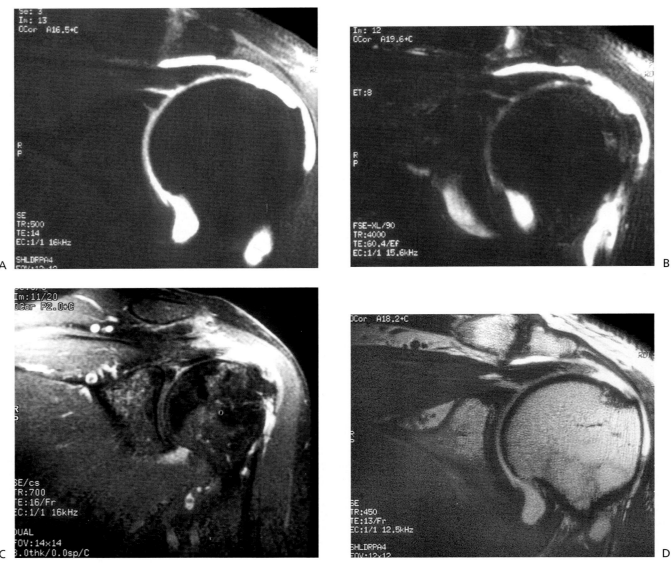

FIGURE 6.7. A: Coronal oblique T1-weighted MR arthrogram image with fat suppression. A full-thickness tear is present. **B:** Coronal oblique fast spin echo T2-weighted MR arthrogram with fat suppression in the same patient. **C:** Coronal oblique T1-weighted intravenous (IV) MR arthrogram image with fat suppression. Note the conspicuity of the tendon and bursal changes. **D:** Coronal oblique high-resolution T1-weighted MR arthrogram without fat suppression.

weight is injected gadolinium will diffuse into the joint enhancing any native fluid that is present. After the injection, exercising the joint results in considerable signal intensity increase within the joint cavity by increasing blood flow, allows for the formation of a joint effusion, and facilitates synovial diffusion and allows for the diffusion of gadolinium into the joint. Time delay is usually 15 to 20 minutes. The joint fluid will then be imaged as high-signal, in contrast to the low-signal labrum, capsule, and rotator cuff tendons. It is performed in all three orthogonal planes with fat-saturated T1-weighted images. Advantages of indirect MR arthrography are that the method is less invasive than direct MR arthrography, and it does not require fluoroscopic guidance

or physician participation. Disadvantages are that there is a higher-contrast load and expense (15 to 20 ccs of contrast vs. 0.1 or 0.2). Allman and coworkers (149) performed indirect MR arthrography of the unexercised shoulder. They found that this technique also leads to a diagnostically adequate enhancement of joint fluid and that it represents a more convenient and less time-consuming alternative to indirect MR arthrography after joint exercise.

For shoulder imaging at high field, the field of view is 12 to 14 cm, and the slice thickness is 3 to 4 mm. The matrix size is 256 × 192 for conventional spin echo sequences. For fast spin echo imaging, a matrix of 256 × 256 is employed with an echo train of 4 to 8. The smaller echo trains are used for PD-weighted imaging, to minimize blurring. Higher resolution can be obtained in selected situations such as MR arthrography where slice thicknesses of 2 mm and matrices up to 512 × 512 may be employed (Fig. 6.7C). Higher matrix imaging is also now commonly employed with fast spin echo imaging to decrease image blurring and improve resolution on higher field systems with stronger gradients (20 mT/m or greater).

MRI IMAGING

Bone Changes

Bone changes are observed in patients with rotator cuff disease and impingement. They are more common in patients with advanced disease and in older patients. Once present, they further exacerbate the problem. The most common sec-

ondary bone changes that have been described in association with extrinsic impingement include acromioclavicular joint osteophytes, subacromial spur formation, and cysts and sclerosis in the greater tuberosity.

Subacromial spurs are a less common finding but are more correlative of the presence of rotator cuff alterations and rotator cuff disease than acromioclavicular osteoarthrosis (37) (Fig. 6.8). They are the most specific finding on MR exam for shoulder impingement (40). Small subacromial spurs may appear on MRI exam as a signal void that projects from the acromion tip in a medial and inferior direction, which may be surrounded by a rim of signal void representing cortical bone (23), and these must be distinguished from the insertion of the coracoacromial ligament or the deltoid insertion (150). The inferior tendon slip of the deltoid inserts on the inferolateral acromion, the coracoacromial ligament on the inferomedial acromion (150). Larger spurs frequently contain

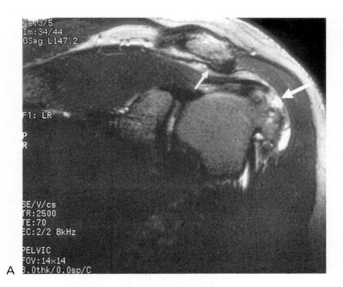

A

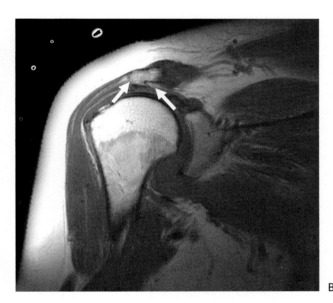

B

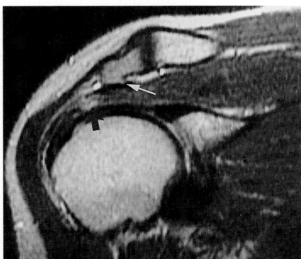

C

FIGURE 6.8. Subacromial spurs. **A:** Immature spur, coronal oblique T2-weighted sequence. Note the low signal focus at the margin of the anterior acromion (*short arrow*). A small anterodistal tear is also identified (*long arrow*). **B, C:** Coronal oblique T1-weighted image in B, Coronal oblique T2-weighted image in C. Mature spurs are noted by the presence of marrow fat signal (*arrows*). A small proximal defect is seen in the tendon in C (*small black arrow*).

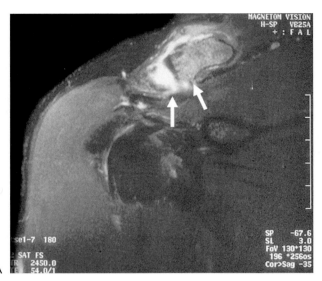
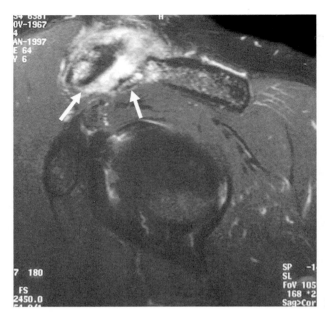

FIGURE 6.9. AC joint OA. Coronal oblique **(A)** and sagittal oblique **(B)** turbo spin echo T2-weighted MR images with fat suppression. The AC joints show advanced degenerative changes with inferiorly projecting spurs and capsular hypertrophy (*arrows*). Signs of AC joint stress in this professional boxer include marginal edema and fluid in the AC joint.

marrow and thus have brighter signal (25). Plain film correlation may be of value if available to distinguish spurs from these anatomic regions. The anterior and inferior location of the spurs are often best shown on sagittal oblique images. Larger spurs may be evident on coronal oblique images.

Degenerative osteophytes of the AC joint have similar appearances. They may be inferiorly projecting. These osteophytes of the AC joint may precede the presence of anterior acromial spurs. Hypertrophy and callus formation of the AC joint capsule may also be visualized, which appears as a rounded mass of medium signal intensity surrounding the joint that often projects inferiorly (151), and may encroach on the bursal surface of the musculotendinous junction of the supraspinatus. These changes can contribute to impingement. Some observers have questioned the relative significance of hypertrophy and callus formation of the AC joint, relative to narrowing of the subacromial space. Even when the contour of the supraspinatus muscle or tendon is deformed by the AC joint, patients may be asymptomatic. Nonetheless, this mass effect by the inferiorly bulging capsule of the AC joint may cause a contour deformity on the superior margin of the supraspinatus, where there are no discrete osteophytes. The relationship of the AC joint arthrosis to the subacromial space and bursal surface of the cuff are best seen on the sagittal oblique and coronal oblique sequences (Fig. 6.9). Fluid may be seen in the AC joint, especially on fat-saturated images, and there may also be increased signal on these fat-saturated images in the bony margins of this joint. The significance of fluid within the AC joint has also been debated, however (152). It is speculated that marginal

edema in the bones about the AC joint may be a marker of this joint as a site or source of pain in patients with this findings. Edema in the distal clavicle alone may be stress related and may be particularly common in athletes such as weight lifters, throwers, and swimmers (Fig. 6.9). Low signal intensity sclerosis, erosions, and subchondral cysts are also identified on MRI images in patients with AC joint arthrosis.

The three types of acromion shape described by Bigliani (21) for plain radiographic exam can be adapted for MRI imaging (Fig. 6.1). Type I has a flat or straight inferior surface. Type II demonstrates a smooth curved inferior surface that approximately parallels the superior humeral head in the sagittal oblique plane. Type III has an inferiorly curved or hook shape (Fig. 6.10), on sagittal images. The latter type is statistically associated with an increased incidence of rotator cuff tears (21). Studies that have used sagittal oblique MRI to determine the presence of hook-shaped anterior acromions have also found an association with clinical impingement (23) and rotator cuff tears (153). Type IV acromion can be appreciated on MR exam when the acromion appears convex near its distal end (Fig. 6.1B) (22).

The shape of the acromion as described on supraspinatus outlet views may also be evaluated on sagittal oblique MRI examinations. Variability has been found, however, among observers when attempting to use the above classification on sagittal oblique MR images (154,155) (Fig. 6.11). This, however, may also be true when attempting to use supraspinatus outlet radiographs to categorize the acromial configuration (154,156), which are very sensitive to mild changes in position. Peh and coworkers (155) concluded that apparent

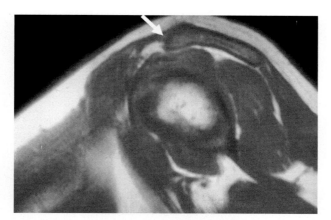

FIGURE 6.10. Type 3 acromion. Sagittal oblique T1-weighted image. Note the deformity of the underlying supraspinatus muscle by the hook shaped anterior acromion (*arrow*).

acromial shape is sensitive to minor changes in MR section viewed. More medial sections closer to the AC joint may falsely produce the appearance of a hooked anterior acromion, which has a flat appearance on more peripheral sagittal oblique images. Reasons for this variability when comparing the MRI appearance to the radiographic correlate have been suggested. The most plausible may be that the radiographic appearance is based on a summation shadow including all parts of the acromion, whereas MR imaging is a tomographic examination in which several sagittal sections of the acromion are evaluated separately. Additionally, it should be noted that the shape of the acromion is evaluated as a continuum, from 1 to 3 (or 4), and therefore there is also bound to be both inter- and intraobserver variability when studying the acromial shape on MR exam.

Lateral or anterior downward sloping of the acromion, or a low-lying acromion, relative to the distal clavicle may contribute to impingement and narrowing of the supraspinatus

outlet, and it can be discerned on MRI images. Impingement related to lateral downsloping of the anterior acromion may cause impingement of the midportion of the supraspinatus tendon. It may cause impingement on the superior aspect of the subscapularis tendon (66,157). This type of acromial position may also be associated with lateral supraspinatus injury near the greater tuberosity insertion, especially in patients who perform forceful abduction of the shoulder (158). Anterior downsloping is best seen on sagittal MR images as well as supraspinatus outlet views and lateral downsloping on coronal MR images. Anterior downsloping of the acromion is present when the anterior inferior cortex of the acromion is more inferiorly located relative to the posterior cortex as assessed on the sagittal oblique images. Lateral downsloping is identified when the inferior surface of the distal acromion is inferior or caudally located, relative to the inferior surface of the more proximal aspect of the acromion, adjacent to the AC joint (Figs. 6.2, 6.12).

MR imaging may also reveal the variability in size and thickness of the coracoacromial ligament. Thickening of the CA ligament may contribute to narrowing of the supraspinatus outlet, and as determined by MRI, it has been associated with rotator cuff tears (23). Thickening of the CA ligament may be best seen on sagittal oblique images (Fig. 6.13). The criteria for determining thickening of the CA ligament on MRI include subjective assessment of its size and whether the thickening is smooth or irregular or the objective criteria of measuring its thickness.

The os acromiale is best identified by reviewing all imaging planes, on superior axial sections that demonstrate the entire acromion (Fig. 6.14A). The synchrondrosis should not be mistaken for the subjacent AC joint. This is most easily discerned with the use of sagittal oblique images (159). When superior axial sections are not available, this pattern of mimicking the AC joint on sagittal and coronal oblique images may also be used to help identify the presence of the os

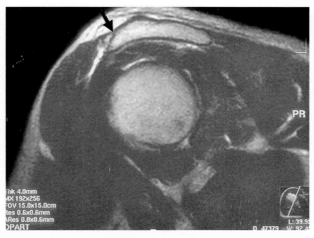
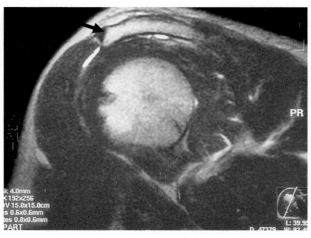

FIGURE 6.11. A, B: Sagittal oblique fast spin echo T2-weighted images. Note how the anterior acromion appears more hook shaped on the more medial image in A (*arrow*) than in B (*arrow*).

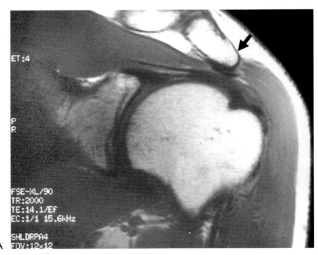
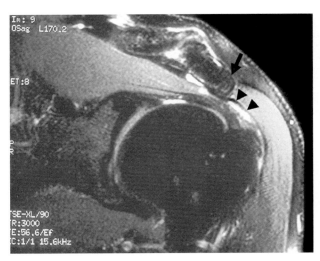

FIGURE 6.12. Lateral downsloping. Coronal oblique fast spin echo proton density– **(A)** and T2-weighted with fat suppression **(B)** images. The anterior distal acromion is projecting inferiorly relative to the AC joint (*arrow*). Note the fluid signal in the subdeltoid bursa in B, consistent with bursal inflammation (*arrowheads*).

acromiale (159) (Fig. 6.14B). Increased signal on adjacent portions of the acromial marrow on either side of the fusion defect may be seen on both STIR and fat-suppressed T2-weighted fast spin echo sequences (Fig. 6.14C). This hyperintensity may correlate with degenerative changes or instability of the os acromiale in symptomatic patients.

It is important to identify the os acromiale not only because of its association with impingement but especially in patients who are being considered for subacromial decompression (49,50). This is because removal of the acromion distal to the synchrondrosis at the time of acromioplasty may further destabilize the synchrondrosis and allow for even greater mobility of the os acromiale after surgery and worsening of the impingement (159).

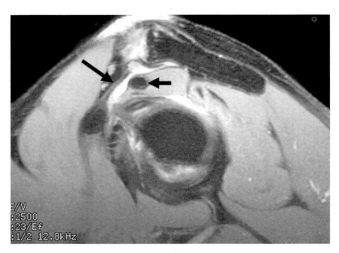

FIGURE 6.13. Sagittal oblique fast spin echo proton density–weighted image. The relationship of the coracoacromial ligament (*larger arrow*) to the supraspinatus muscle and tendon (*smaller arrow*) is best seen in this projection.

Bony sclerosis and an abnormal contour of the underside of the acromion have also been associated with shoulder impingement (160). This condition includes flattening or mild concavity of the facet on the acromion facing the humeral head, and it likely represents bony reaction to traumatization by the greater tuberosity during abduction. An acromion with these derangements is said to more effectively cause impingement, likened to a saw with teeth. On MR exam, the bony remodeling may be better appreciated than on plain radiographs, due to its tomographic nature. The bony sclerosis is manifest as decreased signal in the subchondral bone marrow, which may be less well appreciated on MR (34).

Similar to the acromion changes, on the humeral-side hypertrophic changes or flattening and sclerosis may occur in the region of the greater turberosity in patients with impingement (160). This is likely, as noted earlier to be due to traumatization of the greater tuberosity on the undersurface of the acromion during abduction. These may be appreciated on MR exam as areas of cortical thickening or prominent low signal in the region of the greater tuberosity (34).

Humeral head or greater tuberosity cysts have been associated with shoulder impingement. This is a very common finding on MR exam. More recently these cysts, which can become quite large, have been felt to be nonspecific, and they are as well correlated with increasing age as they are with alterations in the rotator cuff reflective of impingement (39). These cysts are often posteriorly located, at the greater tuberosity, or at its junction with humeral head near the capsular insertion. Cysts may also occur more superiorly or anteriorly as well (34) (Fig. 6.15).

A recent study (161) compared these bone changes of the humerus as identified on plain radiographs to the presence of rotator cuff pathology on MRI. In this study, cortical thickening of the greater tuberosity and subcortical sclerosis

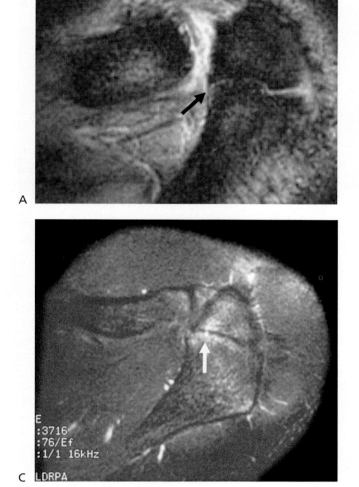

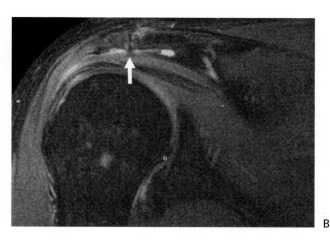

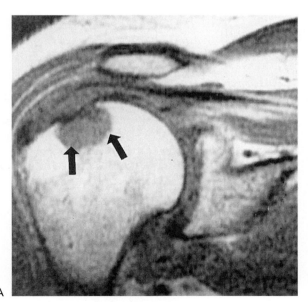

FIGURE 6.14. Os acromiale. **A:** Superior axial section demonstrating the entire acromion. The os acromiale is well seen on this section (*arrow*). **B:** When superior axial sections are not available, the pattern of mimicking the AC joint on coronal oblique images may also be used to help identify the presence of the os acromiale (*arrow*). **C:** Increased signal on adjacent portions of the acromial marrow on either side of the fusion defect may be seen on this fat-suppressed T2-weighted fast spin echo sequence (*arrow*). This may correlate with degenerative changes or instability of the os acromiale.

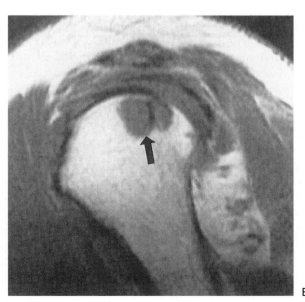

FIGURE 6.15. Posteriorly located humeral head cysts. Coronal oblique T1-weighted image appears in A, sagittal oblique T1-weighted image in B (*arrows*).

were not associated with rotator cuff disease. Identifying cystlike lesions in the greater tuberosity or humeral head was only loosely associated with rotator cuff disease, but there was high interobserver variability and poor positive predictive value in this study for this finding. Sano and coworkers (162) described two distinct types of cystic changes: one at the attachment of the supraspinatus and subscapularis tendons, which they found related to tendon defects, and the other in the bare bone area of the anatomic neck, which they described as being related to aging.

A useful objective criteria on MRI exam that some use to infer anatomic impingement by these bone changes is to evaluate the degree of deformity of the superior portion of the supraspinatus muscle and/or tendon on the oblique coronal or sagittal images, although the relationship of these bony changes to the muscle and tendon is usually best observed on oblique sagittal images, as is any focal thickening of the coracoacromial ligament that may be present (Figs. 6.10, 6.13).

These bone and soft-tissue alterations that have been associated with extrinsic impingement may also be seen in asymptomatic individuals (37), particularly AC joint disease, which was a very common finding in those populations, especially in older patients. This therefore illustrates the importance of clinical correlation in the assessment of patients with such findings on MRI exam. It also emphasizes the point that impingement is a clinical diagnosis and should not be made based on MRI images alone.

One of the problems in the evaluation of patients with clinical evidence of impingement is the fact that with conventional magnets, the size of the imaging gantry only allows imaging with the patient's arm by the side. Ideally, one would like to image in the position of impingement or during motion where the relationships among the cuff, bursa, and biceps tendon would be different than when the arm is positioned by the side (Fig. 6.16). The use of open magnets and dynamic MR imaging evaluation, with or without associated positioning devices (163), may make evaluation of impingement in the positions known to provoke symptoms more feasible, although even at present, they are not in common usage or commonly available. Use of the ABER positioning combined with MRI and MR arthrography may be useful to diagnose posterosuperior glenoid impingement (164).

Graichen et al. (165) described an MR imaging–based technique for three-dimensional determination of the subacromial space width in relation to the rotator cuff in arm abduction. An open MRI scanner was used, with images in seven arm positions, and coronal images were obtained with a gradient echo sequence, and 3D reconstruction of the bones and the supraspinatus was performed. The closest contact between the supraspinatus and the anterior inferior part of the acromion in this study occurred at 90° abduction, in internal rotation.

Shibuta and colleagues (166), to simulate the painful arm position in subacromial impingement syndrome, performed

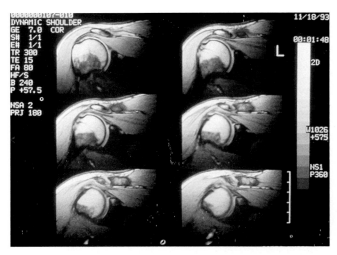

FIGURE 6.16. "Dynamic imaging" of the shoulder. Series of gradient echo images of the shoulder from neutral to abduction.

magnetic resonance imaging of the shoulder with the arms at the sides and at 80° abduction in 20 patients with and 19 patients without clinical findings of subacromial impingement syndrome. When arm position was changed from adduction to abduction, alterations in signal intensity of the rotator cuff were described more often in patients with clinical evidence of impingement (45%) than in those without (26%). Abduction of the arm seemed to cause encroachment of the acromion, especially of the acromioclavicular joint, to the rotator cuff in patients with clinical evidence of subacromial impingement syndrome, even if there were no such findings in the images with the arms at the sides.

Recently the combination of a magnet design allowing shoulder motion and access by the examining physician, real-time MR imaging capability, and a tracking device allowing single image acquisition in a constant imaging plane has made study of shoulder motion during active guided, or physician-guided, motion feasible. In normal abduction, the proximity of the acromion and greater tuberosity during midabduction and the crowding of the subacromial space next to the acromioclavicular joint during full abduction were observed (34). Dynamic demonstration of symptomatic impingement in isolated cases has also been described (34). In a study of asymptomatic volunteers, during normal abduction and adduction the humeral head remained precisely centered in the glenoid fossa over a wide range of motion in asymptomatic individuals (167). Near normal alignment of the glenohumeral joint has also been observed in patients with known supraspinatus tears. This finding supported Burkhart's observations with fluoroscopy in massive cuff tears (168).

Tendinosis

A variety of terms may be used to describe the injured tendon in the absence of a tendon defect. The term most com-

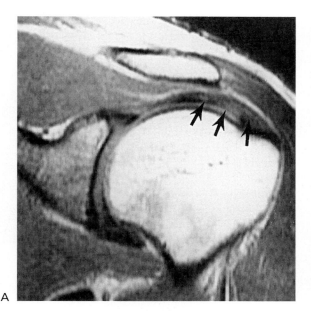
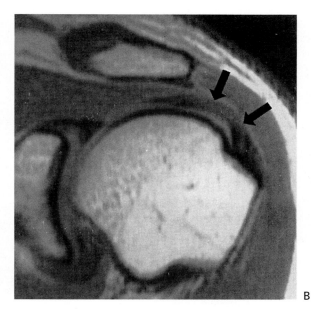

FIGURE 6.17. Tendinosis. **A:** Coronal oblique T1-weighted image. Diffuse increased signal in the distal supraspinatus tendon is seen with some mild thickening (*arrows*). **B:** Coronal oblique T2-weighted image in the same patient as in A. Note that the increased signal identified on the short TR/TE image of the patient seen in A has faded (*arrows*).

monly used (or abused) in the past was *tendonitis*. This is a term often loosely applied to a variety of shoulder problems that lead to focal shoulder pain and tenderness. Often these are patients involved in occupations requiring heavy labor or frequent arm elevation or are individuals or athletes requiring considerable shoulder movement or overhead motion (108). Many authors prefer the term *tendinosis* or *tendinopathy* as the pathologic changes found within such tendons most often do not include inflammation (169, 170), except in the peritendinous tissues (as discussed later). The MRI findings of tendinosis (Fig. 6.17) are moderate increase in signal intensity within the tendon on short TR/TE and proton density images, oriented along the long axis of the tendon, which may be homogeneous (focal, diffuse, or bandlike) (171) or inhomogeneous, which fades or is absent on long TR/TE (T2-weighted images), whether obtained with conventional (125,126,171) or fast spin echo imaging sequences without fat suppression. Fat-suppressed conventional or fast spin echo T2-weighted sequences, or STIR imaging sequences, may make this signal more conspicuous and should be distinguished from true fluid signal as seen in a rotator cuff tear (125) (Figs. 6.18. 6.19). Tendon thickening may be present, and increased and more diffuse thickening may be associated with more advanced tendinosis (34). Mirowitz and coworkers (172) studied the thickness of the supraspinatus tendon with MRI and found it to be 2 to 4 mm in thickness, with a mean of 3.2 mm. It is proposed that persistence of increased signal within the tendon on images with T2 weighting, but less intense than fluid signal may indicate more advanced tendinosis, related to a greater degree of collagen breakdown in the tendon (173). It is postulated

that the increasing disorganization of the tightly bound macromolecules of collagen allows increased absorption of water. The absorbed water is allowed more degrees of freedom, increasing the T2, so that images with relatively short TE show increased signal from the water molecules. In distinction from this, when a tear is present, the signal in the tendon should approach that of fluid. This has been postulated to be related to further disruption of the collagen macromolecules, allowing open spaces to be created that fill with water. This free water has a very long T2 and demonstrates high signal on images with a long TE (173).

On conventional spin echo MRI without fat suppression, peribursal fat plane alterations and fluid in the subdeltoid bursa are less commonly identified, but when present, according to Rafii (171), they may be reflective of bursal inflammation and scarring, which may indicate a more advanced stage of the disease process and indicate a worse prognosis for recovery with conservative therapy alone. Fat-saturated T2-weighted fast spin echo images are more sensitive to the presence of fluid in the subdeltoid bursa (39) (Figs. 6.19–6.21). With the use of the sequences, identifying fluid in the subdeltoid bursa region is a more common correlate of disease at this stage than previously thought (125,126). When evident, this condition is also felt to be indicative of associated subdeltoid bursal inflammation. Persistent low signal intensity in a thickened subacromial subdeltoid bursa on imaging sequences with both T1 and T2 contrast has also been described (171,174), and it is said to indicate proliferative chronic subdeltoid bursitis, but this appearance is more difficult to discern on MR imaging studies.

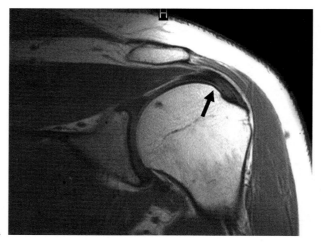

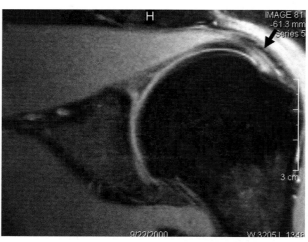

FIGURE 6.18. Tendinosis and fat suppression. **A:** Coronal oblique T1-weighted image. Diffuse increased signal in the supraspinatus tendon is present (*arrow*). The articular and bursal surfaces of the tendon are intact. **B:** Coronal oblique FSE proton density–weighted sequence with fat suppression. Note the relative increase in tendon signal, which does not approach that of fluid (*arrow*).

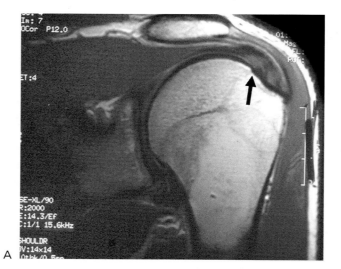

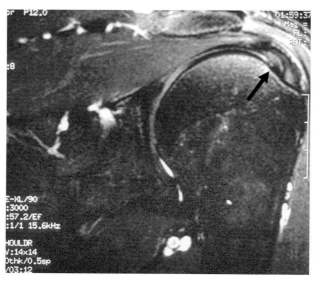

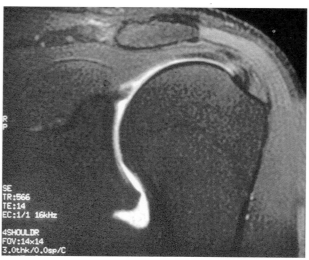

FIGURE 6.19. Tendinosis, fat suppression, and MR arthrography. **A:** Coronal oblique FSE proton density–weighted image. Diffuse increased signal in the supraspinatus tendon is noted (*arrow*). The articular and bursal surfaces of the tendon are smooth. **B:** Coronal oblique FSE T2–weighted sequence with fat suppression. Note the somewhat inhomogeneous increase in tendon signal, which does not, however, approach that of fluid (*arrow*). Mild increased signal in the overlying subdeltoid bursa may reflect bursal inflammation. **C:** Coronal oblique T1–weighted MR arthrogram image, with fat suppression. No contrast-filled tendon defect is seen.

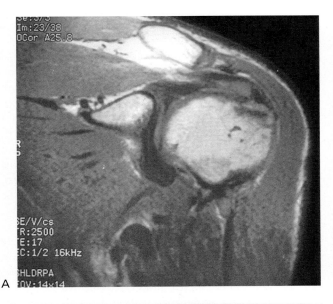
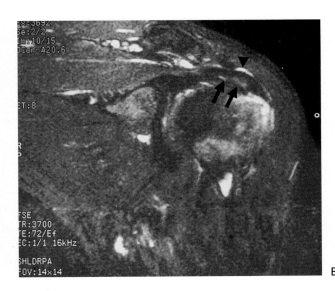

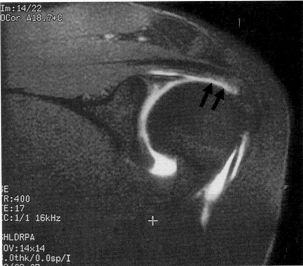

FIGURE 6.20. Tendinosis, articular surface fraying/fibrillation, and MR arthrography. **A:** Coronal oblique FSE proton density–weighted image; **B:** FSE T2-weighted sequence with fat suppression. Moderate tendinosis is seen in the supraspinatus tendon, and there is undersurface fraying and irregularity (*arrows*). A small amount of fluid is seen in the subdeltoid bursa, likely reflective of bursal inflammation (*arrowhead*). Coronal oblique T1-weighted MR arthrogram image, with fat suppression **(C)**, outlines the undersurface fraying and irregularity (*arrows*), but no focal tendon defect is seen.

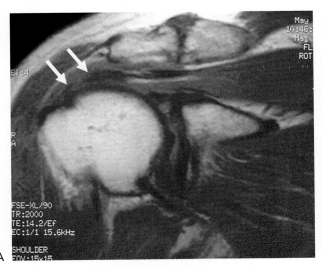
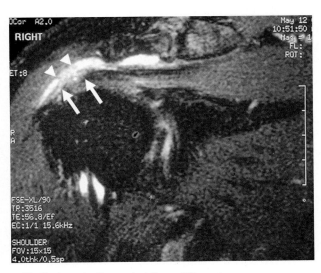

FIGURE 6.21. Tendinosis and bursal surface fraying/fibrillation. **A:** Coronal oblique FSE proton density–weighted image. **B:** FSE T2-weighted sequence with fat suppression. Moderate tendinosis is seen in the supraspinatus tendon, and there is bursal surface fraying and irregularity (*arrows*). A moderate amount of fluid is seen in the subdeltoid bursa (*arrowheads*), reflective of bursal inflammation.

The arthroscopic findings in patients with these MRI findings is hyperemia of the tendon surface and bursal scarring and inflammation (126). Biopsy of the tendon in patients with MRI findings consistent with tendinosis has been carried out in a small number of patients. In these cases, mucoid degenerative changes and some inflammation were found (175). Histological sectioning in cadavers with similar MRI findings reveals eosinophilic, mucoid, and fibrillary degeneration (106,176). These findings are similar to those found in the elbow in patients with overuse syndromes (177,178).

Although routine MR images are generally sufficient at this stage of disease, if MR arthrography is employed in these patients (Fig. 6.19C), its role is to confirm the integrity of the articular surface of the cuff, where partial tears most commonly occur. In patients with tendinosis, the articular surface should be linear in contour and low in signal intensity (182).

Anzilloti and colleagues (180) described a subset of young patients (< 35 years) with acute, posttraumatic insults to the rotator cuff that mimic the signal intensity changes of tendinosis. In this study, patients younger than 35 years had signal intensity that was similar to tendinosis, but more localized in atypical locations of the supraspinatus tendon, and were associated with bone bruise, suggesting the possibility of posttraumatic strain.

Tendons with a similar MRI appearance to tendinosis have also been detected in a frequent number of asymptomatic individuals (132,181). In a recent study of 100 asymptomatic volunteers between 19 and 88 years of age (132), 18% had findings similar to those described as tendinopathy, although this was most common in the 19- to 39-year-old age group (30%). Miniaci (182) and colleagues also found signal alterations in the tendons of young (mean age 29) asymptomatic volunteers using MRI. The clinical significance of these findings is therefore not entirely clear. Thus, careful clinical correlation is important before deciding on types and length of treatment regimes and especially surgery based on these MRI findings. Similar MRI findings have also been seen at histopathologic correlation in patients with tendon scars (176).

The signal intensity changes seen in patients with findings reflective of tendinosis should also be distinguished from problematic artifacts and pitfalls arising from normal anatomic variants and partial volume averaging effects (183,184).

The majority of these causes of altered signal are seen as intermediate signal on short TR/TE and proton density images. They should be distinguished from advanced rotator disease and rotator cuff tears as they are not associated with morphological alterations and do not brighten like fluid on long TR/TE images.

In a study of these tendon signal alterations with histopathologic correlation (184), intermediate signal located in the tendon just prior to the anterior rotator interval was the most common. Owing to the anterior curvature of the humeral head as well as the supraspinatus tendon, partial volume averaging of the superficial fibrofatty or membranous tissues (185) may cause this increased signal, although other structures may contribute as well, such as the biceps tendon sheath (183). Other proposed explanations for this signal are that it represents the critical zone (150,185) or that it is due to magic angle effects (150). If there is fluid in the biceps sheath, this may simulate a small tear if partial volume averaged with the anterior supraspinatus tendon. Misinterpretation of this cause of increased signal may be limited if thin sections are utilized or with MR arthrography. Sagittal oblique images also help distinguish fluid signal in this region from that in the tendon. In this same study (184), anatomic correlation of the second most common cause of intermediate signal on short TR/TE and proton density images indicated that it occurred due to a prominent region of hyaline articular cartilage beneath the mid-supraspinatus tendon. Histologic examination revealed that the transitional zone of articular accounted for the majority of the increase in thickness. The transitional zone is responsible for the highest signal from cartilage on MR imaging (186). Signal isointense to muscle on all pulse sequences can also be identified on more posterior coronal oblique sections in place of the expected signal void of the rotator cuff tendons. The proposed explanation for this cause of intermediate intratendinous signal is that in these cases muscle bundles extend more laterally over the humeral head in the space between the supraspinatus and infraspinatus tendons, as they diverge toward their insertions on the humeral head (184). This finding was corroborated by the appearance of these structures on axial images as well as gross dissection in one cadaver, but it was not confirmed histologically. Vahlensieck and coworkers (186) have described a posterior straplike portion of the supraspinatus tendon, with several shorter tendinous slips arising from muscle fibers separate from those forming the anterior dominant tendon. Imaging of this seemingly different posterior portion of the tendon is another possible explanation for this appearance of interposed muscle tissue. Another similar potential cause of increased signal in the rotator cuff on short TR/TE and proton density–weighted images is overriding of the infraspinatus tendon over the supraspinatus tendon, seen with internal rotation of the shoulder (135).

Magic angle effects have also been shown to be a cause of increased signal in the rotator cuff tendons (187–189). This is due to the presence of angular anisotropy that produces increased signal intensity in normal tendons at a 55° angle from the static magnetic field on short TE sequences. This signal alteration can also be differentiated by repositioning the patient in the magnet, where the position of the altered signal may change, or by observing decrease in its signal intensity on images obtained with a longer TE, thereby differentiating it from a rotator cuff tear.

Other causes of elevated signal in an intact supraspinatus tendon (190) include motion or pulsation artifacts, chemical shift misregistration artifact between the rotator cuff and fat, recent injection of medication, recent surgery, and metal artifacts from prior surgery (see Chapter 9 on the postoperative shoulder).

With respect to injected fluid from an impingement test, in a study by Bergman and colleagues (191), 3 days after the injection, fluid in the bursa and adjacent soft tissues had returned to preinjection levels. To avoid misinterpretations, a delay of 3 days after injection is recommended before a shoulder MR examination is carried out.

Other MRI changes beyond those of simple tendinosis, not indicative of either a partial or complete tear but considered abnormal, include tendon thinning or irregularity of the tendon surface (Figs. 6.20, 6.21). Although these changes may be more common on the bursal side of the tendon, MR arthrography will outline those findings that occur on the articular side. Such irregularities in contour and signal intensity indicate fraying of the superficial fibers of the tendon. At arthroscopy, the tendon surface is described as showing "fraying, roughening or degeneration" (125,126). On the bursal side of the tendon when T2-weighted images are obtained, especially with fat suppression, some fluid will be seen in the subdeltoid bursa, likely reflecting bursal and peribursal inflammation. As noted earlier, the presence of bursal and peribursal changes in association with an abnormal but intact tendon may imply a poorer prognosis (171) and a greater chance of failure of conservative measures. The presence of the aforementioned changes of the tendon surface may also imply a similar phenomenon. These findings may be reflective of the wear and tear on the tendon of impingement. The distinction between this stage of disease and early partial-thickness tears may be difficult to define both

by MRI and at arthroscopy, although by definition fraying or degeneration of the tendinous surface should not be considered a partial tear (110). To describe a partial tear, a discrete tendon defect should be seen.

Partial Tears

Partial tears are more difficult to diagnose than complete tears with diagnostic imaging techniques. Using conventional MRI, the diagnosis of partial tears is less sensitive and accurate than for complete tears (125,126,144,171, 190–192). A partial tear can be diagnosed when there is a defect in tendon that is intrasubstance or extends to one surface only, either the articular surface (Fig. 6.22), which is more common, or the bursal surface, and that shows increased signal on long TR/TE images or on other imaging sequences with T2 contrast. When the increased signal is that of fluid, the diagnosis can be made with confidence. Tears of the bursal surface and of the undersurface will be perpendicular to the long axis of the tendon on coronal oblique imaging sequences, whereas those in the tendon substance are parallel to the long axis of the tendon (Fig. 6.4).

Some partial tears may be partially healed or quite small; therefore, the signal increase may not be as strong. In such situations they may be difficult to distinguish from tendinosis. Fat saturation, or STIR images, may help (136,185, 192–195) (Fig. 6.22B). T2-weighted fast spin echo techniques with fat saturation can obtain this type of contrast in a more efficient manner (136,194,195). STIR imaging has also been suggested to increase diagnostic performance (194). Partial tears may less commonly be manifested by significant loss of tendon thickness.

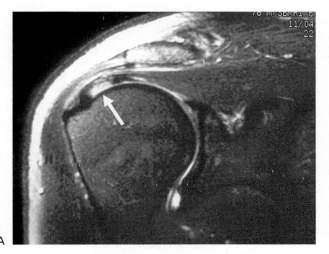
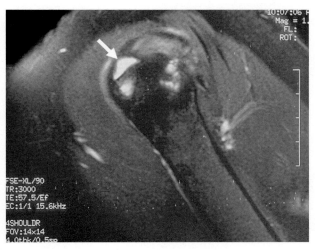

FIGURE 6.22. Partial tears, articular surface. **A:** Coronal oblique T2-weighted image. High-grade partial tear of the supraspinatus tendon undersurface is seen. Note the focal tendon defect, outlined by fluid signal (*arrow*). **B:** Sagittal oblique fast spin echo T2-weighted image, with fat suppression. A deep articular surface defect is again identified, in another patient. The addition of fat suppression increases the conspicuity of the lesion (*arrow*). A cystic area beneath the partial defect may relate to an area of chronic impaction.

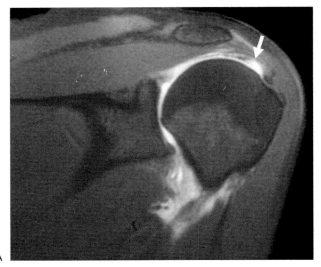
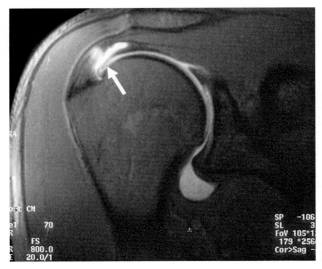

FIGURE 6.23. Partial tears and MR arthrography. **A:** Coronal oblique T1-weighted MR arthrogram image, with fat saturation. An intermediate-grade articular surface partial-thickness tear of the supraspinatus tendon is identified (*arrow*). **B:** Coronal oblique T1-weighted MR arthrogram image, with fat saturation. High-grade articular surface partial-thickness tear of the supraspinatus tendon is present in this patient (*arrow*).

In those patients in whom it is important to make a diagnosis of partial-thickness tears, and in whom partial tears would be subject to repair, such as younger patients with higher demands on the shoulder, including athletes, T1-weighted images with fat saturation after the intraarticular injection of GD DTPA are of considerable value in the diagnosis of partial tears of the articular surface of the tendon (61,179,196–200) (Fig. 6.23). In this situation, MR arth-

rography maximizes anatomic resolution and diagnostic confidence. Partial tears occur and begin commonly along the anterodistal insertion of the cuff along the undersurface, near the "critical zone," and therefore evaluating this region of the cuff undersurface with MR arthrography is of considerable importance in the differentiation between a normal cuff and cuff tendinosis, and one with a partial tear (Fig. 6.24). On MR arthrography, a partial-thickness tear is diag-

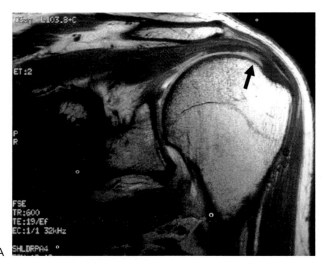
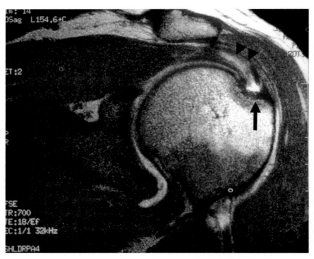

FIGURE 6.24. Partial tears and MR arthrography, high-resolution technique. **A:** Coronal oblique T1-weighted FSE MR arthrogram image, without fat saturation. (Imaging parameters include 12 cm FOV, 2-mm slice thickness, and a 512 × 384 matrix.) A low-grade partial tear of the more posterior supraspinatus articular surface is seen (*arrow*). **B:** Coronal oblique T1-weighted FSE MR arthrogram image, without fat saturation (same imaging parameters as for the patient in A). MR arthrography outlines a distal insertional partial tear in the supraspinatus tendon (*arrow*). The defect extends longitudinally into the tendon substance (*arrowheads*).

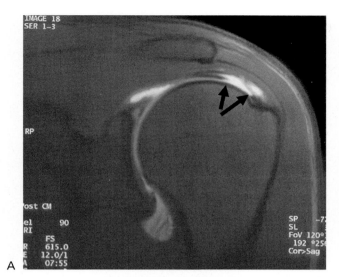 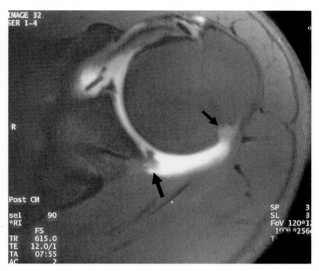

FIGURE 6.25. Subglenoid impingement. **A:** Coronal oblique T1-weighted MR arthrogram image, with fat saturation Note the flaplike areas of undersurface deep partial tearing of the supraspinatus tendon (*arrows*). **B:** Coronal oblique T1-weighted MR arthrogram image, with fat saturation. There is fraying of the posterosuperior labrum (*arrow*). Note the subtle area of flattening of the posterosuperior humeral head (*small arrow*).

nosed when contrast extends in a focal manner into a tendon defect but does not extend into the subacromial subdeltoid bursa (179). MR arthrography is also very effective at depicting the extent of morphological alterations and their depth of involvement by showing contrast imbition and the depth of loss of tendon thickness (Fig. 6.23). This is again helpful in distinguishing these alterations from those associated with tendinosis and tendon surface degeneration. Some studies have shown an increased sensitivity for undersurface partial tears with MR arthrography, over conventional T2-weighted MR imaging (196,199). The use of higher-resolution techniques may improve the visualization of partial tears, with and without MR arthrography (Fig. 6.24).

Partial tears associated with posterosuperior subglenoid impingement may have areas of delamination of the rotator cuff undersurface, and loose flaps of cuff tissue may be seen on the cuff undersurface (Fig. 6.25). These partial tears, which commonly occur posteriorly at the junction of the supraspinatus and infraspinatus, are sometimes referred to as *posterior interval tears* (164).

Additional detection of these types of undersurface tears have been described with the combination of MR arthrography and the arm placed in abduction and external rotation (ABER position) (164,201). This position allows the tendon undersurface to be depicted free from the superior surface of the humerus and promotes separation of the torn edges of the tendon undersurface. Although difficult to obtain on a routine basis, this position is felt to be particularly useful in such patients (164,201).

The ABER position may also demonstrate the contact in these patients with posterosuperior subglenoid impingement of the humeral head and posterosuperior glenoid and allow

for demonstration of some tears of the undersurface of the posterior supraspinatus and infraspinatus tendons not seen in the adducted position (161,164). This position also allows better depiction of the other lesions in the spectrum of this process, including the osteochondral compression fracture of the posterosuperior humeral head (which may simulate a Hill-Sachs lesion), degenerative fraying or tear of the posterosuperior glenoid labrum and alterations of the subjacent glenoid, and the less common involvement of the inferior glenohumeral ligament and anterior inferior labrum.

A recent study with MRI arthrography in the ABER position of the throwing and nonthrowing shoulders of college baseball players (62) revealed that physical contact between the rotator cuff undersurface and the subjacent labrum can be seen in the ABER position in such individuals in the absence of symptoms. Abnormalities of the rotator cuff and superior labrum may also be seen in asymptomatic throwing shoulders but not nonthrowing shoulders of these players. These authors concluded that MRI abnormalities consistent with internal impingement can be seen in asymptomatic patients; therefore, treatment of these abnormalities in young throwing athletes should be approached with caution.

Partial tears along the bursal side of the cuff (Fig. 6.26) and intrasubstance partial tears (Fig. 6.27) are less common than those on the rotator cuff undersurface (202) and may be evaluated with pre- or postcontrast T2-weighted sequences, often best done with fat-suppressed FSE sequences. These latter sequences may also be helpful in the identification of extraarticular fluid collections or periarticular masses (179).

Intrasubstance partial tears are difficult to confirm with either surgery or arthroscopy, unless the tendon is incised. This diagnosis is considered on MR images when fluid signal

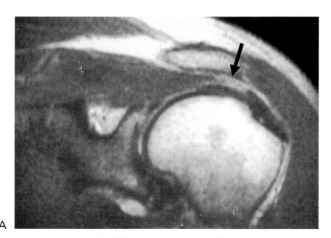

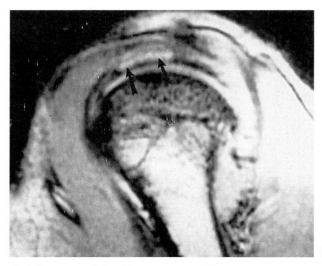

FIGURE 6.26. Bursal surface partial tears. **A:** Coronal oblique T2-weighted image. Intermediate-grade partial tear of the supraspinatus tendon superior surface is seen. A focal tendon defect, outlined by fluid signal, is seen (*arrow*). **B:** Coronal oblique 2D T2-weighted gradient echo image. Note fluid signal outlining a bursal surface partial tear of the central portion of the supraspinatus tendon (*arrows*).

is present on long TR/TE images in the substance of the tendon—that is, parallel to the long axis of the tendon, not extending to either the bursal or articular surface (Fig. 6.27). Fat suppression may make areas of tendinosis more prominent than when observed with non-fat-suppressed images; therefore, the diagnosis of intrasubstance partial tears should be made with caution if increased signal as opposed to fluid signal is seen on these images. Acute tendinitis or tendon contusions after trauma can theoretically have a similar pattern of increased signal as well. Combinations of partial tears may also be seen. Fluid in the subdeltoid bursa may commonly be identified in bursal-side partial-thickness tears and may make it easier to assess the size and depth of bursal-side partial tears (35). Such tears cannot be identified with MR arthrography from the articular side (Fig. 6.28). Preliminary work with MR bursography has the potential to improve the accuracy for diagnosis of bursal side partial tears, but as yet it has not been used very often in clinical practice.

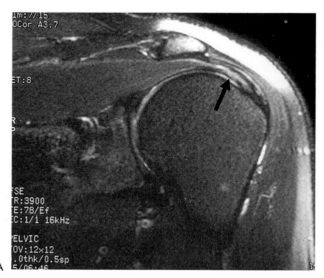

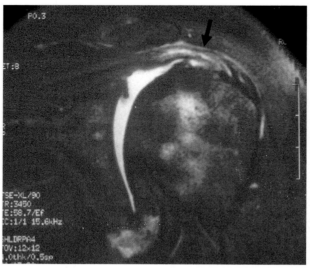

FIGURE 6.27. Intrasubstance partial tears. **A:** Coronal oblique FSE T2-weighted image with fat saturation. Longitudinal increased signal in the tendon substance approaching that of fluid is seen (*arrow*). The signal is oriented parallel to the tendon. **B:** Coronal oblique FSE T2-weighted image with fat saturation. Similar findings to those seen in A are present in the supraspinatus tendon also reflective of an intrasubstance partial tear (*arrow*). There is additional evidence of surface fraying of both tendon surfaces. Note is also made of glenohumeral joint DJD.

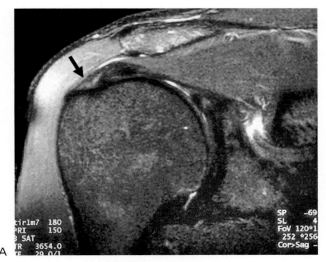 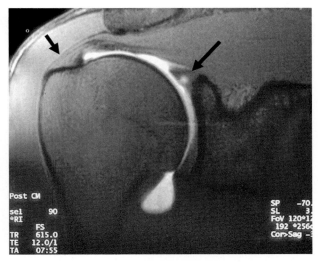

FIGURE 6.28. Intrasubstance partial tears and MR arthrography. **A:** Coronal oblique TSE inversion recovery weighted image prearthrography. A small intrasubstance partial defect is seen (*arrow*). **B:** Coronal oblique T1-weighted MR arthrogram image with fat saturation. The tendon signal is homogenous (*short arrow*). No tendon defect can be seen. Intrasubstance partial tears will be missed if MR arthrography is not accompanied by a pre- or postcontrast image sequence with some type of T2 or fluid contrast. Note the superior labral tear better seen on the MR arthrogram (*long arrow*).

Retraction of tendinous fibers from the distal insertion into the greater tuberosity may also be considered a partial tear (Fig. 6.29). Torres and associates (203) found this not uncommonly in the throwing athlete, specifically baseball players. These were characteristically visualized as small regions of high signal intensity on long TR/TE images in this location, with associated bony defects on the greater tuberosity.

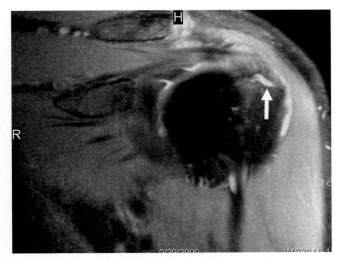

FIGURE 6.29. Insertional partial tear. Coronal oblique FSE proton–density weighted image with fat saturation. A fluid-filled insertional defect is seen at the supraspinatus tendon insertion into the greater tuberosity (*arrow*).

In addition, in many patients partial tears of differing size and nature may coexist in different portions of the rotator cuff or at the posterior margin of a larger tear.

Full-thickness Tears

In most situations, the diagnosis of a complete cuff tear can be made on conventional MRI without the use of intraarticular injection. This diagnosis is made with the visualization of a complete defect in the tendon, extending from the articular to the bursal surface of the tendon, most commonly involving the supraspinatus tendon. The defects in the rotator cuff are filled with fluid, granulation tissue, or hypertrophied synovium (204), and therefore in the majority of cases (80% or greater) with a cuff defect, fluidlike signal is present within the defect on long TR/TE images (106,205), which can be made more conspicuous with the use of fast spin echo sequences with fat suppression (136,192,195) or fast inversion recovery sequences (STIR). The presence of a tendon defect filled with fluid is the most direct and definite sign of a rotator cuff tear (Figs. 6.30–6.40).

In the presence of a full-thickness tear, especially larger tears, tendon retraction may be present, and the supraspinatus may take on a more globular configuration (205) (Fig. 6.33). In the study by Farley and coworkers (206), tendon retraction was a specific sign of a rotator cuff tear. In this study it was determined that the musculotendinous junction could be used as a marker for tendon retraction. The authors determined that the musculotendinous junction should lie no further than 15° from a line drawn through the

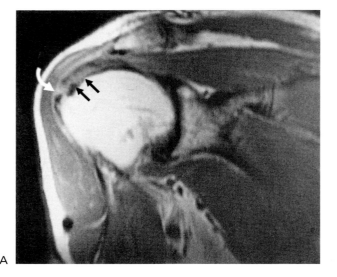
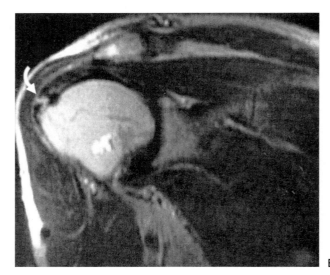

A

B

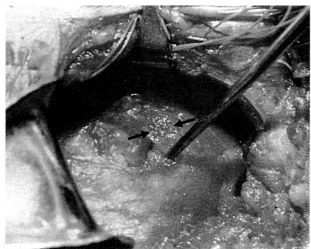

C

FIGURE 6.30. Combined partial and small complete tear. **A:** Coronal oblique image proton density–weighted image. Note the thinned, irregular inferior surface of the supraspinatus tendon (*black arrows*), consistent with a nondiscrete low-grade undersurface partial tear. At the distal tendon, just prior to its insertion, there is a small discrete full-thickness defect seen, extending to both surfaces of the tendon (*curved white arrow*). **B:** Coronal oblique T2-weighted image. Fluid signal further outlines the small distal complete tear (*curved white arrow*). **C:** Surgical photograph. The black arrows demonstrate the more proximal partial tear. The metal probe is in the more distal triangular-shaped complete tear.

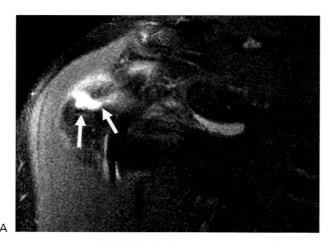
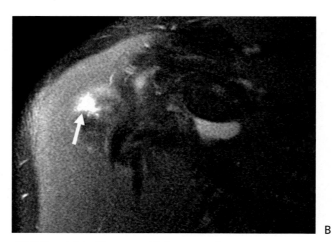

A

B

FIGURE 6.31. Small complete tear. Coronal oblique FSE T2-weighted images with fat saturation. A small fluid-filled defect is identified in the anterior distal tendon insertion (*arrows*). It is occurring just proximal to the rotator interval.

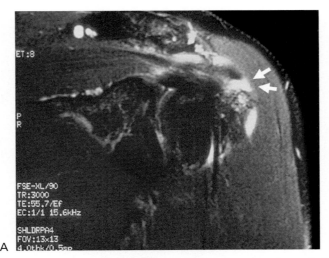

A

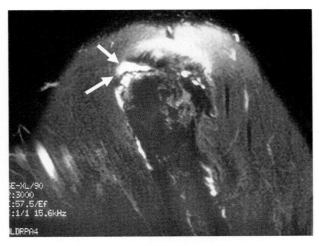

B

FIGURE 6.32. Small complete tear. Coronal oblique **(A)** and sagittal oblique **(B)** FSE T2-weighted images with fat saturation. Again note the small rotator cuff tear outlined by fluid signal (*arrows*). Small tears tend to begin and occur at the anterior distal supraspinatus tendon near its insertion. Also note the small cystic areas in the greater tuberosity, beneath the tendon defects.

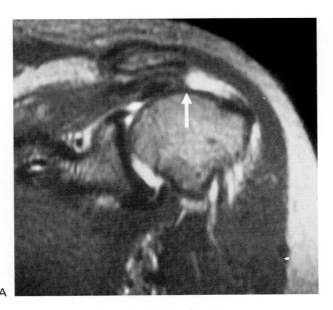

A

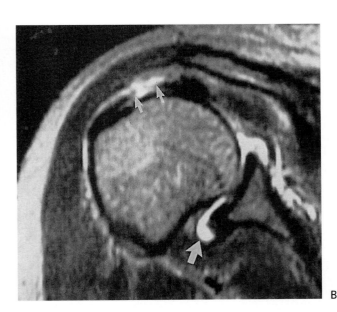

B

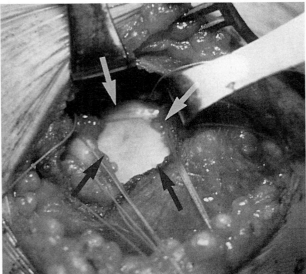

C

FIGURE 6.33. Moderate-size full-thickness tear. **A:** Coronal oblique T2-weighted image. The tendon is retracted to the mid-one-third of the humeral head (*arrow*). The tendon edges have a globular configuration. The tendon defect is filled with fluid. **B:** Coronal oblique T2-weighted image, more posteriorly. The defect is wider anteriorly but does extend to the infraspinatus tendon (*small white arrows*). There is a moderate effusion (*larger white arrow*). **C:** Surgical photograph in C reveals the extent of the cuff defect.

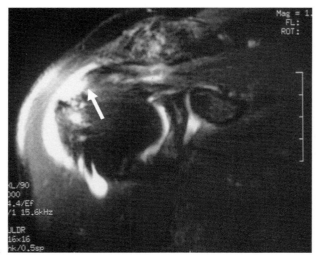
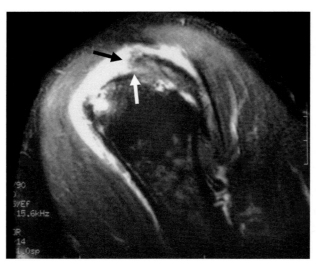

FIGURE 6.34. Moderate-size full-thickness tear. Coronal oblique **(A)** and sagittal oblique **(B)** FSE T2-weighted images with fat saturation. The tendon is retracted to the mid-one-third of the humeral head in A (*arrow*). Sagittal oblique images in B indicate the central and anterior aspect of the supraspinatus tendon is involved (*arrows*). The remaining portions of the rotator cuff reveal advanced tendinosis. There is moderate muscle atrophy, and the tendon edges are mildly frayed. Fluid is present in the subdeltoid bursa. There is cystic change in the greater tuberosity and more posterosuperiorly in the humeral head. Moderate to severe AC joint osteoarthritis and a moderate joint effusion are seen.

12 o'clock position of the humeral head (206). It should be remembered, however, that the location of the musculotendinous junction can vary even in asymptomatic individuals and depending on the position of the arm during the MR examination. Therefore, the use of retraction of the musculotendinous junction alone as a direct sign of a rotator cuff tear, in the absence of a clear tendon defect, is not recommended. In large to massive tears, the tendon may retract as far as the medial glenoid margin (Fig. 6.40).

MR arthrography is most helpful in distinguishing small tears (Fig. 6.41) from partial tears and tendinosis, and in assessing the reparability of the cuff and the postoperative prognosis in larger cuff tears. MR arthrography is helpful in determining the size and location of cuff tears and in assessing the status of the torn tendon edges (Figs. 6.35, 6.42). The diagnosis of a full-thickness rotator cuff tear on MR arthrography is made when contrast extends through a defect in the tendon, from the cuff undersurface into the subacromial-subdeltoid bursa (Figs. 6.35, 6.41, 6.42). The retracted tendon margins may be thickened in response to healing or attenuated in more chronic tears. The uninvolved areas of tendon adjacent to the tear site may demonstrate changes of degeneration or partial-thickness tear. The quality of the retracted tendon edges can be assessed on conventional MRI by assessing their appearance and describing them as noted in the classification scheme discussed earlier as good, fair, or poor (126) and at MR arthrography by evaluating for the presence of contrast imbition (179,199). Contrast imbition is determined by seeing increased signal intensity in the tendon on MR arthrographic images, indicating diffusion of gadolinium into the substance of the tendon edges (Fig. 6.42). This occurs most commonly at the posterior edge of a cuff tear. It is indicative of swelling and friability of the tendon edges, which must be debrided prior to repair (199).

Additional secondary signs (125,205) of rotator cuff tears have been described in the literature. These secondary signs

FIGURE 6.35. Moderate-size full-thickness tear and MR arthrography. Coronal oblique T1-weighted MR arthrogram image with fat saturation. High signal contrast outlines a defect in the supraspinatus tendon. The tendon edges are mildly frayed (*arrow*).

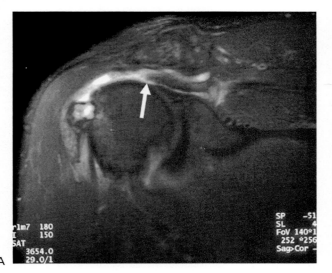
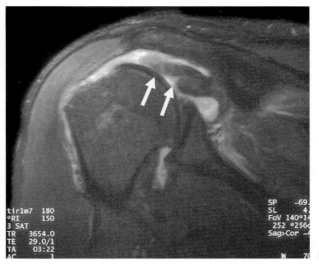

FIGURE 6.36. Large full-thickness tear, posterior extension. **A, B:** Coronal oblique TSE inversion recovery weighted images. The tendon defect is retracted to the medial one-third of the humeral head (*arrow in A*). In B, the posterior extension of the tear into the infraspinatus tendon is seen (*arrows*). The retracted tendon edges are globular in character in B.

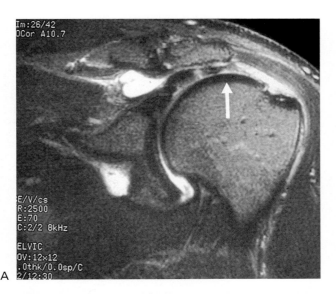
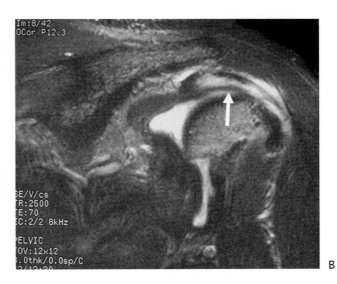
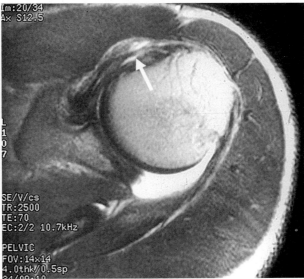

FIGURE 6.37. Large full-thickness tear, anterior and posterior extension. **A:** Coronal oblique T2-weighted image. The supraspinatus tendon is retracted to the medial one-third of the humeral head (*arrow*). The tendon edges are thin, and there is moderate muscle atrophy. **B:** Coronal oblique T2-weighted image, more posteriorly. The defect extends posteriorly to the infraspinatus tendon, in a fluid-filled longitudinal cleavage plane (*arrow*). **C:** Axial T2-weighted image. The tendon lesion extends anteriorly across the rotator interval to involve the superodistal subscapularis tendon (*arrow*).

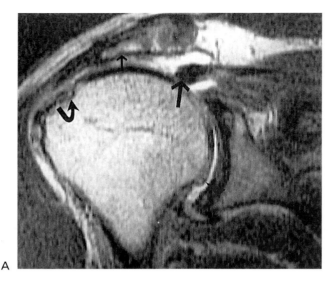

A

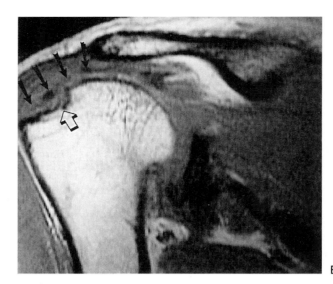

B

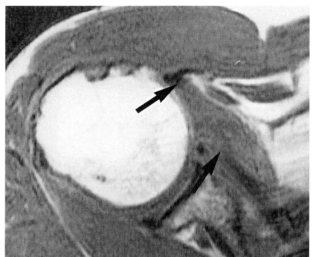

C

FIGURE 6.38. Large to massive tear, anterior and posterior extension. **A:** Coronal oblique T2-weighted image. The tendon is retracted to the medial glenoid margin (*large black arrow*). **B:** Coronal oblique T1-weighted image. The defect extends posteriorly to the infraspinatus tendon (*black arrows*). Early cuff arthropathy is present in A and B manifested by early scalloping of the acromial undersurface (*small arrow in A*) and the alterations on the humeral head (*curved arrow in A, open arrow in B*). **C:** Axial T1-weighted image. The subscapularis is torn and retracted medially (*arrows*).

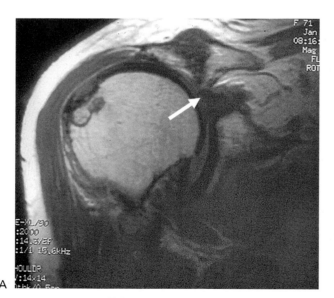

A

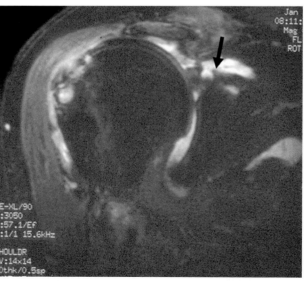

B

FIGURE 6.39. Large to massive tear, retraction to glenoid margin, and severe atrophy. Coronal oblique FSE proton density–weighted image **(A)** and FSE T2-weighted images with fat saturation **(B)**. The supraspinatus tendon is retracted medially to the glenoid margin (*arrow*). There is severe muscle atrophy. Also note advanced AC joint osteoarthritis, early rotator cuff arthropathy, and mild glenohumeral joint osteoarthritis.

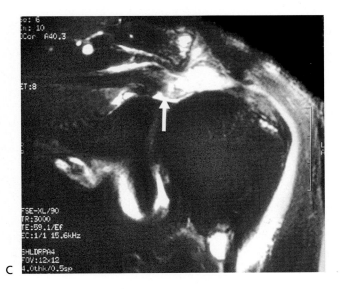

C

FIGURE 6.39 *(continued).* **C:** Coronal oblique FSE T2-weighted image with fat saturation A similar degree of tendon retraction is seen in another patient (*arrow*). Note the thickened irregular tendon edges. Tears retracted this medially may not be repairable.

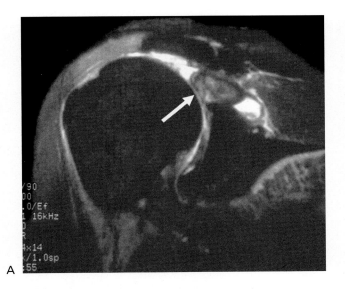

A

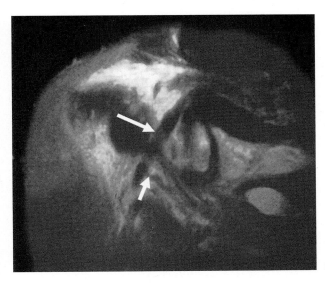

B

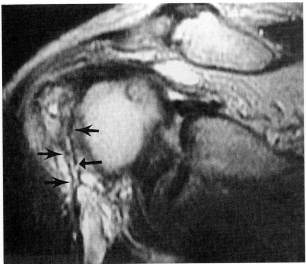

C

FIGURE 6.40. Large to massive tears and biceps tendon involvement. **A, B:** Coronal oblique TSE inversion recovery weighted images and posttraumatic rupture of the supraspinatus tendon. The supraspinatus tendon is retracted to the medial glenoid margin in A, with a fragment of bone avulsed more posteriorly (*arrow*). In B there is evidence of a destabilized biceps tendon, dislocated medially into the glenohumeral joint (*larger arrow*). This is accompanied by a subscapularis tendon rupture (*smaller arrow*). **C:** The supraspinatus tendon is retracted to the medial glenoid margin. There is severe atrophy. The biceps tendon is nearly completely disrupted, with only a thin outline that remains (*arrows*).

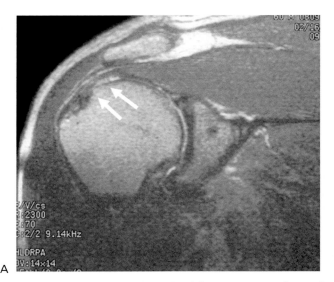 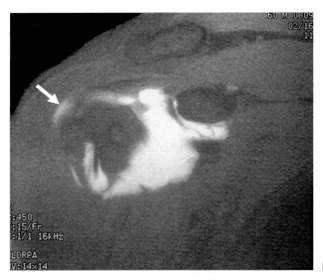

A   B

FIGURE 6.41. Partial tear versus small complete tear and MR arthrography. **A:** Coronal oblique T2-weighted image. In this case, the tendon appears thinned from the undersurface (*arrows*), with undersurface irregularity, but a distinct full-thickness defect is not seen. **B:** Coronal oblique T1-weighted MR arthrogram image with fat saturation. Although a distinct defect is not discerned on this MR image, contrast is clearly present in the subdeltoid bursa, indicating that a full-thickness tear must be present (*arrow*).

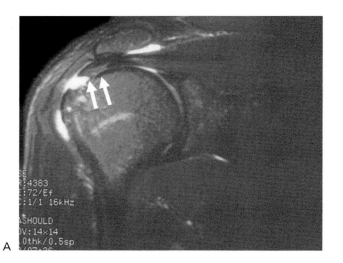 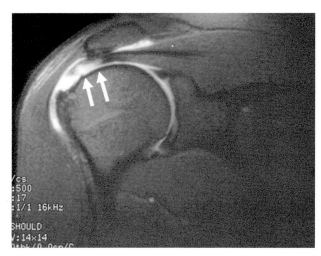

A   B

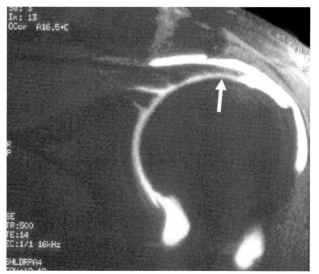

C

FIGURE 6.42. Complete tears, status of tendon edges, and MR arthrography. **A:** Coronal oblique FSE T2-weighted images with fat saturation. A full-thickness defect is seen, outlined by fluid signal (*arrows*). **B:** Coronal oblique T1-weighted MR arthrogram image with fat saturation. High signal contrast imbibes more medial into the torn tendon edges, indicating greater disruption of tendon integrity than may be appreciated on the noncontrast MR images (*arrows*). **C:** Coronal oblique T1-weighted MR arthrogram image with fat saturation in another patient. High signal contrast outlines the full-thickness defect and the thinned edges of the torn tendon (*arrow*).

were of considerable aid in the earlier years of MR imaging, prior to the more common usage of higher-resolution imaging, fat suppression, and MR arthrography, where the tendon defect was more difficult to discern. They are not used in interpretation very commonly currently, with increased experience of those interpreting the images and the better depiction of tendon defects with the aforementioned techniques. They include diffuse loss of the peribursal fat plane and the presence of fluid in the subdeltoid bursa. According to some studies, these are present in 92% of patients with complete tears (205). The loss of the peribursal fat plane when it occurs in association with a rotator cuff tear is most likely related to the presence of bursal fluid and/or inflammatory change, granulation, or scar tissue (207).

A large amount of fluid in the subdeltoid bursa is believed to represent extension of joint fluid through the capsule and tendon defect into the bursa. It has been felt to be a more specific finding of a complete cuff tear, particularly if a large volume of liquid signal is present (Figs. 6.30–6.40) (205).

In past years, these secondary signs have been the subject of controversy in the literature as they have also been observed in asymptomatic individuals (25,106,152,181,185, 205,207–209). One study encompassing 100 asymptomatic volunteers (37) found that although they were common among asymptomatic individuals, so were tendon abnormalities, including partial and complete tendon defects. The secondary signs were, however, associated with these tendon abnormalities and fluid in the subdeltoid bursa specifically with tendon defects (37). This study concluded that while these secondary signs were indeed common findings in the overall asymptomatic population, as a whole, they maintained a close association with an increasing severity of MR-evident cuff abnormalities. The authors felt that this fact would support their usefulness as markers of MR-evident cuff "abnormalities," if not of symptomatic cuff pathology.

Nonetheless, while the presence of these secondary signs should cause the reader to look for the presence of tendon abnormalities, they should never be interpreted as being indicative of a rotator cuff tear in isolation, if a tendon defect is not visualized. In addition, it is quite clear that these secondary signs, especially smaller amounts of fluid in the subdeltoid bursa, can be identified quite commonly in patients without a tendon defect, especially on fat-suppressed images; and in the case of subdeltoid bursa fluid, they may be indicative of bursal inflammation, as discussed earlier (Figs. 6.19–6.21). Fluid in the subdeltoid bursa may also be seen in patients with partial tears, especially those on the bursal surface (Fig. 6.26). Although less common, large amounts of fluid in the subdeltoid bursa may also be identified with primary subdeltoid bursitis in patients with calcium hydroxyapatite deposition disease (HADD) (discussed later) and other inflammatory causes (106). Monu and colleagues retrospectively reviewed and correlated the MR features with arthroscopic findings in 21 symptomatic patients who had fluid in the subacromial bursa on MR imaging without

demonstrable rotator cuff tear. Rotator cuff impingement was the most frequent surgical finding (42.9%). Other frequent surgical observations were glenoid labrum abnormality (28.6%), bursitis (19%), and supraspinatus tendinitis (14.3%).

Other secondary signs of rotator cuff tears include muscle atrophy and fluid in the glenohumeral joint. Fluid in the glenohumeral joint in small amounts is commonly observed in intact tendons and in asymptomatic volunteers (37). Large glenohumeral joint effusions are associated with advanced MR-evident rotator cuff tendon changes, including tears, and are a secondary sign but nonspecific as well, and they may occur in patients with synovitis and arthritis. The presence of fluid in the bursa and in the joint may be more specific than either alone but again may be seen in patients with inflammatory and articular and bursal processes such as rheumatoid arthritis, and therefore it would not be diagnostic of a cuff tear in the absence of visualization of a tendon defect.

Muscle atrophy is a secondary sign seen especially in association with large tears and chronic tears (Figs. 6.37, 6.39) (210). It is best identified on T1- and proton density–weighted images and not easily seen on fat-suppressed imaging sequences. Atrophy may, however, be seen in association with neurological compromise, adhesive capsulitis, and other conditions in which shoulder movement is restricted or absent; therefore, of itself, it is also not diagnostic of tendon disruption.

Other findings associated with large or chronic rotator cuff tears include decrease in the acromial humeral distance less than 7 mm and the presence of AC joint cysts. Decrease in the acromiohumeral distance is a finding available on plain radiographs as well, but if associated with a tear, MRI can be helpful to assess the extent of the defect. AC joint cysts are associated with full-thickness tears, usually large to massive, and occur when a high-riding humeral head impacts on the overlying AC joint. This leads to wear on the inferior aspect of the AC joint capsule, with resultant tear. Fluid from the joint can then extend through the tear, and subdeltoid bursa, into the AC joint. Removal of the cyst only must be avoided because the condition tends to recur if the cuff tear is not repaired. The rotator cuff should be repaired, and the cyst excised (211). Large joint effusions may also accompany rotator cuff tears. This is a nonspecific finding. A recent study revealed the relationship between intramuscular cysts of the rotator cuff and tears of the rotator cuff (212). This series revealed that intramuscular cysts of the rotator cuff are associated with small, full-thickness tears or partial undersurface tears of the rotator cuff. These cysts are best identified on imaging sequences with T2-weighted contrast.

In more chronic tears, a discrete tendon defect can be more difficult to discern due to partial or complete obliteration of the tear due to scarring (Fig. 6.43). Severe morphological changes, a decrease in the acromial-humeral distance, atrophy, and peribursal and bursal changes can help in recognition of these lesions on conventional MR images

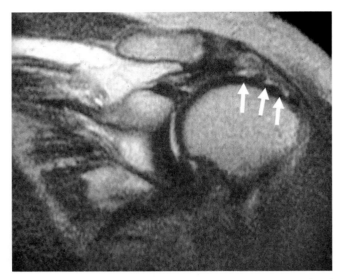

FIGURE 6.43. Chronic atrophic tear. Coronal oblique T2-weighted image. A fluid-filled defect is more difficult to discern in a more chronic lesion (*arrows*), due to the lack of a more discrete fluid-filled defect. Also note the advance muscle atrophy, altered tendon morphology, and decrease in the acromiohumeral distance.

(106). MR arthrography may be helpful in selected such cases if doubt remains about the presence and extent of such tears, if surgery is contemplated.

MRI can also accurately determine the size of the tendon defects (125,126) (Fig. 6.44), including the amount of medial retraction, the anteroposterior extent of the defect, as well as the overall cross-sectional area. As noted earlier, the cross-sectional area of the tendon defect may be the most

important in surgical planning. Sagittal and coronal oblique sequences can assess the medial and anteroposterior extent of cuff tears. In conjunction with axial views, they can also determine the number of tendons involved, including supraspinatus, infraspinatus, and subscapularis tendons, as well as the location of the tendon defect.

Fluid signal in the defect or contrast extravasation on coronal and sagittal oblique and axial images can help identify the specific cuff tendons that are involved as well as the site of the tear, whether anterior, mid-, or posterior and proximal or distal. As mentioned earlier, this is most commonly the supraspinatus tendon. Small full-thickness tears are often found in the anterior portion of the distal supraspinatus tendon, near its insertion into the greater tuberosity, at the junction with the biceps and subscapularis tendon (near the rotator interval). They are therefore best seen on far anterior coronal oblique images (151) (Figs. 6.30–6.32) or on lateral sagittal oblique images (Fig. 6.32B). Partial-thickness tears show a predilection for this area as well (106). When larger, the tears extend to involve the infraspinatus tendon from anterior to posterior (Figs. 6.36–6.38, 6.45). The component of the tear involving the infraspinatus is seen on the more posterior coronal oblique images or on sagittal oblique images. Anterior tears and larger tears may extend to involve the rotator interval capsule and the subscapularis tendon (213) (Figs. 6.37, 6.40) (118), or there will be an associated lesion of the biceps tendon (Fig. 6.40). The biceps tendon is often implicated in these situations since it lies beneath the anterior aspect of the

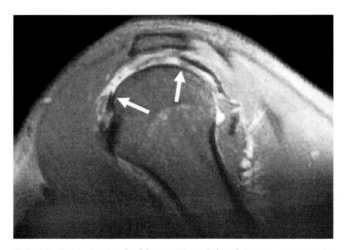

FIGURE 6.44. Sagittal oblique T2-weighted image. Images in multiple planes aid in assessing the site and size of rotator cuff tears. Sagittal oblique images reveal the extent of tendon defects from anterior to posterior. The defect in this patient extends from the anterior rotator interval to the infraspinatus tendon (*arrows*).

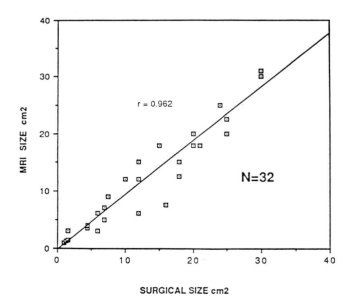

FIGURE 6.45. Linear regression plot of size of cuff tears at MRI versus that found at surgery. The correlation between the surface area estimated at MRI to that found at surgery is high (*R* value = .96). (From Iannotti JP, Zlatkin MB, Esterhai JL, Kressel HY, Dalinka MK, Spindler KP. Magnetic resonance imaging of the shoulder. *J Bone Joint Surg Am* 1991;73:17–29, with permission.)

supraspinatus tendon, which then subjects it to even further impingement between the humeral head and acromion when the supraspinatus tendon is torn (214). A rare occurrence that has been described in association with massive cuff tears is deltoid muscle rupture (35). Subscapularis and infraspinatus tears may also be visualized in the sagittal oblique and axial plane images in addition to the coronal oblique plane where the supraspinatus tendon defects are best seen (Figs. 6.37, 6.45). In larger tears and anterior tears of the supraspinatus tendon, axial images superior to the glenohumeral joint may also demonstrate the fluid-filled tendinous gap.

As noted previously, muscle atrophy may be present, especially in larger tears and more chronic tears (125,126) (Figs. 6.39, 6.43). The presence of muscle atrophy is, as also noted earlier, a secondary sign associated with a rotator cuff tear (206), and the degree and presence of muscle atrophy are highly correlative with the size of the tear (125,126). Muscle atrophy has importance in determining surgical outcome with regard to return of muscle strength (215,216). Atrophy is identified as a decrease in muscle bulk and size. There will be an increase in fat signal within the muscle belly, often appearing as linear bands of high signal on T1- and proton density–weighted images, although other patterns may be seen (25,151,210,217). Images with fat suppression only are less helpful in evaluating muscle atrophy except for visualization of a decrease in muscle bulk. Thomazeau et al. (210) developed a ratio using an image in the oblique sagittal plane that crosses the scapula through the medial border of the coracoid process. They stated that this view allowed a reliable measurement of supraspinatus muscle atrophy by the calculation of an occupation ratio (R), which was the ratio between the surface area of the cross-section of the muscle belly and that of the supraspinous fossa. Using this ratio, they were able to establish a significant difference in the presence of muscle atrophy between surgically confirmed rotator cuff tears and intact rotator cuffs. Zanetti and coworkers (218) describe the use of standardized cross-sectional areas for quantitative assessment of the muscles bulk of the rotator cuff with magnetic resonance imaging. This work was based on a study of asymptomatic patients and patients with different stages of rotator cuff tears. Standardized cross-sectional areas were determined by the rotator cuff muscle areas divided by the area of the supraspinatus fossa. They also described a tangent sign that is based on their assumption that a healthy supraspinatus muscle crosses a line (tangent) drawn through the superior borders of the scapular spine and the superior margin of the coracoid. Sagittal T1-weighted turbo spin echo images of the shoulder were utilized. In this study, the standardized cross-sectional areas did discriminate patients with different stages of rotator cuff tears from asymptomatic subjects. The tangent sign was negative in all asymptomatic subjects but positive in four and nine of ten patients with medium and large rotator cuff tears, respectively.

As noted, the assessment of the status of the torn tendon edges is also important information for the operating surgeon in preoperative evaluation. MRI and, as discussed earlier, MR arthrography can be used to assess the appearance of the torn tendon edges and to indicate whether they are of good quality, whether they are frayed or fragmented and of poor quality (Figs. 6.33–6.38) (125,205), or whether they imbibe contrast and are degenerated as determined by MR arthrography (Fig. 6.42) (199).

The options available to the surgeon in repairing the rotator cuff defects include repairing the tendon defects primarily by suturing tendon to tendon or tendon into a trough in bone. Less commonly, if a tear is large or massive, the surgeon will move local tissue into the deficient area such as biceps, subscapularis, or other tendons or insert an allograft or prosthetic material (87,219,220). This choice is most often predicated by the site and size of the cuff defect, the status of the tendon edges, and the degree of muscle atrophy. Therefore, this information available from MRI and MR arthrography is of considerable value to the surgeon, as it may allow him or her to predict preoperatively the degree of difficulty of the repair and may help decide the type of repair to perform.

Gscwend and coworkers (221) have also demonstrated that the size and site of tears has a significant influence on clinical symptomatology, as well as influencing the postoperative result, particularly with regard to recovery of range of motion and strength. The degree and presence of muscle atrophy also plays a role in this prognosis and clinical decision making (222,223). These findings must therefore be discussed and described in detail on every MR report in addition to the diagnosis of a cuff tear (224). In addition, this information is helpful to the surgeon in choosing the most appropriate surgical candidates, as well as in deciding on the best type of incision to make. Many tears, especially small tears, are now repaired arthroscopically, with a combined approach or mini–open incisions; therefore, this information helps in this decision as well. Additionally, some surgeons when confronted with a severely degenerated and retracted tendon, particularly if there is advanced muscle atrophy, may elect not to repair but instead to debride the remaining cuff tissue, and they then carry out a decompression of the subacromial space for pain relief (108). In patients with massive tears, if surgeons decide to repair the cuff, they may choose a posterior approach, to allow better mobilization of the supraspinatus.

Diagnostic Performance

The diagnostic performance of MRI imaging in rotator cuff disease has been studied (23,125,126,225,226). In Kneeland et al.'s (204) study of 25 patients with known or suspected tears of the rotator cuff, MR visualized the tears in 20 of the 22 cases diagnosed as such by arthrography or surgery. Evancho and coworkers (226) found a sensitivity, specificity, and accuracy of 80%, 94%, and 89% for complete rotator cuff tears and 69%, 94%, and 84% for all tears (partial and complete). Zlatkin, Iannotti, and coworkers evaluated a series (125) of 32 surgically confirmed cases and eight normal volunteers. In this series, a sensitivity, specificity, and accuracy of 91%, 88%, and 89% for all tears (partial and complete), respectively, were found. These results were later confirmed in a larger study by this same group in 91 patients who had surgery and/or arthroscopy (126). In the former study (125), MRI was also found to more sensitive than arthrography, particularly in the diagnosis of small tears in the anterior aspect of the supraspinatus tendon.

In addition, Burk and coworkers (225) compared MRI to arthrography, ultrasound, and surgery in a smaller series of surgically confirmed cases. They found MRI and arthrography to have a similar but better sensitivity and specificity (92% and 100%) than ultrasound (63% and 50%). Rafii and coworkers (106) assessed the diagnostic performance of MRI in 80 consecutive patients who underwent MR imaging. In the evaluation of full-thickness tears, the sensitivity was 97%; the specificity, 94%; and the accuracy, 95%. For partial-thickness tears, the sensitivity was 89%; the specificity, 84%; and the accuracy, 85%. Tuite and associates (227), in a study of 87 patients with combined spin echo T2-weighted images and T2* gradient echo images, found a sensitivity of 91% and specificity of 95% for full-thickness tears and sensitivity of 74% and specificity of 87% for partial-thickness tears. Quinn and coworkers (228) studied 100 patients with fat-suppressed MR imaging, correlated with arthroscopy. For all rotator cuff tears, both partial and complete, they found a sensitivity of 84% and a specificity of 97%. Reinus and coworkers (192) demonstrated an im-provement in detection of rotator cuff tears, both partial and complete with the use of fat suppression techniques.

More recently, other investigators have tested the diagnostic performance of fast (turbo) spin echo techniques in the evaluation of rotator cuff tears, finding them to be similarly efficacious. Singson and coworkers (195), using MR imaging with surgical correlation in 43 patients, showed 86% specificity for intact tendons and 100% sensitivity for full-thickness tears on T2-weighted fast spin echo imaging, both without and with fat suppression. For partial tears, because of increased lesion conspicuity, fat suppression performed better in the diagnosis of partial tears. MR imaging showed a sensitivity of 92% with fat suppression and 67% without fat suppression. In a study of 26 patients with surgical correlation, Sonin et al. (229) found 100% correlation between conventional spin echo and turbo spin echo sequences in the evaluation of rotator cuff integrity. For full-thickness rotator cuff tears, the sensitivity was 89%, specificity was 94%, and diagnostic accuracy was 92%. The potential benefits of the fast imaging sequences included time saving, increased spatial resolution, and, according to this study, improved signal-to-noise ratio.

Needell and Zlatkin (136) compared the diagnostic performance of fast spin echo (FSE) and conventional spin echo (CSE) in 50 surgically confirmed MR shoulder examinations. They found that FSE was 100% sensitive and 94% specific in detection of full-thickness tears ($n = 19$) and 73% sensitive and 97% specific in the detection of partial-thickness rotator cuff tears ($n = 13$). There was no statistically significant difference in the performance of FSE with fat saturation compared with CSE. Their findings suggest that

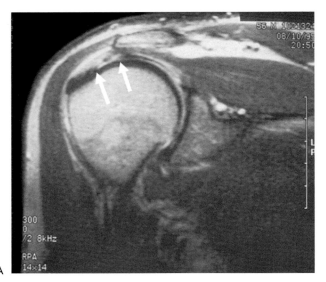 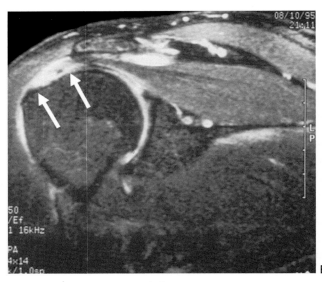

FIGURE 6.46. Convention spin echo (CSE) versus fast spin echo (FSE). **A:** Coronal oblique CSE T2-weighted image of the shoulder. A full-thickness defect in the supraspinatus tendon is identified (*arrows*). **B:** Coronal oblique T2-weighted FSE image with fat saturation. The tendon defect is well seen as well and the addition of fat suppression in fact makes the moderate-sized defect in the supraspinatus tendon more conspicuous (*arrows*).

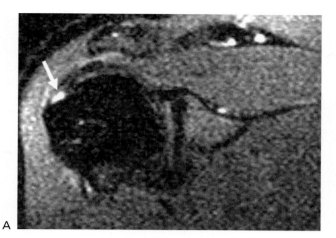
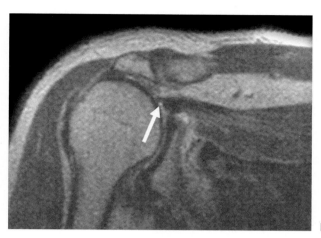

FIGURE 6.47. Rotator cuff tears, 0.2 T extremity magnet. **A:** Coronal oblique STIR image. Small anterior undersurface partial tear (*arrow*). **B:** Coronal oblique T2-weighted image. Full-thickness tear of the supraspinatus tendon, retracted medially, near the gelnoid margin (*arrow*).

fat saturation FSE imaging can effectively replace CSE imaging in the evaluation of rotator cuff pathology (Fig. 6.46).

Carrino and coworkers (230) studied 126 patients who had undergone MR imaging with conventional SE and non-fat-suppressed fast SE sequences (65 patients) or conventional SE and fat-suppressed fast SE sequences (61 patients). They found that fast SE sequences yield similar interpretations as those obtained with a conventional SE sequence for evaluation of the rotator cuff, although they did not obtain surgical correlation in a large number of patients, nor did they calculate sensitivities and specificities in this study.

Recently the assessment of the rotator cuff with low-field extremity magnets has come into increased usage. Preliminary results using these techniques with experienced musculoskeletal radiologists approach that of higher field systems (Shellock F, personal communication), although larger studies are under way to test this finding further (Fig. 6.47).

Sahin-Akyar and coworkers (231) used gradient echo and fat-suppressed fast spin echo MR imaging in the evaluation of rotator cuff tears. The sensitivity for detecting full-thickness tears was 83% to 100% for four different observers for both sequences. Interobserver agreement was good in this study.

Robertson and colleagues (232) studied the intraobserver and interobserver error and found that full-thickness tears of the rotator cuff can be accurately identified at MR imaging with little observer variation, and with an accuracy of greater than 90%, for experienced observers. Consistent differentiation of normal rotator cuff, tendinosis, and partial-thickness tears is more difficult (126,232). The diagnostic performance for partial-thickness tear is less than that for full-thickness tears for all observers. Diagnostic pitfalls causing the most difficulty may include normal alterations in signal intensity at the attachment site of the supraspinatus and at the rotator interval, the presence of articular cartilage of the humeral head beneath the distal portion of the supraspinatus tendon, and the occurrence of muscle fibers between the supraspina-

tus and infraspinatus tendons (233). Furthermore, the discovery of a rotator cuff tear on MRI, especially in older patients, does not indicate with certainty that it is the cause of the patient's shoulder symptoms (132).

According to some studies, MR arthrography can improve the diagnostic performance and confidence in the evaluation of rotator cuff tears (196) over conventional T2-weighted MRI, particularly in the evaluation of partial-thickness tears of the undersurface (200). It may have no added benefit over standard MR imaging in the evaluation of full-thickness tears (200). It is not useful in the assessment of partial-thickness tears confined to the bursal side of the cuff or intrasubstance tears, unless postcontrast images with T2 weighting are employed. The use of abduction and external rotation (ABER) may improve the diagnostic performance of MR arthrography in certain clinical circumstances as well (61). The sensitivity and specificity of MR arthrography in the evaluation of complete tears approach 100% (179). The diagnostic performance of MR arthrography is improved with the use of fat suppression (197,199). Fat suppression helps in confirming that the high signal above the tendon in the subacromial-subdeltoid bursa region is contrast and not fat in the peribursal fat plane (Fig. 6.41). In patients with contrast outlining tendon defects, persistent high signal intensity above the tendon in the subacromial-subdeltoid space indicates a full-thickness tear, but low signal, implying the suppression of fat, indicates a partial tear (179). Fat suppression also improves the diagnostic accuracy of detecting small partial tears of the undersurface (199).

A recent study of 38 cases with surgical correlation (234) compared MR arthrography at low field (0.2 T) and high field (1.5 T). The results of this study revealed that low-field MRI compares favorably to high-field MRI in the detection of full-thickness rotator cuff tears when MR arthrography is used. Disadvantages are the increased duration of the examination and because of this the risk of reduced image quality caused by motion artifacts.

MR arthrography may also have a significant effect on clinical decision making. In a study by Zanetti and coworkers (235), 34 percent of the pre-MR imaging diagnoses were changed after review of the MR arthrography findings, and new diagnoses were made after MR arthrography in 13% of the cases. Confidence in the orthopedic surgeons' clinical diagnosis increased significantly after MR imaging for supraspinatus and infraspinatus lesions. Changes in the therapeutic management after MR arthrography were noted in 36 of the 73 patients (49%). In 23 patients, more invasive therapeutic procedures were initiated after MR arthrographic imaging, and more conservative treatment was implemented for 13 patients. Agreement of the MR arthrographic diagnoses with those of surgery was 94% for supraspinatus tears, 87% for infraspinatus tears, 77% for subscapularis tears, and 81% for biceps tendon lesions. Agreement of the clinical diagnoses with surgery was 56%, 83%, 50%, and 64%, respectively. The authors concluded that MR arthrography of the shoulder has a major effect on diagnostic thinking and therapeutic decisions by orthopedic shoulder surgeons.

The diagnostic performance of indirect MR arthrography (147) is still under question. The results are more inconsistent in that there is less reliable joint opacification, no joint distension, and opacification of vessels. It may be inconvenient for the patient as well as present problems in arranging scanning time, as it requires a time delay. Early results claim comparable sensitivities and specificities for rotator cuff and glenoid labrum pathology. Rudolph and associates (236) studied 63 patients with rotator cuff pathology with indirect MR arthrography. They found there was a significant perceptual increase in contrast enhancement in patients with rotator cuff pathology. While they found indirect MR arthrography was 100% sensitive to complete tear, it was less accurate in evaluating partial tears with a sensitivity of 75% and a specificity of 50%. Partial tears were difficult to distinguish from "degeneration" changes. Allman and coworkers (149) carried out indirect MR arthrography without exercise and found that it also leads to a "diagnostically efficient enhancement of joint fluid." They stated that characterization of rotator cuff tears was significantly improved by using enhanced fat-suppressed T1-weighted gradient echo sequences compared with conventional MR imaging and that this technique represents a more convenient and less time-consuming alternative to indirect MR arthrography after joint exercise.

There is also excellent correlation between the size of the rotator cuff tears determined by MRI and that found at surgery (106,125,126). When the surface area of complete tears as determined by MRI was compared to that found at surgery, the correlation between MRI and surgery was excellent. These were categorized as poor, fair, or good. When the linear regression curve was plotted, an R value of 0.96 was obtained (Fig. 6.44). The correlation between MRI

and surgery in the evaluation of the status of the torn tendon edges was also found to be excellent. These were categorized as poor, fair, or good.

The degree of rotator cuff atrophy has also been directly correlated with the size of the cuff tear, in patients with chronic tears (128). Patients without atrophy or mild atrophy had a mean cuff tear size of 4.6 cm², versus 19.3 cm² for patients with moderate to severe atrophy.

Tears of the Subscapularis Tendon

Situations involving tears of the subscapularis tendon have been discussed in the preceding paragraphs. Involvement of the subscapularis tendon is relatively uncommon but being recognized more frequently with better understanding of the causes of injury and improved imaging techniques. Codman reported 3.5% involvement of the subscapularis tendon in his series of rotator cuff tears (13). In a more recent study of rotator cuff tears, tears of the subscapularis were recognized in 8% of patients (93), in association with tearing of other components of the rotator cuff.

Injury to the subscapularis may also occur with larger tears of the rotator cuff, as well as anterior tears. Incomplete tears of the subscapularis tendon may also occur in conjunction with small or medium-sized tears of the supraspinatus tendon. In a study of 46 cadaver shoulders (237), 20 shoulders had a tear of the supraspinatus tendon, and 17 had a tear of the subscapularis tendon. The majority were articular-side incomplete tears, on the upper portion. Lesions of the long head of the biceps brachii were identified in 14 (30.4%) shoulders. On magnetic resonance imaging, these articular side partial tears were identified as an area of high signal intensity on axial T2-weighted images.

Degeneration and tearing of the subscapularis (as well as the rotator interval capsule) may also occur in patients with subcoracoid impingement (66,67,116,238,239). Subcoracoid impingement leads to subscapularis tendon impingement pathology, visible on MR exam, similar to that described with the stages of supraspinatus impingement (34) (Fig. 6.48). Thickening and fluid may also be present in the subcoracoid bursa (68). Fluid in the subcoracoid space, revealed on MR imaging of the shoulder, may lie in the subcoracoid bursa or the subscapularis recess. Subcoracoid effusions may also be associated with anterior rotator cuff tears, including tears of the rotator interval (240).

Isolated injury of the subscapularis is uncommon. Acute isolated ruptures of the subscapularis can occur with severe trauma (118). Traumatic injury of the subscapularis is caused by either forceful hyperextension or external rotation of the adducted arm (93,94,118,241). The patients complain of anterior shoulder pain and weakness of the arm when it was used above and below the shoulder level. Such injury may also occur in elderly patients with recurrent anterior dislocation (88,242).

On MRI exam, the spectrum of pathology in the subscapularis may range from advanced thickening and

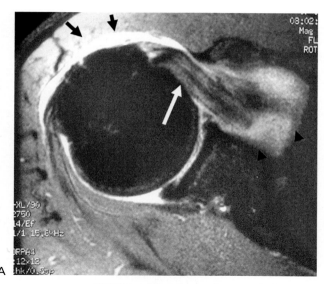 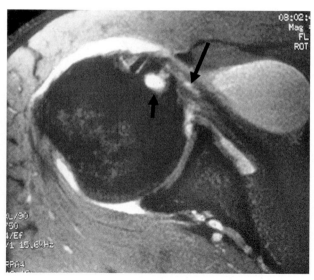

FIGURE 6.48. Subscapularis tendinosis/partial tear and subcoracoid impingement. **A:** Axial FSE images with fat saturation. The subscapularis tendon is thickened and shows increased signal in its substance (*large arrow*). There is a large amount of fluid in the subscapularis bursa (*arrowheads*) and in the subdeltoid bursa (*small arrows*). **B:** Axial FSE proton density–weighted images with fat saturation. Note the cyst in the lesser tuberosity (*small arrow*). There is some longitudinal increased signal approaching fluid in the subscapularis tendon substance (*large arrow*), indicating an intrasubstance partial tear. The coracoid process is lateral and mildly prominent.

increased signal on images with T1- and proton density–weighted contrast, reflective of tendinosis, to partial-thickness tears in the substance and in the superior distal insertion (Figs. 6.48, 6.49). Full-thickness tendon tears are associated with fluid signal on images with T2-weighted contrast and with medial tendon retraction (Fig. 6.50). Less

commonly fluid may extend into the subdeltoid bursa. Use of both the sagittal and axial images aid in the assessment of tears of the subscapularis tendon (35,93).

As rotator cuff lesions propagate anteriorly into the subscapularis or in association with subscapularis tendon rupture, they may be associated with disruption of the stabilizers

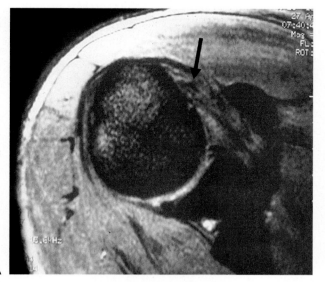 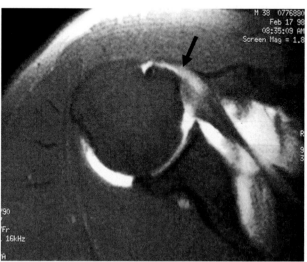

FIGURE 6.49. **A:** Subscapularis tendinosis, intrasubstance partial tear. Medial migration of the biceps tendon. Axial T2-weighted sequence with fat saturation. The subscapularis tendon is thickened. There is increased signal approaching fluid in the distal portion of the tendon. The biceps tendon is displaced medially into the substance of the subscapularis partial defect (*arrow*). **B:** Subscapularis tendon intrasubstance partial tear and MR arthrography. Axial T1-weighted MR arthrogram image with fat saturation. The distal subscapularis tendon is thickened. High signal contrast imbibes into the tendon substance outlining a partial-thickness defect (*arrow*).

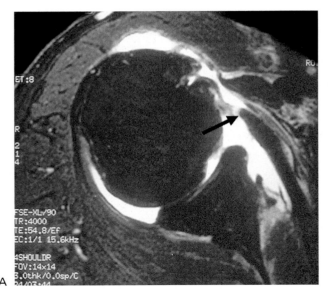 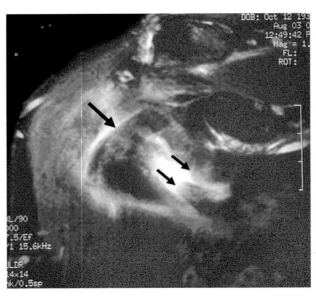

FIGURE 6.50. Subscapularis complete tear, no biceps dislocation. **A:** Axial T2-weighted FSE sequence with fat saturation. There is a complete tendon defect in the subscapularis with medial retraction (*arrow*). B: Coronal oblique T2-weighted FSE image with fat saturation. The fluid-filled defect in the subscapularis tendon is seen (*small arrows*). A thickened biceps tendon remains within the intertubercular groove (*larger arrow*).

of the biceps, such as the transverse humeral ligament. This may then result in medial subluxation or dislocation of the biceps tendon (213), and it is best seen on axial images (Fig. 6.51). This is discussed further later in this chapter and in Chapter 8.

Li and coworkers (243) studied the MR appearance of tears of the subscapularis tendon and assessed the association of subscapularis tears with other rotator cuff tears and injuries of the biceps tendon. In their study 2% of rotator cuff tears involved the subscapularis, 27% were partial and 73%

were complete tears. Tears were best seen in the sagittal oblique plane. Almost all subscapularis tears in this study were an extension of typical rotator cuff tears: supraspinatus 79%, extending into infraspinatus tears in 56% and into teres minor tears in 4% (two patients). Bicipital dislocations were seen in 49%, and three complete tears of the biceps (7%) were noted as well.

Pfirrmann (244) studied the value of MR arthrography in evaluation of the subscapularis tendon in 50 consecutive patients with arthroscopic or surgical confirmation. The diag-

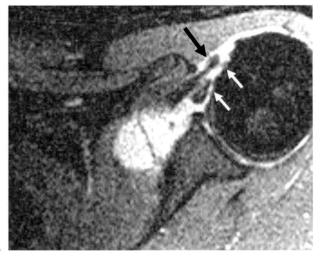 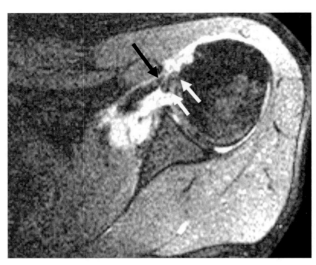

FIGURE 6.51. Subscapularis complete tear and medial subluxation of biceps tendon. **A, B:** Axial T2-weighted images. The subscapularis tendon is torn and retracted medially (*larger arrow*). The biceps tendon is destabilized and is retracted medially toward the glenohumeral joint (*smaller white arrows*).

nosis was established on findings from axial and/or sagittal images (Fig. 6.49B). With combined axial and sagittal images, sensitivity was 91%, and the specificity was 86%. Several signs at MR arthrography were specific (90%–100%) but insensitive (29%–62%); these included leakage of contrast material onto the lesser tuberosity, fatty degeneration of the subscapularis muscle, and abnormality in the course of the long head of the biceps tendon (subluxation). They concluded that MR arthrography is accurate in the evaluation of subscapularis tendon lesions. The specificity of findings on axial images was improved by including indirect signs and findings on sagittal images.

Infraspinatus and Teres Minor injuries

As noted, most tears of the infraspinatus tendon occur in association with large tears of the supraspinatus tendon. It may occur in association with injury to the teres minor tendon in posterior dislocation (122). Isolated injury of the infraspinatus tendon is not that common. It may occur in younger patients who subject this area to stress in overhead motion. It may occur as part of the posterosuperior subglenoid impingement syndrome (62). Full-thickness tendon defects may be seen in all three imaging planes, and the criteria are similar to those for tears of the supraspinatus tendon, with the lesion appearing as a fluid-filled defect on images with T2-type contrast (Fig. 6.52).

Linker, Helms, and Fritz (245) described the MR findings in isolated teres minor muscle denervation injury in middle-aged patients. This occurred 6 to 12 months after abduction and external rotation injury. Injuries of the teres minor without other rotator cuff injury may be identified with MR imaging (Fig. 6.53) and MR arthrography (122). This may occur after posterior dislocation in association with posterior capsular tears and may occur without the typ-

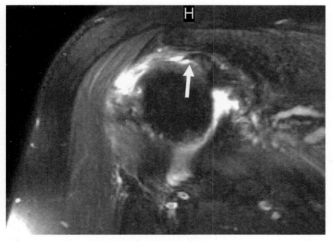

FIGURE 6.52. Isolated complete tear of the infraspinatus tendon, coronal oblique turbo spin echo image with fat suppression. The tendon is torn and retracted medially (*arrow*).

ical reverse Bankart lesion. Injuries may range from muscle edema to partial and complete tendon tears. Tendon tears are manifested by tendon discontinuity on MR imaging exam. The tendon may be avulsed from its insertion into the greater tuberosity. The other rotator cuff tendons should not be involved, but injury to the posterior inferior infraspinatus may be less commonly seen. MR imaging findings of posterior capsule injury include disruption or irregularity of the normally continuous hypointense line representing the posterior capsule. Edema and hemorrhage behind the shoulder joint may also be seen. MR arthrography may also reveal extravasation of contrast material behind the shoulder joint (122). Isolated teres minor muscle tears seen on MR imaging after posterior dislocation may cause pain. These lesions seen on MR images may be treated either surgically or conservatively, depending on the clinical situation and/or the orientation of the treating surgeon.

Rotator Interval Lesions

Rotator interval tears are an uncommon but clinically important subtype of rotator cuff tear. Tears of this region may be difficult to diagnose with MRI. Differentiation of a true rotator interval tear from normal synovium and capsule in this space may often not be possible with MRI, and symptoms may be referred and misleading. It is therefore important to correlate the MR findings with the clinical history and physical examination when this injury is suspected (245).

The rotator interval is defined as the space between the superior border of the subscapularis muscle and tendon below and the supraspinatus muscle and tendon (183,247, 248) above. It is a complex region and can be conceptualized in layers (249,250). The outermost layer consists of fibrofatty tissue, and beneath this fibrofatty tissue is the coracohumeral ligament, the joint capsule, and then the superior glenohumeral ligament. The deepest structure in the anterior interval is the long head of biceps tendon. Surgeons may enter the joint through this region for an arthrotomy. It is through this interval that the long head of the biceps tendon enters the shoulder joint from the proximal bicipital groove to extend to the superior labral-biceps anchor and the supraglenoid tubercle attachment. The interval is bridged by the rotator interval capsule (251). The fused rotator interval capsule and the coracohumeral ligament may be seen as a roof over the biceps tendon, and they are important anterior supporting structures for shoulder function.

As previously discussed, partial volume averaging of some of the structures in this region may lead to intermediate signal at the anterior margin of the supraspinatus tendon. In addition, synovium and joint capsule can herniate into this space, which may give rise to high signal in this region on T2-weighted images as well, not to be mistaken for a rotator cuff tear. This may be best discerned on sagittal oblique T2-weighted imaging sequences with fat suppression (190).

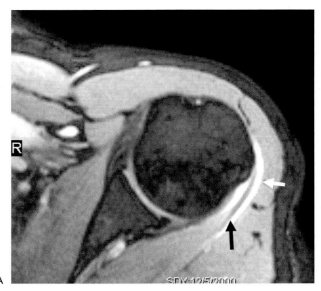
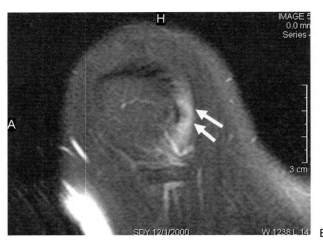

FIGURE 6.53. Injury to the teres minor. **A, B:** Axial and sagittal oblique fast spin echo T2-weighted images with fat suppression. Edema is seen in and about the teres minor tendon (*arrows*) compatible with a tendinous and peritendinous injury in this patient injured in a motor vehicle accident.

Chung and coworkers (252) studied the rotator interval in 32 cadaveric shoulders. The rotator cuff interval, rotator interval capsule, and crossing structures were best evaluated by MR arthrography. The anteroposterior dimension of the rotator interval capsule could also be best depicted on postarthrogram MR images.

It is believed that injury or deficiency of the rotator interval capsule and coracohumeral ligament may lead to posterior inferior laxity and instability (251). Lesions of the rotator interval may also be seen in association with shoulder subluxations and dislocations, where this region may be an area of relative weakness, susceptible to injury, and therefore during which time this region may be torn or enlarged. Therefore, many surgeons believe this area should be repaired or reinforced during stabilization procedures for instability.

Injuries to this interval may also occur in individuals without a history of instability (247). In such a case, there may also be an anterior tear of the supraspinatus tendon as well as tear of the superior subscapularis tendon, in association with the tear of the interval. Isolated lesions of the rotator interval appear thin and longitudinal and are not associated with muscle retraction (246). Tears of the rotator interval may cause communication with the subdeltoid bursa, and fluid or contrast may be seen in this region on conventional MRI and MR arthrography. This may be identified along with altered signal in the region of the interval involving such structures as the coracohumeral ligament and the long head of biceps tendon, without necessarily involving the supraspinatus tendon. This may be confusing if this anatomy and lesion are not understood. Lesions of the rotator interval may often be best discerned on sagittal oblique

T2-weighted imaging sequences with fat suppression or with MR arthrography.

In addition to the concepts and lesions discussed earlier, a further understanding of the importance of the anatomic and functional region of the rotator interval has come to the forefront more recently. This includes the understanding that injury to this area may occur as a complex or spectrum of injuries and that the structures of this region are intimately associated. The structures that contribute to the functional anatomy of this region, or may be injured in association, include the anatomic structures alluded to previously, including the anterior margin of the supraspinatus tendon, the distal superior margin of the subscapularis tendon, the coracohumeral ligament, the rotator interval capsule, the superior glenohumeral ligament, and the long head of the biceps tendon. It is also associated with the superior labrum and labral biceps anchor. It also takes into account the ligamentous reflection pulley for the long head of biceps tendon formed by these structures at the lateral margin of the rotator interval, extending to the lesser tuberosity and proximal bicipital groove. It also includes the transverse humeral ligament extending between the greater and lesser tuberosities.

The lesions may be acute, as after a dislocation, or chronic, as in overuse injuries. If acute, the alterations may be identified as areas of edema, fluid signal, and synovitis and have high signal on T2-weighted images; if chronic, they show areas of thickening and scarring, revealed as areas of low to intermediate signal in the region of the interval, including the coracohumeral ligament and capsule (Fig. 6.54). Other associated injuries may occur to the biceps tendon, includ-

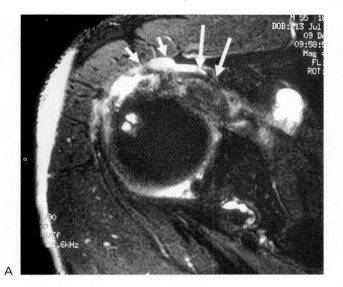

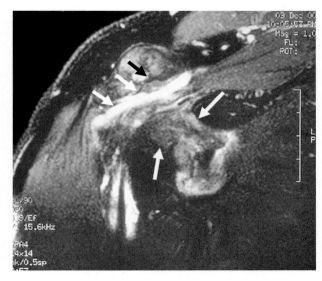

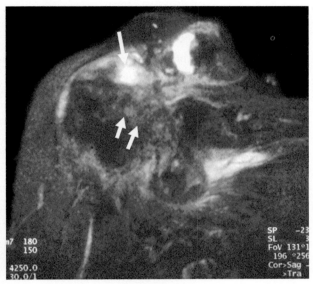

FIGURE 6.54. Rotator interval injury. Axial **(A)** and coronal oblique **(B)** T2-weighted fast spin echo sequences with fat saturation. Fluid signal on T2-weighted images due to edema and synovitis, as well as areas of thickening and scarring, revealed as areas of low to intermediate signal in the region of the rotator interval, are noted (*arrows*). Fluid is also present in the anterior aspect of the subdeltoid bursa (*small arrows*). **C:** Coronal oblique turbo spin echo images with fat saturation. Similar findings are also present in this patient (*small arrows*). Also note the anterior, fluid-filled defect in the supraspinatus tendon (*larger arrow*).

ing inflammation and tear, or with disruption of the transverse humeral ligament or tear of the subscapularis tendon at the lateral superior margin, at its attachment to the lesser tuberosity, biceps instability, including medial dislocation. With interval disruption tearing of the distal anterior supraspinatus tendon at its insertion into the greater tuberosity, "the anterior or leading edge," at the lateral rotator interval may also occur (213). Owing to the course of the long head of biceps through the interval to the superior labrum, SLAP lesions may also occur and should be searched for as well (253).

These lesions may not be as well identified on coronal oblique sections and are often better recognized on sagittal oblique sections or axial sections, acquired as either T2-weighted FSE imaging with fat suppression or with MR arthrography. When any one of the spectrum of these associated injuries is suspected or found, all of the other possible

associated injuries should be searched for both clinically and on MR examination (253).

Biceps Tendon

This topic is discussed more fully in Chapter 8. As noted earlier, however, the biceps tendon may also become involved in patients with impingement and rotator cuff tears, and the pathology that is seen on MRI in these patients (254–257) should be reviewed again briefly. In general, the extent of disease in the biceps is less severe than that in the cuff, but it follows the progression seen. A small amount of fluid may be observed in the biceps tendon sheath even in asymptomatic individuals (39). Since the tendon sheath communicates with the joint, it may fill with fluid when a shoulder joint effusion is present for some other cause; therefore, this is a nonspecific finding. Tenosynovitis can be

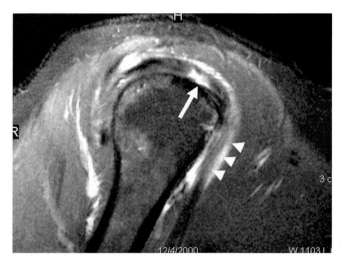

FIGURE 6.55. Partial-thickness rotator cuff tear and biceps tendinosis. Sagittal oblique T2-weighted turbo spin echo image with fat saturation. A deep partial tear of the more central to anterior supraspinatus tendon is identified (*arrow*). Note the increased signal in the proximal biceps tendon, associated with tendon thickening, reflective of tendinosis (*arrowheads*).

diagnosed when the amount of fluid in the tendon sheath is out of proportion to that in the joint.

Tendinosis of the biceps tendon may be manifested by increase in the tendon size and increased signal in its substance on T1- and proton density–weighted images (Fig. 6.55). With T2-weighted FSE with fat suppression or FSE STIR, the increased signal may persist or mildly increase.

In shoulders with tears of the rotator cuff, the biceps also becomes an active depressor of the head of the humerus (258). On MRI examination the biceps may enlarge as a response to this increased workload. This is sometimes termed *tendonization.*

Partial-thickness tears may be more easily discerned when there is alteration in morphology such as thinning, irregularity, or splitting of the tendon. Biceps tendon ruptures may be seen with anterior tears of the rotator cuff (Fig. 6.40). Up to 7% of large rotator cuff tears are also accompanied by biceps tendon rupture. After a tear, the intracapsular portion of the tendon lies free in the joint cavity, while the extraarticular portion is pulled distally. With MRI, the tendon is absent from the groove, which is filled with fluid. Distal retraction of the muscle and tendon may be seen, best identified in longitudinal planes of section. Occasionally the intertubercular groove may fill with scar tissue of low signal and may cause a false-negative diagnosis.

Medial dislocation of the biceps tendon may also result from chronic impingement, associated with a large anterior cuff tear (256,257). There is tearing of the secondary biceps stabilizers, including the anterior supraspinatus and subscapularis tendons and the coracohumeral ligament. The low-signal tendon is displaced medially outside the intertubercular groove (Figs. 6.40, 6.49, 6.51). This is best seen on

axial views. There may be an extraarticular tendon dislocation with an intact subscapularis. With rupture of the subscapularis tendon either posttraumatic or with a large or massive cuff tear, then the biceps tendon may also dislocate intraarticularly. The biceps tendon may then extend into and be entrapped in the joint.

A lesion of the common insertion of the coracohumeral and the superior glenohumeral ligaments and the superior border of the subscapularis tendon, which predisposes to biceps tendon subluxation and subsequent degeneration, is known as a *pulley lesion.* MR arthrography may be helpful in detecting this lesion. Abnormalities of the superior border of the subscapularis tendon on axial and parasagittal images, an extraarticular contrast collection, and biceps tendon subluxation are the MR arthrographic findings of a pulley lesion (259). Differentiation from an isolated lesion of the superior border of the subscapularis tendon may not always be possible in these cases.

Rotator Cuff Tear Arthropathy

The pathophysiology of rotator cuff tear arthropathy has been discussed earlier (17). This generally occurs in the setting of large to massive tears (Figs. 6.38, 6.39, 6.56). In addition to the presence of the advanced disruption of the cuff, there is abrasion of the humeral head articular cartilage against the coracoacromial arch, causing subacromial im-

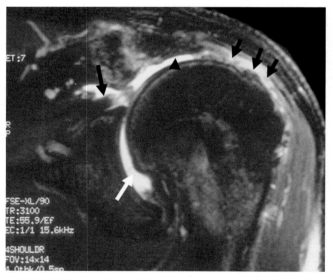

FIGURE 6.56. Rotator cuff arthropathy, coronal oblique fast spin echo T2-weighted image with fat saturation. In this patient with a large retracted full-thickness tear (*large arrow*), changes of rotator cuff arthropathy are seen. Note the decrease in the acromiohumeral distance, scalloping and resorption of the undersurface of the anterior acromion (*arrowhead*), and fraying and thinning of the articular cartilage of the humeral head (*small arrows*). There is early glenohumeral joint degenerative arthritis. Note the head neck osteophyte at the humeral head/neck junction (*white arrow*).

pingement that in time erodes the anterior portion of the acromion and the acromioclavicular joint. There may be collapse of the soft, atrophic humeral head (17), with eventual erosion of the glenoid and coracoid. While many of these findings may be visible on plain radiographs, MRI can help assess the full extent of bone and soft-tissue involvement. This process should be recognized and described at the time of MRI evaluation, as the best treatment for this may be total shoulder replacement with, if possible, rotator cuff reconstruction. Recognition of this entity is also a factor for the surgeon to consider when deciding whether a documented tear of the rotator cuff should or can be surgically repaired (17).

Calcium Hydroxyapatite Deposition Disease (HADD)

The shoulder is the most common site of involvement with calcium hydroxyapatite crystal deposition disease (HADD). Patients may often be asymptomatic, but clinical symptoms occur in 30% to 45% of patients in whom calcifications are present. The disorder occurs in both males and females, usually between the ages of 40 and 70. The pathogenesis of hydroxyapatite crystal deposition is unknown, although trauma, ischemia, or other systemic factors may induce abnormalities in the connective tissue, leading to crystal deposition (260,261). Crystal deposition most commonly occurs in the tendinous and bursal structures about the shoulder, particularly the supraspinatus tendon (Fig. 6.57) (52%). It may become bilateral in up to 50% of patients (262). In the supraspinatus tendon, it may target the critical zone, as this may be an area of both altered vascularity and mechanical

pressure, which therefore may predispose it to hydroxyapatite crystal deposition. It may also occur in the other tendons of the rotator cuff or in the biceps tendon. Bursal calcification is most common in the subacromial-subdeltoid bursa (Fig. 6.58). These crystals incite a synovitis, tendonitis, or bursitis and periarticular inflammation. The calcification alone may not be the inciting agent, but symptoms may occur with the dissolution of the calcium. With rupture of a calcific deposit, hydroxyapatite crystals are spilled into the surrounding soft-tissue space or bursa, setting off an acute inflammatory response. McCarty and coworkers (263) has described an entity known as *Milwaukee shoulder*, which consists of a destructive arthropathy, hydroxyapatite deposits, high collagenase activity in the synovial fluid, and rotator cuff tears.

The nodular calcific deposits in HADD can usually be easily seen with plain radiographs and the combination of radiographs, and the characteristic history is usually sufficient for diagnosis and subsequent therapy. When MRI is obtained in these patients, the calcific densities, usually of low signal intensity, may be difficult to see, especially when small, due to the lack of contrast with the low signal of the tendons (Fig. 6.57). They are difficult to differentiate from a thickened tendon without calcification (264). It may be difficult to distinguish a calcified tendon from a thickened tendon without calcification. They may be more easily identified when they are large or, if there is subjacent high signal on images with T2-type contrast, related to peritendinous edema and inflammation. T2-gradient echo images may also enhance visualization by providing a blooming effect. Although areas of high signal intensity may be observed about foci of calcification in tendons and bursae on

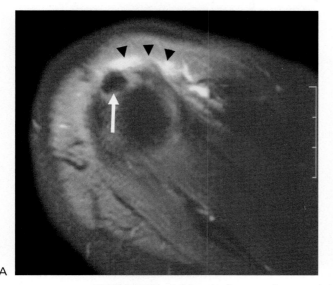
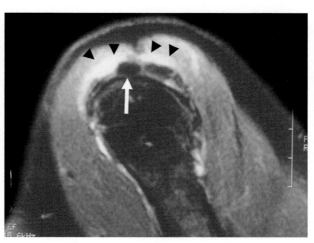

A   B

FIGURE 6.57. Calcium hydroxyapatite crystal deposition disease (HADD). Coronal **(A)** and sagittal oblique **(B)** fast spin echo T2-weighted images with fat saturation. There is a nodular focus of low signal consistent with calcium in the central aspect of the supraspinatus tendon (*arrow*). Fluid is also seen in the subdeltoid bursa (*arrowheads*).

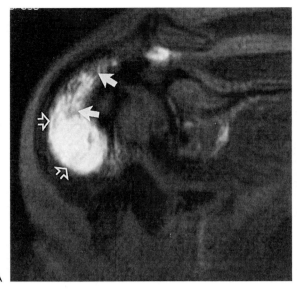
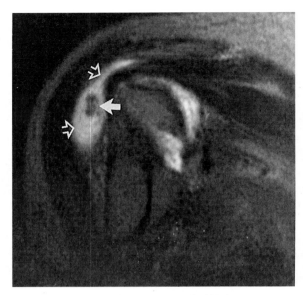

FIGURE 6.58. Calcium hydroxyapatite crystal deposition disease (HADD). **A, B:** Coronal oblique T2-weighted images. A large amount of fluid is seen in the subdeltoid bursa (*open white arrows*), with nodular areas of low signal within it (*white arrows*), representing calcium hydroxyapatite deposition.

T2-weighted spin echo MR images and after injection of gadolinium intravenously, the correlation of such findings to calcific tendinitis and bursitis has not been proven (42).

When the calcifications are seen, MRI (120) can localize the specific tendons or bursa involved and document associated changes such as tendinitis or the less common tears. Tears of the rotator cuff can occur in association with calcific

tendonitis, although the mechanism is not yet clear. It may relate to localized hyperemia in the tendon, which may lead to impingement.

The presence of effusions in the subacromial-subdeltoid bursa can be identified, particularly after extrusion of the calcifications into the bursa (Figs. 6.57, 6.58). MRI may also be helpful in these patients to exclude other causes of shoul-

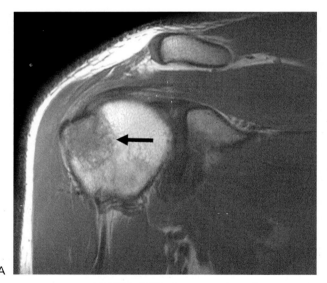
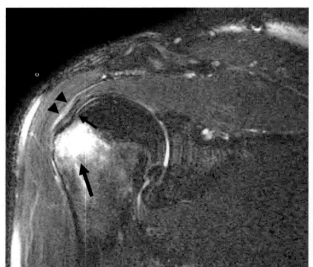

FIGURE 6.59. Greater tuberosity contusion. Coronal T1 **(A)** and turbo inversion recovery weighted images **(B)**, reveal a greater tuberosity contusion (*large arrow*). Also note there is mild increased signal in the supraspinatus tendon, which could reflect posttraumatic strain or contusion (*small arrow*). The small amount of fluid in the subdeltoid bursa may indicate some posttraumatic bursitis (*arrowheads*).

der pain. In patients with Milwaukee shoulder, the extent of joint destruction may be determined, and the presence of a rotator cuff tear, as well as its extent, can be documented.

Treatment consists of rest, antiinflammatory therapy, and, where appropriate, local steroid injection. If recalcitrant, they may be removed with flouroscopically or ultrasound guided needle aspiration (farin) or surgically, either via an open technique or, as shown more recently, arthroscopically (265,266). Extracorporeal shockwave therapy has also been shown to be an effective method for treating chronic calcific tendinitis of the shoulder (267).

Bone Injuries

Occult fractures about the proximal humerus are discussed in Chapter 8. Nondisplaced fractures and bone contusions about the humeral head (Fig. 6.59) and greater tuberosity, however, may result in pain and associated contusion-like injuries of rotator cuff that may mimic pain due to rotator cuff tears. Anzilloti and colleagues (268) found that this tended to occur in younger patients and in atypical locations of the supraspinatus tendon. This posttraumatic strain of the rotator cuff was typically associated with a bone bruise in this study (268).

CONCLUSIONS

In summary, MRI can diagnose rotator cuff abnormalities due to chronic impingement. Tendon abnormalities can be seen in patients without cuff tears. Complete cuff tears can be reliably identified. The size and extent of rotator cuff tears and the degree of muscle atrophy can also be depicted. The ability to distinguish between tendonitis and tendon degeneration, partial-, and small full-thickness tears may not prove possible in all cases. However, disease of the rotator cuff represents a continuum, and no doubt there will be some overlap of the MRI appearance of these entities.

REFERENCES

1. Kronberg M, Nemeth G, Brostrom LA. Muscle activity and coordination in the normal shoulder: an electromyographic study. *Clin Orthop* 1990;(257):76–85.
2. Howell SM, Galinat BJ, Renzi AJ, Marone PJ. Normal and abnormal mechanics of the glenohumeral joint in the horizontal plane. *J Bone Joint Surg Am* 1988;70(2):227–232.
3. Howell SM, Imobersteg AM, Seger DH, Marone PJ. Clarification of the role of the supraspinatus muscle in shoulder function. *J Bone Joint Surg Am* 1986;68:398–404.
4. Colachis SC, Strohm BR. Effect of suprascapular and axillary nerve blocks on muscle force in the upper extremity. *Arch Phys Med Rehabil* 1971;52:22–29.
5. Colachis SC, Strohm BR, Brechner VL. Effects of axillary nerve block on muscle force in the upper extremity. *Arch Phys Med Rehabil* 1969;50:647–654.
6. Otis JC, Jiang CC, Wickiewicz TL, Peterson MG, Warren RF, Santner TJ. Changes in the moment arms of the rotator cuff and deltoid muscles with abduction and rotation. *J Bone Joint Surg Am* 1994;76:667–676.
7. Poppen NK, Walker PS. Forces at the glenohumeral joint in abduction. *Clin Orthop* 1978;135:165–170.
8. Sher JS. Anatomy, biomechanics and pathophysiology of rotator cuff disease. In: Iannotti JP, Williams GR Jr., eds. *Disorders of the shoulder: diagnosis and management*. Philadelphia: Lippincott, Williams and Wilkins, 1999: chap. 1.
9. Sharkey NA, Marder RA, Hansen PB. The entire rotator cuff contributes to elevation of the arm. *J Orthop Res* 1994;12:699–708.
10. Matsen FA, Artnz CT. Subacromial impingement. In: Rockwood CE, Matsen FA, eds. The shoulder. Philadelphia: WB Saunders, 1990: chap. 15.
11. Harryman DT, Clark JH. Anatomy of the rotator cuff. In: Burkhead WZ, ed. Rotator cuff disorders. Baltimore: Williams and Wilkins, 1996: chap. 2.
12. Codman EA, Akerson TB. The pathology associated with rupture of the supraspinatus tendon. *Ann Surg* 93:354–359.
13. Codman EA. The shoulder, rupture of the supraspinatus tendon and other lesions in or about the subacromial bursa. Boston: Thomas Todd, 1934.
14. Codman EA. Rupture of the supraspinatus, 1834–1934. *J Bone Joint Surg* 1937;19:643–652.
15. Brems JJ. Rotator cuff tear: evaluation and treatment. *Orthopaedics* 1988;11:69–81.
16. Meyer AW. Chronic functional lesions of the shoulder. *Arch Surg* 1937; 35:646–674.
17. Neer CS III. Impingement lesions. *Clin Orthop* 1983;173:70–77.
18. Neer CS III. Anterior acromioplasty for the chronic impingement syndrome of the shoulder: a preliminary report. *J Bone Joint Surg Am* 1972;54A:41–50.
19. Laumann U. Decompression of the subacromial space: an anatomical study. In: Bayley I, Kessel L, eds. Shoulder surgery. Berlin: Springer, 1982:14–21.
20. Peterson CJ, Gentz CF. Ruptures of the supraspinatus tendon: the significance of distally pointing acromioclavicular osteophytes. *Clin Orthop* 1983;174:143–148.
21. Bigliani Lu, Morrison DS, April EW. The morphology of the acromion and its relationship to rotator cuff tears. *Orthop Trans* 1986;10:228.
22. Vanarthos WJ, Monu JU. Type 4 acromion: a new classification. *Contemp Orthop* 1995;30:227–229.
23. Farley TE, Neumann CH, Steinbach LS, Peterson SA. The coracoacromial arch: MR evaluation and correlation with rotator cuff pathology. *Skeletal Radiol* 1994;23:641–645.
24. Bigliani Lu, Morrison DS, April EW. The morphology of the acromion and its relationship to rotator cuff tears. *Orthop Trans* 1986;10:228.
25. Seeger LL, Gold RH, Bassett LW, Ellman H. Shoulder impingement syndrome: MR findings in 53 shoulder. *AJR* 1988;50:343–347.
26. Morrison DS, Bigliani LU. The clinical significance of variations in the acromial morphology. *Orthop Trans* 1986;11:234.
27. Edelson JG. The "hooked" acromion revisited. *J Bone Joint Surg* 1995;77B:284–287.
28. Tuite TJ, Toivonen DA, Orvin JF, et al. Acromial angle on radiographs of the shoulder: correlation with the impingement syndrome and rotator cuff tears. *AJR* 1995;165:609–612.
29. Getz JD, Recht MP, Piraino DW, et al. Acromial morphology: relation to sex, age, symmetry, and subacromial enthesophytes. *Radiology* 1996;199:737–741.
30. Edelson JG, Taitz C. Anatomy of the coraco-acromial arch: relation to degeneration of the acromion. *J Bone Joint Surg Br* 1992; 74:589–594.

31. Fritts HM. MRI and shoulder imaging. *Lippincott's Reviews in Radiology* 1992;1:373.
32. Yao L, Lee HY, Gentili A, Shapiro MM. Lateral down-sloping of the acromion: a useful MR sign? *Clin Radiol* 1996;51:869–872.
33. Farley TE, Neumann CH, Steinbach LS, Peterson SA. The coracoacromial arch: MR evaluation and correlation with rotator cuff pathology. *Skeletal Radiol* 1994;23:641–645.
34. Bergman AG. Rotator cuff impingement: pathogenesis, MR imaging characteristics, and early dynamic MR results. *Magn Reson Imaging Clin N Am* 1997;5:705–819.
35. Fritz RC, Stoller DW. MR imaging of the rotator cuff. *MRI Clin N Am* 1997;5:735–754.
36. Kessel L, Watson M. The painful arc syndrome. *J Bone Joint Surg* 1977;59:B166–172.
37. Needel S, Zlatkin MB, Sher J, Uribe J, Murphy B. MR Imaging of the rotator cuff: peritendinous and bony abnormalities in an asymptomatic population. *AJR* 1996; 166:863–867.
38. Jim YF, Chang CY, Wu JJ, Chang T. Shoulder impingement syndrome: impingement view and arthrography study based on 100 cases. *Skeletal Radiol* 1992;21:449–451.
39. Deleted in text.
40. Resnick D, Kang HS. Shoulder. In: Resnick D, Kang HS, eds. *Internal derangement of joints*. Philadelphia: WB Saunders, 1997:163–334.
41. Burns WC, Whipple TL. Anatomic relationships in the shoulder impingement syndrome. *Clin Orthop Rel Res* 1993;294:96–102.
42. Morrimoto K, Mori E, Nakagawa Y. Calcification of the coracoacromial ligament: a case report of the shoulder impingement syndrome. *Am J Sports Med* 1988;16:80.
43. Gallino M, Battiston B. Annartone G, Terragnoli F. Coracoacromial ligament: a comparative arthroscopic and anatomic study. *Arthroscopy* 1995;11:564–567.
44. Sarkar K, Taine W, Uthoff HK. The ultrastructure of the coracoacromial ligament in patients with chromic impingement syndrome. *Clin Orthop Rel Res* 1990;254:49–54.
45. Mudge MK, Wood VE, Frykman GK. Rotator cuff tears associated with os-acromiale. *J Bone Joint Surg Am* 1984;66:427–429.
46. Park JG, Lee JK, Phelps CT. Os acromiale associated with rotator cuff impingement: MR imaging of the shoulder. *Radiology* 1994; 193:255–257.
47. Neer CS. Rotator cuff tears associated with os acromiale. *J Bone Joint Surg Am* 1984;66:1320–1321.
48. Norris TR, Fisher J, Bigliani LU, Neer CS II. The unfused acromial epiphysis and its relationship to the impingement syndrome. *Orthop Trans* 1983;7:505–506.
49. Edelson JG, Zuckerman J, Hershkowitz I. Os acromiale: anatomy and surgical implications. *J Bone Joint Surg* 1993;74B:551–555.
50. Hutchinson MR, Veenstra MA. Arthroscopic decompression of shoulder impingement secondary to os acromiale. *Arthroscopy* 1993;9(1):28–32.
51. Gold RH, Seeger LL, Yao L. Imaging shoulder impingement. *Skeletal Radiol* 1993:22:555–561.
52. Fu FH, Harner CD, Klein AH. Shoulder impingement syndrome: a critical review. *Clin Orthop* 1991;269:162–173.
53. Ticker JB, Fealy JS, Fu FH. Instability and impingement in the athlete's shoulder. *Sports Med* 1995;19:418–422.
54. Hawkins RJ, Kunkel Sanford S. Rotator cuff tears. In: Torg JS, Welsh RP, Shepherd RJ, eds. *Current therapy in sports medicine–2*. Toronto: BC Decker, 1990.
55. Jobe FW. Impingement problems in the athlete. *Instr Course Lect* 1989;15:205–209.
56. Jobe FW, Kvitne RS, Giangarra CE. Shoulder pain in the overhand or throwing athlete: the relationship of anterior instability and rotator cuff impingement. *Orthop Rev* 1989;18:963–975.
57. Jobe FW, Bradley JP, Pink M. Impingement syndrome in overhead athletes. *Surg Rounds Orthop* 1990;4:19–24.
58. Giombini A, Rossi F, Pettrone FA, Dragoni S. Posterosuperior glenoid rim impingement as a cause of shoulder pain in top level waterpolo players. *J Sports Med Phys Fitness* 1997;37:273–238.
59. Davidson PA, Elattrache NS, Jobe CM, et al. Rotator cuff and posterosuperior glenoid labrum injury associated with increased glenohumeral motion: a new site of impingement. *J Shoulder Elbow Surg* 1995;4:384–390.
60. Jobe CM. Posterior superior glenoid impingement: expanded spectrum. *Arthroscopy* 1995;11:530–536.
61. Tirman TFJ, Bost FW, Steinbach LS, et al. MR arthrographic depiction of tears of the rotator cuff: benefit of abduction and external rotation of the arm. *Radiology* 1994:192:851–856.
62. Halbrecht JL, Tirman P, Atkin D. Internal impingement of the shoulder: comparison of findings between the throwing and non-throwing shoulders of college baseball players. *Arthroscopy* 1999; 15:253–258.
63. Walch G, Boileau P, Noel E, et al. Impingement of the deep surface of the supraspinatus tendon on the posterior superior glenoid rim: an arthroscopic study. *J Shoulder Elbow Surg* 1992;1:238–245.
64. Liu SH, Boynton E. Posterior superior impingement of the rotator cuff on the glenoid rim as a cause of shoulder pain in the overhead athlete. *Arthroscopy* 1993;9:697–701.
65. Edelson G, Teitz C. Internal impingement in the shoulder. *J Shoulder Elbow Surg* 2000;9:308–315.
66. Gerber CH, Terrier F, Ganz R. The role of the coracoid process in the chronic impingement syndrome. *J Bone Joint Surg Br* 1985;67:703–708.
67. Dines DM, Warren RF, Inglis AE, Pavlov H. The coracoid impingement syndrome. *J Bone Joint Surg* 1990;72B:314–316.
68. Bonutti PM, Norfray JF, Friedman RJ, Genez BM. Kinematic MRI of the shoulder. *JCAT* 1993;17:666–669.
69. Rathbun JB, Mcnab I. The microscopic pattern of the rotator cuff. *J Bone Joint Surg Br.* 1970;52B:540–553.
70. Lindblom K. On the pathogenesis of ruptures of the tendon aponeurosis of the shoulder joint. *Acta Radiol* 1939;20:563–567.
71. Rothman HR, Parke W. The vascular anatomy of the rotator cuff. *Clin Orthop* 1965 41;176–186.
72. Uthoff HK, Sarkar K, Hammond DI. An algorithm for shoulder pain caused by soft tissue disorders. *Clin Orthop Rel Res* 1990;254:121–127.
73. Ozaki J, Fujimoto S, Nakagawa Y, Masuhara K, Tamai S. Tears of the rotator cuff of the shoulder associated with pathologic changes in the acromion. *J Bone Joint Surg* 1988;70A:1224–1230.
74. Lohr JF, Uthoff HK. The microvascular pattern of the supraspinatus tendon. *Clin Orthop* 1990;254:35–38
75. Mosely FH, Goldie I. The arterial pattern of the rotator cuff of the shoulder. *J Bone Joint Surg Br* 1963;45:780–789.
76. Pettersson CJ. Rupture of the tendon aponeurosis of the shoulder joint in anterior inferior dislocation: a study on the origin and occurrence of the ruptures. *Acta Chir Scand* 1942:77(suppl):1–187.
77. Kumagai J, Sarkar K, Uhthoff HK. The collagen types in the attachment zone of rotator cuff tendons in the elderly: an immunohistochemical study. *J Rheumatol* 1994;21:2096–2100.
78. Swiontkowski MF, Iannotti JP, Boulas HJ, Esterhai JL. Intraoperative assessment of rotator cuff vascularity using laser Doppler flowmetry. In: Post M, Morrey BF, Hawkins RJ, eds. *Surgery of the shoulder*. St. Louis: Mosby Yearbook, 1990:208–212.
79. Wilson CL. Lesions of the supraspinatus tendon: degeneration, rupture and calcification. *Arch Surg* 1943;46:307–325.
80. Wilson CL, Duff GL. Pathologic study of degeneration and rupture of the supraspinatus tendon. *Arch Surg* 1943;47:121–135.
81. Brooks CH, Revell WJ, Heatley FW. A quantitative histological study of the vascularity of the rotator cuff tendon. *J Bone Joint Surg Br* 1992;74:151–153.
82. Nirschl RP. Rotator cuff tendinitis: basic concepts of pathoetiology. *Instr Course Lect* 1989;38:439–445.

83. Ogata S, Uhthoff HK. Acromial enthesopathy and rotator cuff tear: a radiologic and histologic postmortem investigation of the coracoacromial arch. *Clin Orthop* 1990;254:39–48.

84. Budoff JE, Nirschl RP, Guidi EJ. Debridement of partial thickness tears of the rotator cuff without acromiplasty. *J Bone Joint Surg* 1998;80A:733–748.

85. Burkhead WZ, Burkhart SS, Gerber C, Harryman DT, Morrison DS, Uhthoff HK, Williams GR Jr. Symposium on the rotator cuff: debridement vs repair—part II. *Contemp Orthop* 1995; 31:313–326.

86. Norwood LA, Barrack R, Jacobsen KE. Clinical presentation of complete tears of the rotator cuff. *J Bone Joint Surg* 1989;71A: 499–505.

87. Neviaser RJ. Tears of the rotator cuff. *Orthop Clin North Am* 1980;11;295–303.

88. Neviaser RJ, Neviaser TJ, Neviaser JS. Concurrent rupture of the rotator cuff and anterior dislocation of the shoulder in the older patient. *J Bone Joint Surg* 1988;70A:1308–1311.

89. Neviaser TJ. The anterior labroligamentous periosteal sleeve avulsion injury: a cause of anterior instability of the shoulder. *Arthroscopy* 1993;9:17–21.

90. Ribbans WJ, Mitchell R, Taylor GJ. Computerised arthrotomography of primary anterior dislocation of the shoulder. *J Bone Joint Surg Br* 1990;72:181–185.

91. Tijmes J, Loyd HM, Tullos HS. Arthrography in acute shoulder dislocations. *South Med J* 1979;72:564–567.

92. Pevny T, Hunter RE, Freeman JR. Primary traumatic anterior shoulder dislocation in patients 40 years of age and older. *Arthroscopy* 1998;14:289–294.

93. Deutsch A, Altchek DW, Veltri DM, Potter HG, Warren RF. Traumatic tears of the subscapularis tendon: clinical diagnosis, magnetic resonance imaging findings, and operative treatment. *Am J Sports Med* 1997;25:13–22.

94. Gerber C, Krushell RJ. Isolated rupture of the tendon of the subscapularis muscle: clinical features in 16 cases. *J Bone Joint Surg Br* 1991;73:389–394.

95. McAuliffe TB, Dowd GS. Avulsion of the subscapularis tendon: a case report. *J Bone Joint Surg Am* 1987;69:1454–1455.

96. Itoi E, Tabata S. Rotator cuff tears in anterior dislocation of the shoulder. *Int Orthop* 1993;17:64.

97. Matsen FA, Artnz CT. Subacromial impingement. In: Rockwood CE, Matsen FA, eds. *The shoulder.* Philadelphia: WB Saunders, 1990:chap. 15.

98. Neer CS. Displaced proximal humeral fractures: part 1: classification and evaluation. *J Bone Joint Surg Am* 1970;52:1077–1089.

99. Reinus WR, Hatem SF. Fractures of the greater tuberosity presenting as rotator cuff abnormality: magnetic resonance demonstration. *J Trauma* 1998;44:670–675.

100. Mason BJ, Kier R, Bindleglass DF. Occult fractures of the greater tuberosity of the humerus: radiographic and MR imaging findings. *AJR* 1999;172:469–473.

101. Neer CS II. Cuff tears, biceps lesions, and impingement. In: Neer CS II ed. *Shoulder reconstruction.* Philadelphia: WB Saunders, 1990:63–70.

102. Murthi AM, Vosburgh CL, Neviaser TJ. The incidence of pathologic changes of the long head of the biceps tendon. *J Shoulder Elbow Surg* 2000;9:382–385.

103 Kronberg M, Saric M. Fibrosis in the subacromial bursa and outcome after acromioplasty. *Ann Chir Gynaecol* 1997;86: 45–49.

104. Matsen FA, Artnz CT. Rotator cuff tendon failure. In: Rockwood CE, Matsen FA, eds. *The shoulder.* Philadelphia WB Saunders 1990:chap. 16.

105. Ciepiela MD, Burkhead WZ. Classification of rotator cuff tears. In: Burkhead WZ Jr., ed. *Rotator cuff disorders.* Baltimore: William and Wilkins, 1996:100–110.

106. Rafii M, Firooznia H, Sherman O, et al. Rotator cuff lesions: signal patterns at MR imaging. *Radiology* 1990;177:817–823.

107. Ellman H, Gartsman GM. *Rotator cuff disorders: arthroscopic shoulder surgery and related disorders.* Philadelphia: Lea and Febiger, 1993:98–119.

108. Matsen FA, Artnz CT, Lippitt SB. Rotator cuff. In: Rockwood CE, Matsen FA, eds. *The shoulder.* Philadelphia: WB Saunders 1998:755–795.

109. Wolfgang GL. Surgical repair of tears of the rotator cuff of the shoulder: factors influencing the result. *J Bone Joint Surg Am* 1974;56:14–26.

110. Wolfgang GL. Rupture of the musculotendinous cuff of the shoulder. *Clin Orthop* 1978;134:230–243.

111. Ellman H. Diagnosis and treatment of incomplete rotator cuff tears. *Clin Orthop* 1990; 254:64–74.

112. Ellman H. Surgical treatment of rotator cuff rupture. In: Watson M, ed. *Surgical disorders of the shoulder.* Edinburgh: Churchill Livingstone, 1991:283–284.

113. Iannotti JP, Bernot MP, Kuhlman JR, Kelley MJ, Williams GR. Postoperative assessment of shoulder function: a prospective study of full-thickness rotator cuff tears. *J Shoulder Elbow Surg* 1996;5:449–457.

114. Iannotti JP. Full-thickness rotator cuff tears: factors affecting surgical outcome. *J Am Acad Orthop Surg* 1994;2:87–95.

115. Harryman DT, Mack LA, Wang K, Jackins SE, Richardson ML, Matsen FA. Repairs of the rotator cuff: correlation of functional results with integrity of the cuff. *J Bone Joint Surg Am* 1991:73: 982–989.

116. Patte D. The subcoracoid impingement. *Clin Orthop* 1990;254: 55–59.

117. Tuite MJ, Turnbull JR, Orwin JF. Anterior versus posterior, and rim-rent rotator cuff tears: prevalence and MR sensitivity. *Skeletal Radiol* 1998;27:237–243.

118. Terrier F, Wegmuller H, Vock P, Gerber C. Diagnosis of subscapular lesions in rotator cuff tears: comparison of MR imaging with US. *Radiology* 1989;173(P):438.

119. Patten RM. Tears of the anterior portion of the rotator cuff (the subscapularis tendon): MR imaging findings. *AJR* 1994;162:351.

120. Terrier F, Wegmuller H, Vock P, Gerber C. Diagnosis of subscapular lesions in rotator cuff tears: comparison of MR imaging with US. *Radiology* 173(P):438, 1989.

121. Gartsman GM. Massive, irreparable tears of the rotator cuff. Results of operative debridement and subacromial decompression. *J Bone Joint Surg Am* 1997;79:715–721.

122. Hottya GA, Tirman PF, Bost FW, Montgomery WH, Wolf EM, Genant HK. Tear of the posterior shoulder stabilizers after posterior dislocation: MR imaging and MR arthrographic findings with arthroscopic correlation. *AJR* 1998;171:763–768.

123. Ovesen J, Sojbjerg JO. Posterior shoulder dislocation: muscle and capsular lesions in cadaver experiments. *Acta Orthop Scand* 1986;57:535–539.

124. Blazar PE, Williams GR, Iannotti JP. Spontaneous detachment of the deltoid muscle origin. *J Shoulder Elbow Surg* 1998;7: 389–392.

125. Zlatkin MB, Iannotti JP, Roberts MC, Esterhai JC, Dalinka MK, Kressel HY, Lenkinski R. Rotator cuff disease: diagnostic performance of MR imaging: comparison with arthrography and correlation with surgery. *Radiology* 1989;172:223–229.

126. Iannotti JP, Zlatkin MB, Esterhai JL, Kressel HY, Dalinka MK, Spindler KP. Magnetic resonance imaging of the shoulder. *J Bone Joint Surg Am* 1991;73:17–29.

127. Ellman H. Diagnosis and treatment of incomplete rotator cuff tears. *Clin Orthop* 1990; 254:64–74.

128. Wilson CL. Lesions of the supraspinatus tendon: degeneration, rupture and calcification. *Arch Surg* 1943;46:307–325.

129. Wilson CL, Duff GL. Pathologic study of degeneration and rupture of the supraspinatus tendon. *Arch Surg* 1943;47:121–135.

130. Fukuda H, Mikasa M, Ogawa K, et al. The partial thickness tear of the rotator cuff. *Ortho Trans* 1983;7:137.

131. Depalma AF. *Surgery of the shoulder*. Philadelphia: JP Lippincott, 1983;47–64.

132. Sher JS, Uribe JW, Posada A, Murphy BJ, Zlatkin MB. Abnormal magnetic resonance images in asymptomatic shoulders. *JBJS* 1994;77A:10–16.

133. Frost P, Andersen JH, Lundorf E. Is supraspinatus pathology as defined by magnetic resonance imaging associated with clinical signs of shoulder impingement? *J Shoulder Elbow Surg* 1999;8: 565–568.

134. Sasaki M, Ehara S, Nakasato T, Tamakawa Y, Kuboya Y, Sugisawa M, Sato T. MR of the shoulder with a 0.2-T permanent-magnet unit. *AJR* 1990;154:777–778.

135. Davis SJ, Teresi LM, Bradley WG, Ressler JA, Eto RT. Effect of arm rotation on MR imaging of the rotator cuff. *Radiology* 1991;181:265–268.

136. Needel SD, Zlatkin MB. Comparison of fat-saturation fast spin echo versus conventional spin-echo MRI in the detection of rotator cuff pathology. *J MRI* 1997;7:674–677.

137. Rand T, Trattnig S, Haller J, Nguyen NK, Imhof H. MR imaging in shoulder trauma: value of STIR images. *Acta Radiol* 1998; 39:273–275.

138. Petersilge CA, Lewin JS, Duerk JL, Hatem SF. MR arthrography of the shoulder: rethinking traditional imaging procedures to meet the technical requirements of MR imaging guidance. *AJR* 1997;169:1453–1457.

139. Hajek PC, Sartoris DJ, Gylys-Morin V, et al. The effect of intra-articular gadolinium DTPA on synovial membrane and cartilage. *Invest Radiol* 1990;25:179–183.

140. Stiles RG, Resnick D, Sartoris DJ, Andre MP. Rotator cuff disruption: diagnosis with digital arthrography. *Radiology* 1988; 168(3):705–707.

141. DeMouy EH, Menedez CV Jr. Bodin CJ. Palpation directed saline enhanced MR arthrography of the shoulder. *AJR* 1997; 169:229.

142. Valls R, Melloni P. Sonographic guidance of needle position for MR arthrography of joints. *AJR* 1997;169:845–847.

143. Trattnig S, Breitenseher M, Rand T, Bassalamah A, Schick S, Imhof H, Petersilge CA. MR imaging-guided MR arthrography of the shoulder: clinical experience on a conventional closed high-field system. *AJR* 1999;172:1572–1574.

144. Zanetti M, Hodler J. Contrast media in MR arthrography of the glenohumeral joint: intra-articular gadopentetate vs saline: preliminary results. *Eur Radiol* 1997;7:498–502.

145. Tirman PFJ, Stauffer AE, Crues JV, et al. Saline magnetic resonance arthrography in the evaluation of glenohumeral instability. *Arthroscopy* 1993;9:550–559.

146. Brenner ML, Morrison WB, Carrino JA, et al. Direct MR arthrography of the shoulder: is exercise prior to imaging beneficial or detrimental? *Radiology* 2000;215:491–496.

147. Vahlensieck M, Lang P, Sommer T, et al. Indirect MR arthrography: techniques and applications. *Semin US CT MR* 1997;18: 302–306.

148. Winalski CS, Aliabadi P, Wright RJ, et al. Enhancement of joint fluid with intravenously administered gadopentetate dimeglumine: technique, rationale, and implications. *Radiology* 1993; 187:179–185.

149. Allmann KH, Schafer O, Hauer M, Winterer J, Laubenberger J, Reichelt A, Uhl M. Indirect MR arthrography of the unexercised glenohumeral joint in patients with rotator cuff tears. *Invest Radiol* 1999;34:435–440.

150. Kaplan PA, Bryans KC, Davick JP, Otte M, Stinson WW, Dussault RG. MR imaging of the normal shoulder: variants and pitfalls. *Radiology* 1992;184:519–524.

151. Seeger LL. Magnetic resonance imaging of the shoulder. *Clin Orthop* 1989;244:48–59.

152. Schweitzer ME, Magbalon, MJ, Frieman BG, Ehrlich S, Epstein RE. Acromioclavicular joint fluid: determination of clinical significance with MR imaging. *Radiology* 1994;192:205–207.

153. Epstein RE, Schweitzer ME, Freiman BG, Fenlin JM, Mitchell DG. Hooked acromion: prevalence on MR images of painful shoulders. *Radiology* 1993;187:479–481.

154. Haygood TM, Langlotz CP, Kneeland JB, Iannotti JP, Williams GR, Dalinka MK. Categorization of acromial shape: interobserver variability with MRI imaging and conventional radiography. *AJR* 1994;162:1377–1382.

155. Peh WCG, Farmer THR, Totty WG. Acromial arch shape: assessment with MRI imaging. *Radiology* 1995;195:501–505.

156. Jacobson SR, Speer KP, Moor JT, et al. Reliability of radiographic assessment of acromial morphology. *J Shoulder Elbow Surg* 1995; 4:449–453.

157. Altchek DW, Dines DM. Shoulder injuries in the throwing athlete. *J Am Acad Orthop Surg* 1995;3:159–165.

158. Crues JV III, Fareed DO. Magnetic resonance imaging of shoulder impingement. *Top Magn Reson Imaging* 1991;3:39–49.

159. Uri DS, Kneeland JB, Herzog R. Os acromiale: evaluation of markers for identification on sagittal and coronal oblique MR images. *Skeletal Radiol* 1997;26:31–34.

160. Cone RO III, Resnick D, Danzig L. Shoulder impingement syndrome: radiographic evaluation. *Radiology* 1984;150:29–33.

161. Huang LF, Rubin DA, Britton CA. Greater tuberosity changes as revealed by radiography: lack of clinical usefulness in patients with rotator cuff disease. *AJR* 1999;172:1381–1388.

162. Sano A, Itoi E, Konno N, et al. Cystic changes of the humeral head on MR imaging: relation to age and cuff-tears. *Acta Orthop Scand* 1998;69:397–400.

163. Brown SM, Rosenbach D, Zlatkin MB. Kinematic MRI of joints. In: Edelman RR, Hesselink JR, Zlatkin MB, eds. *Clinical magnetic resonance imaging*, 2nd ed. Philadelphia: WB Saunders, 1996:2140–2159.

164. Tirman PFJ, Bost FW, Garving GJ, et al. Posterosuperior glenoid impingement of the shoulder: findings at MR imaging and MR arthrography with arthroscopic correlation. *Radiology* 1994; 193:431–437.

165. Graichen H, Bonel H, Stammberger T, Heuck A, Englmeier KH, Reiser M, Eckstein F. A technique for determining the spatial relationship between the rotator cuff and the subacromial space in arm abduction using MRI and 3D image processing. *Magn Reson Med* 1998;40:640–643.

166. Shibuta H, Tamai K, Tabuchi K. Magnetic resonance imaging of the shoulder in abduction. *Clin Orthop* 1998;348:107–113.

167. Beaulieu CF, Hodge DK, Bergman AG, et al. Glenohumeral relationships during physiologic shoulder motion and stress testing: initial experience with open MR imaging and active imaging-plane registration. *Radiology* 1999;212:699–705.

168. Burkhart SS. Fluoroscopic comparison of kinematic patterns in massive rotator cuff tears: a suspension bridge model. *Clin Orthop* 1992;284:144–152.

169. Khan KM, Cook JL, Bonar F, Harcourt P, Astrom M. Histopathology of common tendinopathies: update and implications for clinical management. *Sports Med* 1999;Jun;27(6):393–408.

170. Wolf WB. Shoulder tendinoses. *Clin Sports Med* 1992;11(4): 871–890.

171. Rafii M, Firoozonia H, Sherman O, et al. Rotator cuff lesions: signal patterns at MR imaging. *Radiology* 1990;177:817–823.

172. Mirowitz SA. Normal rotator cuff: MR imaging with conventional and fat-suppression techniques. *Radiology* 1991;180:735–740.

173. Tyson LL, Crues JV III. Pathogenesis of rotator cuff disorders: magnetic resonance imaging characteristics. *Magn Reson Imaging Clin N Am* 1993;1:37–46.

174. Rafii M. The shoulder. In: Firooznia HF, Golimbu C, Rafii M, et al., eds. *MRI and CT of the musculoskeletal system*. St. Louis: Mosby Year Book, 1992:465.

175. Kieft GH, Bloem JL, Rosing PM, Oberman WR. Rotator cuff impingement syndrome: MR imaging. *Radiology* 1988;166: 211–214.

176. Kjellin J, Ho CP, Cervilla V, et al. Alteration of the supraspinatus tendon at MR imaging: correlation with histopathologic findings in cadavers. *Radiology* 1991;181:837–841.

177. Patten RM. Overuse syndromes and injuries involving the elbow: MR imaging findings. *AJR* 1995;164:1205–1211.

178. Potter HG, Hannafin JA, Morwessel RM, et al. Lateral epicondylitis: correlation of MR imaging, surgical and histopathologic findings. *Radiology* 1995;196:43–46.

179. Tirman PFJ, Palmer WE, Feller JF. MR Arthrography of the shoulder. *MRI Clin North Am* 1997;5:811–839.

180. Anzilotti KF Jr., Schweitzer ME, Oliveri M, Marone PJ. Rotator cuff strain: a post-traumatic mimicker of tendonitis on MRI. *Skeletal Radiol* 1996;25:555–558.

181. Neumann CH, Holt RG, Steinbach LS, et al. MR imaging of the shoulder: appearance of the supraspinatus tendon in asymptomatic volunteers. *AJR* 1992;158:1281–1287.

182. Miniaci A, Dowdy PA, Willits KR, Vellet AD. Magnetic resonance imaging evaluation of the rotator cuff tendons in the asymptomatic shoulder. *Am J Sports Med* 1995;23:142–145.

183. Tsai JC, Zlatkin MB. Magnetic resonance imaging of the shoulder. *Radiol Clin North Am* 1990;28:279–291.

184. Falchook FS, Zlatkin MB, Buck BE. Nonpathologic causes of increased signal in the rotator cuff: MR imaging frequency with anatomic and surgical correlation. Presented at the Radiological Society of North American 78th Annual Meeting, Chicago, November 29–December 4, 1992.

185. Mirowitz SA. Normal rotator cuff: MR imaging with conventional and fat suppression techniques. *Radiology* 1991;180: 735–740.

186. Vahlensieck M, Pollack M, Lang P, Grampp S, Genant HK. Two segments of the supraspinatus muscle: cause of high signal at MR imaging? *Radiology* 1993;186:449–454.

187. Erickson SJ, Cox IH, Hyde JS, Carrera GF, Strandt JA, Estkowski LD. Effect of tendon orientation on MR imaging signal intensity: a manifestation of the "magic angle" phenomenon. *Radiology* 1991;181:389–392.

188. Erickson SJ, Prost RW, Timins ME. The "magic angle" effect: background physics and clinical relevance. *Radiology* 1993;188: 23–235.

189. Timins ME, Erickson SJ, Estkowski LD, Carrera GF, Komorowski RA. Increased signal in the normal supraspinatus tendon on MR imaging: diagnostic pitfall caused by the magic-angle effect. *AJR* 1995;165:109–14.

190. Steinbach LS. Rotator cuff disease. In: Steinbach LS, Tirman PFJ, Peterfy CG, Feller JF, eds. *Shoulder magnetic resonance imaging*. Philadelphia: Lippincott-Raven, 1998:99–135.

191. Bergman AG, Fredericson M. Shoulder MRI after impingement test injection. *Skeletal Radiol* 1998;27:365–368.

192. Reinus WR, Shady KL, Mirowitz S, Totty WG. MR diagnosis of rotator cuff tears of the shoulder: value of using T2 weighted fat saturated images. *AJR* 1995;164:1451–1455.

193. Nelson MC, Leather GP, Nirschl RP, Pettrone FA, Freedman MT. Evaluation of the painful shoulder: a prospective comparison of magnetic resonance imaging, computerized tomographic arthrography, ultrasonography, and operative findings. *J Bone Joint Surg Am* 1991;73:707–716.

194. Traughber PD, Goodwin TE. Shoulder MRI: arthroscopic correlation with emphasis on partial tears. *J Comput Assist Tomogr* 1992;16:124–133.

195. Singson RD, Hoang T, Dan S, Friedman M. MR Evaluation of rotator cuff pathology using T2-weighted fast spin-echo technique with and without fat suppression. *AJR* 1996;166:1061–1065.

196. Flanigan BD, Kursonogulu-Brahme S, Snyder S, Karzel R, Del Pizzo W, Resnick DL. MR arthrography of the shoulder: comparison with conventional MR imaging. *AJR* 1990;155;829–832.

197. Fritz RC, Stoller DW. Fat-suppression MR arthrography of the shoulder. *Radiology* 1992;185:614–615.

198. Karzel RP, Snyder SJ. Magnetic resonance arthrography of the shoulder. *Clin Sports Med* 1993;12:123.

199. Palmer WE, Brown JH, Rosenthal DI. Rotator cuff: evaluation with fat suppressed MR arthrography. *Radiology* 1993;188: 683–687.

200. Hodler J, Kursunoglu-Brahme S, Snyder SJ, et al. Rotator cuff disease: assessment with MR arthrography versus standard MR imaging in 36 patients with arthroscopic confirmation. *Radiology* 1992;182:431–436.

201. Walch G, Boileau P, Noel E, et al. Impingement of the deep surface of the supraspinatus tendon on the posterior superior glenoid rim: an arthroscopic study. *J Shoulder Elbow Surg* 1992;1: 238–245.

202. Itoi E, Tabata S. Incomplete rotator cuff tears: results of operative treatment. *Clin Orthop* 1992;284:128–135.

203. Torres JL, Burk DL, Marone P, Mitchell DG, Rifkin MD, Karasick D. MRI of shoulder injuries in professional baseball players. *Magn Reson Imaging* 1990;8:(suppl 1) 77.

204. Kneeland JB, Middleton WD, Carrera GF, et al. MR imaging of the shoulder: diagnosis of rotator cuff tears. *AJR* 1987;149: 333–337.

205. Zlatkin MB, Reicher MA, Kellerhouse LE, McDade W, Vetter L, Resnick D. The painful shoulder: MR imaging of the glenohumeral joint. *J Comput Assist Tomogr* 1988;12:995–1001.

206. Farley TE, Neumann CH, Steinbach LS, Jahnke AJ, Peterson SS. Full-thickness tears of the rotator cuff of the shoulder: diagnosis with MR imaging. *AJR* 1992;158:347–351.

207. Mitchell MJ, Causey G, Berthoty DP, et al. Peribursal fat plane of the shoulder: anatomic study and clinical experience. *Radiology* 1988; 168:699–704.

208. Chadnani VP, Ho C, Gerharter J, Neumann C, Kursunoglu-Brahme S, Sartoris DJ, Resnick D. MR findings in asymptomatic shoulders: a blind analysis using symptomatic shoulders as controls. *Clin Imaging* 1992;16:25–30.

209. Liou JT, Wilson AJ, Totty WG, Brown JJ. The normal shoulder: common variations that simulate pathologic conditions at MR imaging. *Radiology* 1993;186:435–441.

210. Thomazeau H, Rolland Y, Lucas C, et al. Atrophy of the supra spinatus belly: assessment by MRI in 55 patients with rotator cuff pathology. *Acta Orthop Scand* 1996;67:264–268.

211. Postacchini F, Perugia D, Gumina S. Acromioclavicular joint cyst associated with rotator cuff tear: a report of three cases. *Clin Orthop* 1993;294:111–113.

212. Sanders TG, Tirman PF, Feller JF, Genant HK. Association of intramuscular cysts of the rotator cuff with tears of the rotator cuff: magnetic resonance imaging findings and clinical significance. *Arthroscopy* 2000;16:230–235.

213. Walch G, Nove-Josserand L, Levigne C, et al. Tears of the supraspinatus tendon with hidden lesions of the rotator interval. *J Shoulder Elbow Surg* 1994;3:353–360.

214. Neviaser TJ. The role of the biceps tendon in the impingement syndrome. *Orthop Clin North Am* 1987;18:383–386.

215. Zlatkin MB, Iannotti JP, Esterhai JL, Dalinka MK, Kressel HY, Spindler K. Evaluation of rotator cuff disease and glenohumeral

instability with MR imaging: correlation with arthroscopy and arthrotomy in a large population of patients. *Magn Reson Imaging* 1990;8(suppl 1):78(abstr).

216. Iannotti JP, Zlatkin MB, Esterhai JL, Dalinka MK, Kressel HY, Spindler K. Magnetic resonance imaging of the shoulder: sensitivity, specificity and predictive value. *J Bone Joint Surg Am* 1991; 73:17–29.

217. Fuchs B, Weishaupt D, Zanetti M, Hodler J, Gerber C. Fatty degeneration of the muscles of the rotator cuff: assessment by computed tomography versus magnetic resonance imaging. *J Shoulder Elbow Surg* 1999;8:599–605.

218. Zanetti M, Gerber C, Hodler J. Quantitative assessment of the muscles of the rotator cuff with magnetic resonance imaging. *Invest Radiol* 1998;33:163–170.

219. Hawkins RJ. The rotator cuff and biceps tendon. In: Evarts CM, ed. *Surgery of the musculoskeletal system.* New York: Churchill Livingstone, 1983:5–35.

220. Cofield RH. Rotator cuff disease of the shoulder. *J Bone Joint Surg Am* 1985;67A:974–979.

221. Gscwend N, Ivosevic-Radonovic A, Patte D. Rotator cuff tear: relationship between clinical and anatomicopathological findings. *Arch Orthop Trauma Surg* 1988;107:7–15.

222. Nakagaki K, Ozaki J, Tomita Y, Tamai S. Function of the supraspinatus muscle with torn cuff evaluated by magnetic resonance imaging. *Clin Orthop* 1995;318:144–151.

223. Nakagaki K, Ozaki J, Tomita Y, Tamai S. Fatty degeneration in the supraspinatus muscle after rotator cuff tear. *J Shoulder Elbow Surg* 1996;5:194–200.

224. Shellock FG, Stoller D, Crues JV. MRI of the shoulder: a rational approach to the reporting of findings. *J Magn Reson Imaging* 1996;6:268–270.

225. Burk DL, Karasick D, Kurtz AB. et al. Rotator cuff tears: prospective evaluation of MR imaging with arthrography, sonography and surgery. *AJR*:1989;153:87–92.

226. Evancho AM, Stiles RG, Fajman WA, Flower SP, Macha T, Brunner MC, Fleming L. MR imaging diagnosis of rotator cuff tears. *AJR* 1988;151:751–754.

227. Tuite MJ, Yandow DR, DeSmet AA, Orwin JF, Quintana FA. Diagnosis of partial and complete rotator cuff tears using combined gradient echo and spin echo imaging. *Skeletal Radiol* 1994;23:541–545.

228. Quinn SF, Sheley RC, Demlow TA, Szumowski J. Rotator cuff tendon tears: evaluation with fat-suppressed MR imaging with arthroscopic correlation in 100 patients. *Radiology* 1995;195:497–500.

229. Sonin AH, Peduto AJ, Fitzgerald SW, Callahan CM, Bresler ME. MR imaging of the rotator cuff mechanism: comparison of spin-echo and turbo spin-echo sequences. *AJR* 1996;167:333–338.

230. Carrino JA, McCauley TR, Katz LD, Smith RC, Lange RC. Rotator cuff: evaluation with fast spin-echo versus conventional spin-echo MR imaging. *Radiology* 1997 Feb;202(2):533–539.

231. Sahin-Akyar G, Miller TT, Staron RB, McCarthy DM, Feldman F. Gradient-echo versus fat-suppressed fast spin-echo MR imaging of rotator cuff tears. *AJR* 1998;171:223–227.

232. Robertson PL, Schweitzer ME, Mitchell DG, Schlesinger F, Epstein RE, Frieman BG, Fenlin JM. Rotator cuff disorders: interobserver and intraobserver variation in diagnosis with MR imaging. *Radiology* 1995;194:831–835.

233. Zlatkin MB, Falchook F. MRI pathology of the rotator cuff. *Top Magn Reson Imaging* 1994;6:94–121.

234. Loew R, Kreitner KF, Runkel M, Zoellner J, Thelen M. MR arthrography of the shoulder: comparison of low-field (0.2 T) vs high-field (1.5 T) imaging. *Eur Radiol.* 2000;10:989–996.

235. Zanetti M, Jost B, Lustenberger A, Hodler J. Clinical impact of MR arthrography of the shoulder. *Acta Radiol* 1999;40:296–302.

236. Rudolph J, Lorenz M, Schroder R, Sudkamp NP, Felix R, Maurer J. Indirect MR arthrography in the diagnosis of rotator cuff lesions. *Rofo Fortschr Geb Rontgenstr Neuen Bildgeb Verfahr* 2000; 172:686–691.

237. Sakurai G, Ozaki J, Tomita Y, Kondo T, Tamai S. Incomplete tears of the subscapularis tendon associated with tears of the supraspinatus tendon: cadaveric and clinical studies. *Shoulder Elbow Surg* 1998;7:510–515.

238. Gerber C, Terrier F, Zehnder R, Ganz R. The subcoracoid space: an anatomic study. *Clin Orthop* 1987;215:132–138.

239. Sunaga N, Minami A, Kato H. Subcoracoid impingement after surgery for rotator cuff tear. *J Shoulder Elbow Surg* 1997;6(suppl): S250.

240. Grainger AJ, Tirman PF, Elliott JM, Kingzett-Taylor A, Steinbach LS, Genant HK. MR anatomy of the subcoracoid bursa and the association of subcoracoid effusion with tears of the anterior rotator cuff and the rotator interval. *AJR* 2000;174:1377–1380.

241. Patten RM. Tears of the anterior portion of the rotator cuff (the subscapularis tendon): MR imaging findings. *AJR* 1994;162:351.

242. Neviaser RJ, Neviaser TJ, Neviaser JS. Anterior dislocation of the shoulder and rotator cuff rupture. *Clin Orthop* 1993;291:103–106.

243. Li XX, Schweitzer ME, Bifano JA, Lerman J, Manton GL, El-Noueam KI. MR evaluation of subscapularis tears. *J Comput Assist Tomogr* 1999;23:713–717.

244. Pfirrmann CW, Zanetti M, Weishaupt D, Gerber C, Hodler J. Subscapularis tendon tears: detection and grading at MR arthrography. *Radiology* 1999;213:709–714.

245. Linker CS, Helms CA, Fritz RC. Quadrilateral space syndrome: findings at MR imaging. *Radiology* 1993;188:675–676.

246. Seeger LL, Lubowitz J, Thomas BJ. Case report 815: tear of the rotator interval. *Skeletal Radiol* 1993;22:615–617.

247. Nobuhara K, Ikeda H. Rotator interval lesion. *Clin Orthop* 1987; 223:44–50.

248. Post M. Surgical and nonsurgical treatment. In: Post M, ed. *The shoulder.* Philadelphia: Lea and Febiger, 1978.

249. Clark JM, Sidles JA, Matsen FA. The relationship of the glenohumeral joint capsule to the rotator cuff. *Clin Orthop Rel Res* 1990;254:29–34.

250. Clark JM, Harryman DT. Tendons, ligaments and capsule of the rotator cuff: gross and microscopic anatomy. *J Bone Joint Surg* 1992;74A(5):713–725.

251. Harryman DT II, Sidles JA, Harris SL, Matsen FA III. The role of the rotator interval capsule in passive motion and stability of the shoulder. *J Bone Joint Surg Am* 1992;74:53–66.

252. Chung CB, Dwek JR, Cho GJ, Lektrakul N, Trudell D, Resnick D. Rotator cuff interval: evaluation with MR imaging and MR arthrography of the shoulder in 32 cadavers. *J Comput Assist Tomogr* 2000;24:738–743.

253. Ho CP. MR imaging of rotator interval, long biceps, and associated injuries in the overhead-throwing athlete. *Magn Reson Imaging Clin North Am* 1999;7:23–37.

254. Van Leersum M, Schweitzer ME. Magnetic resonance imaging of the biceps complex. *MRI Clin North Am* 1993;1:77–86.

255. Klug JD, Moore SL. MR imaging of the biceps muscle–tendon complex. *Magn Reson Imaging Clin North Am* 1997;5:755–765.

256. Chan TW, Dalinka MK, Kneeland JB, et al. MR imaging of biceps tendon dislocation. *Radiology* 1991;179:649–652.

257. Cervilla V, Shweitzer ME, Ho C, et al. Medial dislocation of the biceps brachii tendon: appearance at MR imaging. *Radiology* 1991;180:523–526.

258. Kido T, Itoi E, Konno N, Sano A, Urayama M, Sato K. The depressor function of biceps on the head of the humerus in shoulders with tears of the rotator cuff. *J Bone Joint Surg Br* 2000; 82:416–419.

259. Weishaupt D, Zanetti M, Tanner A, Gerber C, Hodler J. Lesions of the reflection pulley of the long biceps tendon. MR arthrographic findings. *Invest Radiol* 1999;34:463–469.

260. Greenway GD, Danzig LA, Resnick D, Haghighi P. The painful shoulder. *Med Radiogr Photogr* 1982; 58:22–67.

261. Zlatkin MB, Dalinka MKD. Crystal deposition diseases: current concepts. *Postgrad Radiol* 1988;8:88–98.

262. Arner O, Lindvall N, Rieger A. Calcific tendinitis of shoulder joint. *Acta Chir Scand* 1958;114:319–323.

263. McCarty DJ, Halverson PB, Carrera GF, Brewer BJ, Kozin F. "Milwaukee shoulder"—association of microspheroids containing hydroxyapatite crystals, active collagenase, and neutral protease with rotator cuff defects. I. *Clin Asp Arthritis Rheum* 1981; 24:464–472.

264. Burk DL Jr., Karasick D, Mitchell DG, Rifkin MD. MR imaging of the shoulder: correlation with plain radiography. *AJR* 1990;154:549–553.

265. Uhthoff HK, Sarkar K. Calicifying tendinitis. In: Burkhead WZ Jr., ed. Rotator cuff disorders. Baltimore: William and Wilkins, 1996:210–219.

266. Jerosch J, Strauss JM, Schmiel S. Arthroscopic treatment of calcific tendinitis of the shoulder. *J Shoulder Elbow Surg* 1998;7:30–37.

267. Loew M, Daecke W, Kusnierczak D, Rahmanzadeh M, Ewerbeck V. Shock-wave therapy is effective for chronic calcifying tendinitis of the shoulder. *J Bone Joint Surg Br* 1999;81:863–867.

268. Anzilotti KF Jr, Schweitzer ME, Oliveri M, Marone PJ. Rotator cuff strain: a post-traumatic mimicker of tendonitis on MRI. *Skeletal Radiol* 1996;25:555–558

SHOULDER INSTABILITY

MICHAEL B. ZLATKIN

GENERAL FEATURES

Instability is relatively common in the shoulder, and the shoulder is considered the most unstable joint in the human body. A simple definition of instability indicates that the humeral head slips out of its socket during activities. In the past, it was considered to be present only if a previous dislocation had occurred. Now more subtle degrees of instability are well recognized, including subluxation and instability that results from microtrauma rather than a single large episode of trauma, that may lead to labral injury (1). Although the humeral head may translate a small amount during daily activities, in these more subtle types of instability, movement that then causes pain resulting from spasm, or capsular stretching, is what is then considered instability. The traditional forms of instability should be differentiated from glenohumeral joint laxity, in which asymptomatic passive translation of the humeral head on the glenoid fossa is observed (2). Glenohumeral joint laxity and instability may, however, coexist.

Instability may be classified according to frequency (acute, recurrent, or chronic), degree (subluxation or dislocation), etiology, and direction (3). With respect to degree, in a dislocation no contact remains between the opposing surfaces of the glenoid cavity and humeral head. In a subluxation, abnormal translation of the humeral head in relation to the glenoid cavity is evident, but it is not accompanied by complete separation of the opposing articular surfaces (4). With regard to etiology, instability may result from one specific traumatic episode and be called *traumatic instability*. It may also arise from repetitive microtrauma in activities such as swimming or throwing. In addition, it may occur without any history of trauma at all, neither a single traumatic episode nor repetitive microtrauma, and in this situation, it is termed *atraumatic instability*. This latter type of instability is most often involuntary, but it can be voluntary as well (voluntary subluxation or dislocation) (5). These patients often have a coexistent history of congenital ligamentous laxity. Shoulder instability can also be described by direction as anterior, posterior, or inferior to the glenoid or multidirec-

tional (5,6). Anterior instability is by far the most common type of instability.

Functional instability is another term that has also been used in the description of instability, indicating derangement of the shoulder is caused by damage that may be confined to the glenoid labrum alone (5). This can result in mechanical dysfunction due to interposition of torn labral fragments between the articulating surfaces, causing the shoulder to catch, slip, or lock. In this situation, the shoulder may not exhibit subluxation or dislocation.

Another term that is in current use to define different types of minor instability, similar in some ways to the term *functional instability*, is *microinstability*. This condition is said to occur in some 5% of patients. It is a spectrum of disorders involving the upper half of the shoulder joint, as opposed to more traditional instability, which involves the lower third to half. Involved in the etiology of this process are such entities as a lax rotator interval, and there may also be history of overuse in these patients (7).

A useful classification of traditional glenohumeral stability consists of the acronyms TUBS and AMBRI (8). These separate instability into two broad categories. In the former, the *T* indicates that there has been prior trauma; the *U* that it is unidirectional, most commonly anterior; the *B* that there is a Bankart lesion; and the *S* that surgery is usually required and is successful in treatment. In the latter, *A* refers to atraumatic, *M* that is often in more than one direction (anterior and posterior or multidirectional), and *B* that it is often bilateral. The *R* and *I* refer to the fact that the initial line of treatment is rehabilitation, and if surgery is performed, it is an inferior capsular shift.

Stability of the shoulder is maintained by both the static and dynamic restraints of the glenohumeral joint. The static constraints include the bone outline of the glenohumeral joint but also the capsule and the labroligamentous structures. The dynamic constraints include the muscles and tendons that occur about the glenohumeral joint, in particular those of the rotator cuff (4). The stability of the glenohumeral joint is also affected by the size, shape, and tilt of the glenoid fossa (9,10). In patients with recurrent instability, the glenoid fossa and its contact area may be smaller than those in normal shoulders. In patients with posterior instability, retroversion of the glenoid cavity may be excessive.

ANTERIOR INSTABILITY

Clinical Features

The shoulder is an extremely mobile joint. This mobility thus allows for a considerable range of motion but also results in the joint being inherently unstable. As such, it is extremely prone to traumatic injuries such as subluxations, dislocations, recurrent dislocations, and permanent dislocations. That the shoulder is prone to dislocations has been known for a long time. The most detailed early description of anterior shoulder dislocation belongs to Hippocrates in the fifth century B.C.E. (11).

The presence of a shoulder dislocation implies that the apex of the humeral head circumference moves beyond the anterior lip of the glenoid (12). Anterior dislocations of the glenohumeral joint account for approximately 50% of all dislocations in the body. It is most common in young males. The mechanism is abduction, extension, and external rotation. These forces are applied to the arm, which then transfers them to the anterior capsule and ligaments. Subluxation of the glenohumeral joint indicates that an applied stress causes the humerus to move out of its normal relationship with the glenoid. In distinction to a dislocation, in a subluxation the apex of the humeral head, circumference does not move beyond the rim of the glenoid fossa. As opposed to a dislocation, a subluxation may be a subtle transient event that may be difficult to recognize (13).

Recurrent subluxation or dislocation (shoulder instability) is the most frequent complication of acute traumatic dislocation. When the initial event occurs between the ages of 15 and 35, the dislocations usually become recurrent or habitual. Once a second dislocation has occurred, the patient becomes a "recurrent dislocator." The recurrence rate in the younger age group of patients is very high, possibly as high as 80% to 90% (14). Recurrences usually occur in the first 2 years. The damage to the shoulder seems to occur at the time of the original trauma, although each redislocation may cause further damage. The incidence of recurrence seems to be inversely related to the severity of the initial trauma (13). There does not appear to be a relationship between the length and type of immobilization and the development of redislocation (15–17), although many surgeons still immobilize the shoulders of younger patients for up 6 weeks, in the hope of allowing the damaged tissues to heal (18). Recurrences are more common in men.

After the age of 40, the recurrence rate typically drops to 15% or less (19), although a subset of the older population, which includes those who are active and also have a high degree of generalized joint ligamentous laxity, remain predisposed (20). In older patients, the injury may often be to the more posterior supporting structures, rather than to the anterior structures. In these patients, the spectrum of lesions is different, and there is more often a tear of the rotator cuff or fracture of the greater tuberosity (21). The fractures of the greater tuberosity are often nondisplaced and occult at plain film evaluation, and they should be treated conservatively. One-third of these patients may avulse the subscapularis tendon and joint capsule from the region of the lesser tuberosity. These latter patients may then become unstable as well and may often be considered surgical candidates. The biceps tendon may also dislocate in these patients as a result of disruption of the transverse humeral ligament and other support structures of the biceps tendon in the groove arising in relation to or from the subscapularis.

As described earlier, anterior subluxation may also occur in the absence of a history of prior dislocation, due to repetitive trauma or excessive use, or it may develop without any history of trauma or excessive use as well (22).

Pathologic Lesions

Patients with recurrent subluxations and dislocations incur lesions to the capsular mechanism. Bankart (23) believed the essential lesion is detachment of the glenoid labrum and capsule from the anterior glenoid margin (13,23). Others believed the most important abnormality is a Hill-Sachs defect (24). Fractures of the inferior glenoid margin, insufficiency, stretching, or avulsion of the subscapularis muscle and tendon and stretching rather than actual detachment of the anterior capsule may also be important. Other factors include aplasia or hypoplasia of the glenoid, variations in contour of the glenoid fossa, excessive anteversion of the glenoid, increased anteversion of the humeral head, as well as muscle imbalances (25).

True Bankart lesions are more commonly found in patients with a history of complete traumatic dislocation. Patients with a history of a subluxating shoulder may experience just laxity or redundancy of the capsule, although labral lesions, fractures of the glenoid rim, and articular defects of the posterolateral humeral head may also be seen in these patients, particularly at arthroscopy (26); damage to the glenoid rim and Hill-Sachs lesions are, however, more frequently found in complete traumatic dislocation (27). Arthroscopic findings indicate that the lesion more commonly associated with anterior subluxation without a history of dislocation is caused by stretching of the anteroinferior glenohumeral ligament, which allows anterior translation of the humeral head on the glenoid fossa (28,29). Initially these may be the only abnormalities present. These lesions are difficult to document with imaging, although MR arthrography may be able to document the capsuloligamentous laxity; reliable criteria to assess this condition, however, have not been fully developed and described. With repetitive stress, further damage and involvement of the anteroinferior labrum and impaction of the articular cartilage of the posterolateral humeral head may occur, and these may be more easily visualized with MR and MR arthrography (30).

Bone Abnormalities

The two most common bone abnormalities are Hill-Sachs lesions and fractures of the inferior glenoid margin. A Hill-Sachs lesion is a specific indicator of a prior anterior glenohumeral joint dislocation. In 1940, Hill and Sachs published a clear and detailed review of the available information on the superolateral humeral head compression fracture that now bears their name (31). It is a posterolateral notch defect in the humeral head that is created by impingement of the articular surface of this portion of the humerus against the anteroinferior rim of the glenoid fossa. In Hill and Sach's original article (31), this lesion was found in 74% of their patients with recurrent anterior dislocations. It is most common in patients with recurrent anterior subluxation and dislocation (86%) (32). In patients with anterior subluxation alone, it is less common (25%) (33) and also uncommon in patients with multidirectional instability or patients with labral pathology not associated with recurrent subluxations or dislocations. Although the defect is seen in the majority of patients with acute anterior dislocations, the defect is larger when the humeral head is dislocated for a longer period of time and when the dislocations are recurrent (4). It is also larger with anteroinferior, rather than pure anterior dislocations.

Radiographically, the Hill-Sachs lesion appears as a sharp dense line running downward from the top of the humeral head to the area of the shaft, somewhat lateral to the midline, "a line of condensation" (34) (Fig. 7.1). Plain radio-

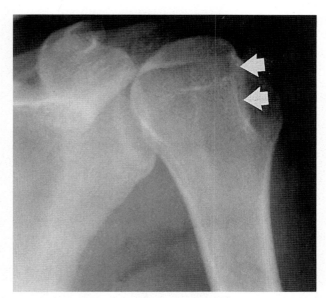

FIGURE 7.1. Plain radiograph in internal rotation demonstrating a large Hill-Sachs lesion. Note the sharp, dense line running downward from the top of the humeral head to the area of the shaft, "a line of condensation" (*white arrows*). Smaller lesions may be difficult to appreciate on conventional plain radiographs.

graphic delineation of these lesions is difficult if they are not large, unless special radiographic views or a combination of views are obtained (34). Many of these special views may be difficult to attain. Pavlov and coworkers indicated that internal rotation views and Stryker notch views were the best method of detailing these abnormalities with plain radiographs (35). A Stryker notch view is obtained by placing the patient supine and elevating the humerus, so that the palm of the hand supports the undersurface of the back of the head. The shaft of the humerus is parallel to the sagittal plane of the body, and the beam is angled 10 degrees cephalad, centered on the coracoid process.

The Hill-Sachs lesion that develops in these patients may be of variable size. When large, it involves the subchondral bone of the humeral head and meets the criteria for an osteochondral fracture. On MRI, Hill-Sachs lesions appear as wedgelike defects on the posterolateral aspect of the humeral head (Fig. 7.2). They are identified above the level of the coracoid process (36–39). They are best seen on axial images but may also be apparent on coronal and sagittal oblique images (Fig. 7.3) (39). Both the larger, more traditional Hill-Sachs lesions and the minor compaction injuries of the humeral articular cartilage and subchondral plates that may be more easily appreciated with arthroscopy (26,40) can be seen (36,37). Hill-Sachs lesions should not be confused with the normal posterolateral flattening seen in the inferior aspect of the humeral head (Fig. 7.4). This is typically present below the level of the coracoid, hence the importance of this landmark. They must also be distinguished from the bony lesions associated with posterosuperior internal glenoid impingement (Fig. 7.5) (see later discussion). Depending on their age, they may be associated with marrow edema (Fig. 7.2) or trabecular sclerosis. They should also be distinguished from cysts or erosions that may occur in a similar location but at the infraspinatus insertion site, as they are more angular in contour and associated with cortical depression (41).

MRI is highly accurate in the detection of Hill-Sachs lesions (42). In one study, MRI imaging was found to have a sensitivity of 97%, a specificity of 91%, and an accuracy of 94% in the detection of a Hill-Sachs lesion (42).

The osseous Bankart lesion (Fig. 7.6) is a defect in the anterior inferior margin of the glenoid rim (43) or ectopic bone formation at this site. This is produced by an anterior or inferior translation of the humeral head against this glenoid rim. These lesions may be difficult to visualize with conventional radiographs, but they can be observed with specialized views such as the West Point and Didier views (35). Cross-sectional imaging with either CT or MRI with or without intraarticular contrast injection can be helpful in depicting these lesions (34,44) and determining their size and location. It is generally thought that a large defect should be treated with bone grafting, but there is a lack of consensus with regard to how large a defect must be in order to necessitate this procedure. Some investigators have proposed that a defect must involve at least one-third of the glenoid surface

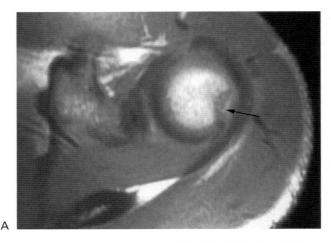

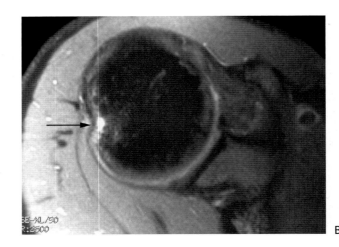

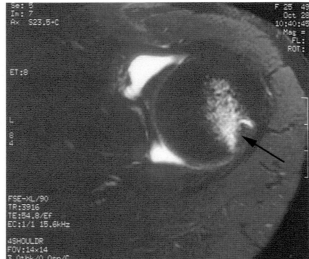

FIGURE 7.2. Hill-Sachs lesions. **A:** Axial T1-weighted image at the level of the coracoid process, TR/TE 800/17. A wedgelike defect is seen at the posterior superior lateral aspect of the humeral head (*arrow*). **B:** Axial fast spin echo proton density lesion with fat suppression in a different patient, TR/TE 2500/13. Similar findings of a wedgelike defect in the posterior lateral aspect of the humeral head are noted (*arrow*). **C:** Acute lesion. Axial fast spin echo T2-weighted image with fat suppression, TR/TE 3000/57. This patient had an acute dislocation a few days prior to this scan. Note the high signal margin of edema arising adjacent to the defect (*arrow*).

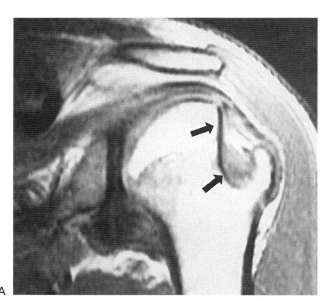

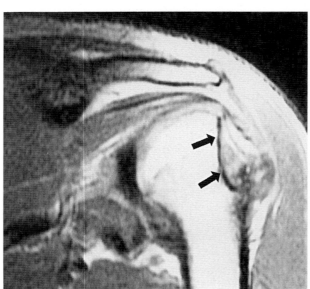

FIGURE 7.3. Hill-Sachs lesion, coronal images. **A, B:** Large Hill-Sachs lesion as seen on coronal oblique T1-weighted images (*black arrows*), TR/TE 800/20.

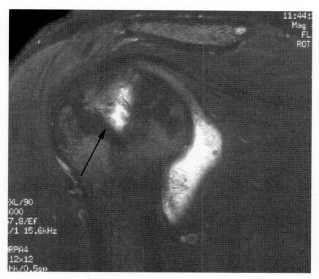

FIGURE 7.3 *(continued)*. C: Coronal oblique fast spin echo T2-weighted image, with fat suppression, TR/TE 3916/54. Similar pattern, large Hill-Sachs lesion with associated marrow edema *(arrow)*.

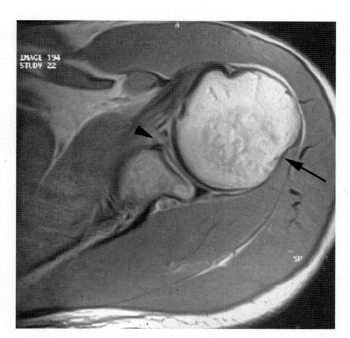

FIGURE 7.4. Normal humeral notch. Axial T1-weighted image, TR/TE 800/20. As distinct from the Hill-Sachs lesions, the normal humeral notch is seen below the level of the coracoid, is more posterior, and is somewhat broader *(arrow)*. A labral tear is present anteriorly *(arrowhead)*.

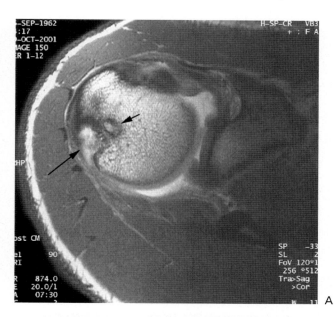

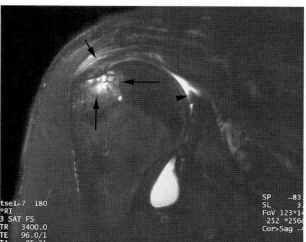

FIGURE 7.5. A, B: Axial image in A, TR/TE 874/20, reveals a small Hill-Sachs-like lesion *(long arrow)*, seen in this patient with posterosuperior subglenoid impingement. Also note the cysts or erosions anterior to this *(short arrow)*, which are also seen on the coronal oblique fast spin echo with fat suppression images in B *(long arrows)*. The marrow edema revealed on the image in B may be reactive to the cysts or due to the repetitive impaction. Note the rotator cuff tendinosis and posterosuperior labral increased signal *(small arrow)*, and contour change *(arrowhead)*.

in order to necessitate bone grafting (43,45). In a more recent study by Itoi and coworkers (43), a cadaveric study, they stated that an osseous defect with a width that is at least 21% of the glenoid length may cause instability and limit the range of motion of the shoulder after Bankart repair.

When large, the bony Bankart lesions may lead to reversal of the normal pear shape of the glenoid surface, a situation that promotes recurrent dislocations, CT scanning may reveal (44) periosteal reaction, fracture, bone erosion, and glenoid osseous rim attrition. The bony glenoid rim lesions may be easier to interpret with CT, especially fractures and ectopic ossification, although lesions in the subchondral bone and marrow are more easily identified with MRI. On

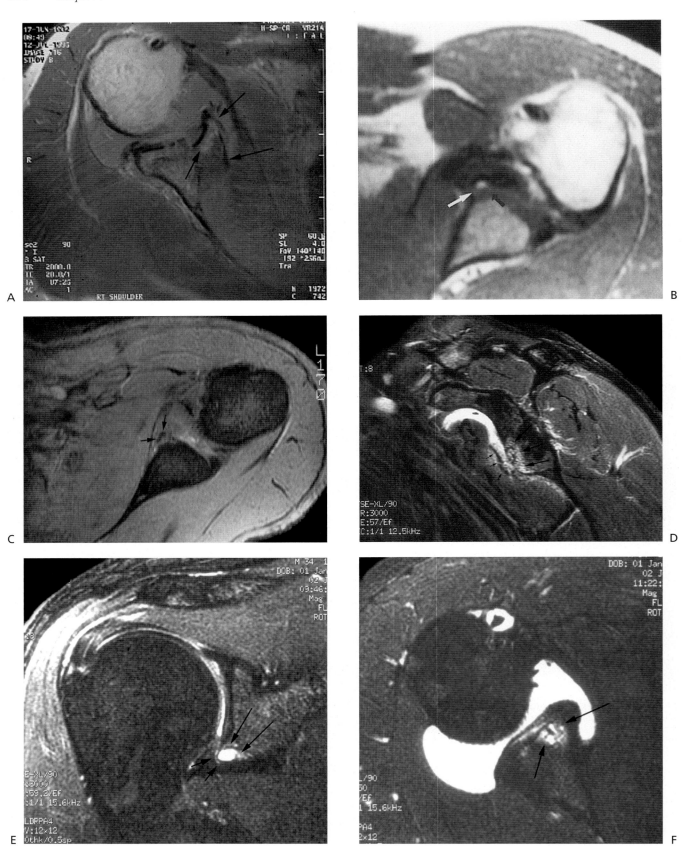

MRI, cystic change and sclerosis may be seen. STIR images and/or intermediate or T2-weighted MRI images with fat suppression in the sagittal oblique plane may particularly well depict bone and marrow alterations associated with Bankart lesions (Fig. 7.6).

LABRAL AND CAPSULAR AND LIAGAMENTOUS LESIONS

General Features

The soft-tissue lesions associated with recurrent anterior subluxation and dislocation include damage to the anterior glenoid labrum, associated glenohumeral ligaments (labroligamentous complex), anterior capsule, or both (46). Specifically, the "cartilaginous" lesion as originally described by Bankart has been considered to be an avulsion or tear of the glenoid labrum and/or stripping of the joint capsule (23). Rowe et al. (46) observed detachment of the capsule from the anterior glenoid rim in 85% of patients who underwent Bankart repair for recurrent anterior dislocation, and virtually all had some form of damage to the anterior glenoid labrum. The damage to the anterior labrum that is seen at surgery, however, may vary from detachment of the labrum from the glenoid rim, tears of the substance of the labrum, to a completely destroyed or absent labrum (46).

More recently, the term *injury* or *avulsion of the anterior inferior labroligamentous complex* has been used to describe the spectrum of soft-tissue injury associated with anterior instability. Cases of anterior glenohumeral joint instability are usually related to this region and, in particular, to the region of the anterior band of the inferior glenohumeral ligament. Failure of this complex may occur at its glenoid insertion site (70%–75%). The labrum tears as it is avulsed by the glenohumeral ligaments at the time of injury. Failure of this complex may also occur at its humeral insertion site (5%–10% of cases) or in its substance (15%–20%), whereby there will be capsular failure due to tear or laxity. Those associated with glenoid-sided failure include the Bankart lesion described earlier but also includes its variants, the Perthes lesion and the anterior labroligamentous periosteal sleeve avulsion (ALPSA lesion). Lesions associated with humeral failure include humeral avulsion of the glenohumeral ligament (HAGL) and its bone counterpart (BHAGL) lesion. Failure of this ligament

at both its glenoid and humeral insertion destabilizes both ends of the anterior band of the inferior glenohumeral ligament (floating avulsion of the inferior glenohumeral ligament AIGHL). These lesions are discussed in more detail later.

The current pathologic description of the anatomic lesion considered to be typical Bankart lesion would be an avulsion of the labroligamentous complex from the anteroinferior portion of the glenoid (47–49). In this lesion, the periosteum of the scapula is lifted and disrupted. It occurs at the 3 to 6 o'clock position but, as noted, may extend upward, and the free labroligamentous tissue may extend superiorly as well. The avulsed tissue may later adhere to its site of origin with fibrosis and scar formation. As noted previously, the soft-tissue lesion may be avulsed along with a piece of bone, the bony Bankart lesion, along the anteroinferior aspect of the glenoid rim. It may be displaced or nondisplaced and may heal back to the parent bone in a normal or malunited position.

Labral Lesions

Lesions of the glenoid labrum are considered to be a reliable sign of instability. When evaluating the glenoid labrum, one has to consider the variability in its shape and signal intensity. Normal variations of the attachments of the labrum, especially those that occur in the superior portion from the 11 to 3 o'clock position, have to be taken into consideration as well, including the sublabral foramen and the Buford complex. This has been discussed at length in Chapter 5 on anatomy. Nonetheless, pathology that occurs in the labrum associated with anterior instability typically occurs from the 3 to the 6 o'clock position. One also has to consider the intermediate signal that occurs in the sublabral zone, between the articular cartilage of the glenoid and the mainly dense fibrous tissue of the labrum itself. This region has been labeled the *transitional zone* (50), and its presence may cause diagnostic difficulty (Fig. 7.7). Another cause of difficulty is the occurrence of magic angle phenomena in the labrum, which can cause increased signal intensity on short TE, MR imaging sequences.

The criteria used to diagnose an abnormality of the glenoid labrum include alterations in its morphology and/or signal intensity or a combination of both (Fig. 7.8). The criteria may include labra that are visibly torn or ones that are

---

FIGURE 7.6. Glenoid margin alterations ("bony Bankart lesions"). **A:** Axial proton density–weighted image, TR/TE 2000/20. A large fracture fragment from the mid- to anterior inferior glenoid is seen in this patient, after anterior dislocation (*arrows*). **B:** Axial T1-weighted image, TR/TE 800/20. Small linear fracture at the anterior inferior glenoid margin (*arrows*), slightly displaced. **C:** Axial 2D gradient echo image, TR/TE 600/15, flip angle 70°. A small glenoid margin fracture is seen (*arrows*). **D:** Sagittal oblique T2-weighted fast spin echo image with fat suppression, TR/TE 3000/57. A large area of marrow edema of the anterior more inferior glenoid (*longer arrows*) parallels the labroligamentous avulsion anterior to it (*shorter arrows*). **E, F:** Coronal oblique **(E)** and axial **(F)** T2-weighted fast spin echo image with fat suppression, TR/TE 3000/57. There is anterior inferior glenoid marginal cystic change and edema, best seen in E (*longer arrows*). A small collection of fluid outlines the anterior inferior labral separation in E (*shorter arrows*).

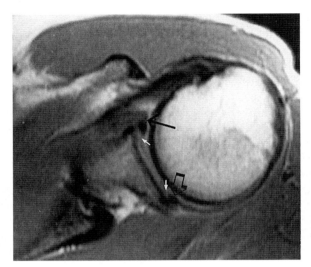

FIGURE 7.7. Axial MR image, TR/TE 2500/25. Note the low signal glenoid labrum that is triangular anteriorly (*black arrow*) and more round in appearance posteriorly (*open black arrow*). Note the normal appearance of the intermediate signal articular cartilage at the base of the labrum anteriorly and posteriorly (*small white arrows*), which should not be mistaken for a labral tear or detachment. This is the transitional zone. This appearance has also been termed *articular cartilage undercutting*.

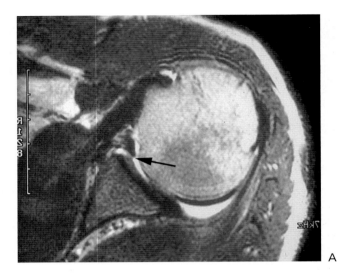

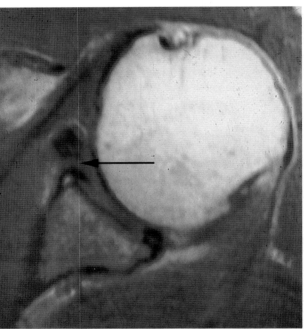

FIGURE 7.8. Labral lesions associated with anterior instability. **A:** Anterior labral separation outlined by fluid signal on an axial T2-weighted image (*arrow*), TR/TE 2500/70. **B:** Axial T1-weighted image, TR/TE 800/20. Chronic anterior labral detachment, with a globular thickened anterior labrum (*arrow*).

truncated or absent (51). A classification scheme has been developed for use on MRI. Although not commonly used, it may be helpful in diagnosis and in understanding the varied MRI appearances of the labrum in patients with chronic anterior instability. The labral lesions are generally not isolated findings but may occur in accompaniment with other pathology associated with Bankart lesions and their variants, including capsular lesions, and the bony defects described and discussed earlier. In this schema, the labral appearance is divided into four types, to aid in diagnosis (52). This schema may also, however, be applied in situations in which the labral pathology is not associated with a Bankart lesion. Increased signal within the labrum but not extending to the surface is type 1 and is consistent with the findings of internal labral degeneration (52) (Fig. 7.9). Histologically, there is evidence of eosinophilic and mucoid degeneration (50). A type 2 labrum is one whose signal is normal but shows significant morphological abnormalities whereby the labrum may be blunted, eroded, or frayed and irregular. A type 3 labrum has moderate or intense increased signal on short TR/TE, density-weighted, or gradient echo images, extending to the surface of the labrum, and it brightens on images with T2-weighted contrast or with fat-suppressed proton density images (Fig. 7.8A) or imbibe contrast into the defect at MR arthrography (Fig. 7.10). A type 4 labrum has the combined features of types 2 and 3. Labra with the signal and morphological alterations seen in types 2 through 4 are considered pathologic. Labral tears and altered labral morphology may be

highlighted on T1-weighted images with fat saturation following intraarticular gadolinium administration (30,47,53–56).

In the study by Goss (12), pathologic labra were classified as torn (type 1) when a line or band of intermediate signal intensity extended to the labral surface; degenerative (type 2) if the margin was ill defined, or abnormal signal intensity was present in the labral substance that did not extend to the labral surface; or eroded (type 3) when the labra were abnormally small or completely absent. Using these criteria, Gross

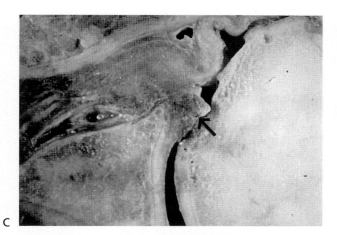

C

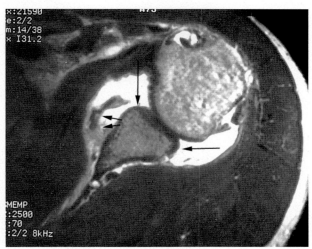

E

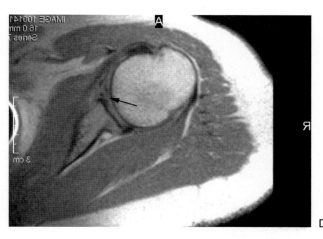

D

FIGURE 7.8 *(continued).* C: Axial cadaver section reveals a linear labral tear in the labral substance (*arrow*). **D:** Axial T1-weighted image, TR/TE 600/25, performed on a dedicated extremity magnet. There is a complex tear in the labral substance (*arrow*). **E:** Axial T2-weighted image, TR/TE 2500/70. The labrum is completely eroded anteriorly as well as posteriorly (*longer arrows*). Also note the capsule and inferior glenohumeral ligament is avulsed and attenuated (*shorter arrows*).

achieved a sensitivity of 90.6%, a specificity of 68.8%, and an overall accuracy of 83.3% in the evaluation of labral tears. According to the author, limited use of T2 may have contributed to the poorer specificity results.

Another morphological alteration of the labrum that may occur in patients with chronic instability is the development of a thick, low signal–displaced anterior labral fragment, which takes on a globular masslike appearance and may migrate anterosuperiorly and act like a loose body (Fig. 7.8B). Legan and coworkers (51) coined the term *GLOM sign* to refer to this glenoid labrum ovoid mass.

With gadolinium MR arthrography, contrast will extend into a labral defect (Fig. 7.10). This is the most specific finding for a labral tear. MR arthrography will also help outline morphological alterations of the labrum and will imbibe into areas of labral fraying in more degenerative type labral lesions. MR arthrography also best depicts labral detachment (Fig. 7.10), by allowing contrast to outline directly and distend out these abnormalities and increase the conspicuity of the labral separation. The diagnostic performance of MR

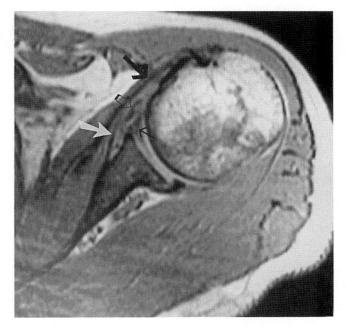

FIGURE 7.9. Axial 3D volume spoiled gradient echo image (SPGR), TR/TE 35/10, flip angle 50°. Increased signal in the labrum is not extending to the surface (*small black arrow*), reflective of internal degeneration. Such increased signal may also be difficult to distinguish from magic angle effects. The middle glenohumeral ligament is seen (*open black arrow*), separate from the labrum, and anterior capsule (*white arrow*) (*large black arrow*, subscapularis tendon).

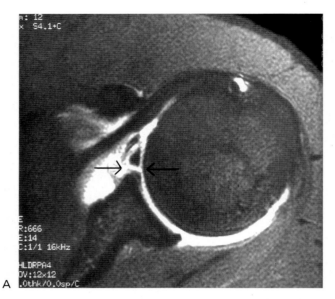

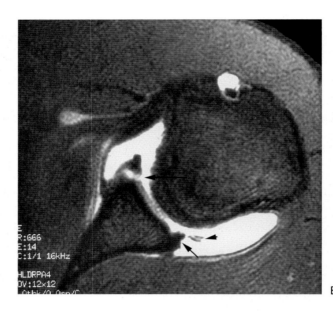

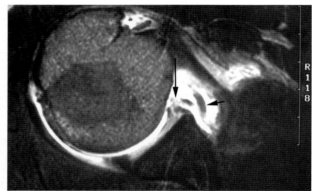

FIGURE 7.10. MR arthrography and labral lesions. **A, B:** Axial T1-weighted MRI arthrogram images, TR/TE (666/14). A tear and detachment of the anterior mid- to inferior labrum is seen, outlined by the high signal contrast (*longer arrows*). Also note the blunted irregular posterior labrum in B (*shorter arrow*), with an associated small displaced fragment (*arrowhead*). **C:** Axial T1-weighted MRI arthrogram image, TR/TE (800/20). In another patient, contrast outlines and imbibes into a complex tear in the anterior labrum (*longer arrow*). Note the attenuated glenohumeral ligament (*middle*) anterior to this (*shorter arrow*).

imaging for labral tears indicates a high sensitivity and specificity, although MR arthrography is better at distinguishing labral separations and detachments (50,52,53,57,58). MR arthrography in the axial oblique plane performed with abduction and external rotation (ABER) may improve the sensitivity of MRI to anterior glenoid labral tears in some situations, including nondetached tears near the attachment of the inferior glenohumeral ligament (59).

The labrum has been divided into six quadrants: I, superior; II, anterior superior; III, anterior inferior; IV, inferior; V, posterior inferior; VI, posterior superior (Fig. 7.11). As noted, labral tears associated with anterior instability usually occur in the anterior inferior portion, related to the inferior glenohumeral ligament—thus the term the *labral capsular ligamentous complex* (60). This complex is best depicted with MR arthrography (30,47,56,61,62). It should be noted, however, that not uncommonly the labral tear may then extend superiorly along the entire anterior glenoid margin (63, 64), beyond the regions of insertion of the superior and middle glenohumeral ligament, to the region of the biceps labral complex (Fig. 7.12). In one study of 45 patients using

MR arthrography, 9 of 27 labral tears associated with anterior instability had this distribution (30). Isolated anterosuperior or superior quadrant labral tears (discussed later) including SLAP lesions are not usually seen in patients with recurrent anterior subluxation or dislocation; although they may cause pain and a sensation of instability with throwing (65), they are generally considered to be more stable lesions or related to functional instability. However, some SLAP lesions may be seen in patients with instability.

The diagnostic performance of MRI and MR arthrography in the evaluation of labral tears has been evaluated in other studies. Iannotti, Zlatkin, and coworkers (52), in a study of 39 patients using conventional MRI and correlating with arthroscopy and surgery, found MRI to have a sensitivity of 93% and a specificity 87%. Conversely, Garneau (52a), in a small study relying only on axial images using two observers, found that one observer achieved a sensitivity of 44.4% and a specificity of 66.7%; the second observer had a sensitivity of 77.8% and a specificity of 66.7%. Gusmer, Potter, and coworkers (57) in a more recent larger study of 103 patients, also using conventional MRI, found a sensitivity of

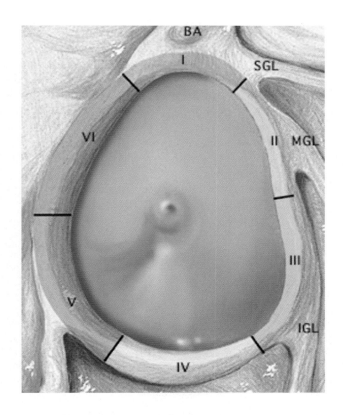

FIGURE 7.11. Sagittal diagram outlining the labral quadrants: superior, anterior, inferior, and posterior. Since the anterior and posterior aspects of the labrum are also divided into superior and inferior segments, there are six segments in total: I, superior; II, anterior superior; III, anterior inferior; IV, inferior; V, posterior inferior; VI, posterior superior. BA, biceps anchor; SGL, superior glenohumeral ligament; MGL, middle glenohumeral ligament; IGL, anterior band inferior glenohumeral ligament.

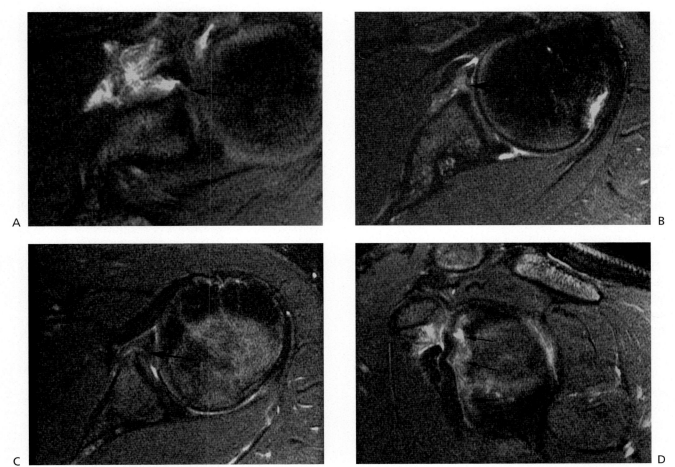

FIGURE 7.12. Anterior inferior labral tear extending into the anterior superior segment (*arrows*) (Bankart lesion with superior extension). **A–C:** Axial fast spin echo T2-weighted image with fat suppression, TR/TE 3100/55. **D:** Sagittal oblique fast spin echo image with fat suppression, TR/TE 2800/57.

89% and a specificity of 97%. MRI was found to be most sensitive in the evaluation of anterior labral tears and less sensitive in superior and posterior tears. Chandnani and co-workers (53) studied 30 patients who underwent MR imaging, followed by MR arthrography after intraarticular injection of 25 ml of a dilute solution of gadopentetate dimeglumine. Twenty-eight of 30 patients also underwent CT arthrography after intraarticular injection of air and radiographic contrast material, and the researchers compared their findings to arthroscopy and surgery. At surgery, labral tears were found in 28 patients; a detached fragment was found in 26 patients. The labrum was found to be degenerated in 18. A labral tear was detected on MR images in 93%, on MR arthrograms in 96%, and on CT arthrograms in 73%. A detached labral fragment was detected on MR images in 46%, on MR arthrograms in 96%, and on CT arthrograms in 52%. Labral degeneration was detected on MR images in 11%, on MR arthrograms in 56%, and on CT arthrograms in 24%. MR arthrography was the best of the three imaging techniques for showing the inferior part of the glenoid labrum and inferior glenohumeral ligament. They concluded that MR arthrography and MR imaging both showed labral tears with greater sensitivity than CT arthrography did. In addition, MR arthrography was the most sensitive of the three techniques for detecting a detached labral fragment and labral degeneration. In a study of 65 patients, using MRI arthrography, Tirman and coworkers (56) found a sensitivity of 89% and a specificity of 98% in the evaluation of labral tears. Similarly, Palmer and coworkers (30), in a study of 48 patients also using MR arthrography, found a sensitivity of 91% and a specificity of 93%.

Capsular Lesions

In patients with shoulder instability after one or repeated dislocations and or subluxations, there may be traumatic avulsion of the capsule from its glenoid insertion. In the latter circumstance, the capsule would be peeled back to the neck of the scapula with the first and subsequent dislocation. This is described as *capsular stripping* or *shearing*.

The insertion of the anterior capsule has been described as being of three types. Type 1 inserts in or near the labrum, types 2 and 3 more broadly along the scapular neck (66). The normal posterior capsule inserts directly into the labrum. The variations of capsular insertions (2 and 3) have been considered to be either developmental by some or pathologic by others, related to traumatic avulsion. Differentiation of "normal variation" in the appearance of the capsule from stripping related to traumatic avulsion on imaging studies may be determined by observing a disruption of the soft-tissue mantle that extends from the site of capsular attachment to the glenoid labrum. In addition, this abnormal appearance of the capsule tends to occur more inferiorly than a medial capsule that occurs as a variant of normal. Earlier studies

found an association of type 2 and 3 capsules with recurrent anterior dislocations (52). More recent studies using MR arthrography questioned the usefulness of the type 3 capsule as a predictor of anterior instability (55,56,58). These studies found no correlation in the perceived capsular insertion type and glenohumeral instability as found on subsequent examination under anesthesia or as implied by the lesions discovered at surgery.

The anterior inferior capsule and associated glenohumeral ligaments (especially the anterior band of the inferior glenohumeral ligament) can often be best seen in nonarthro-

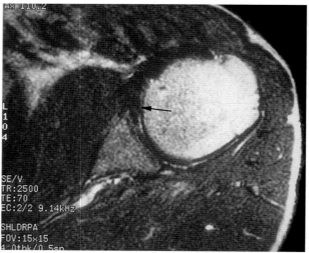

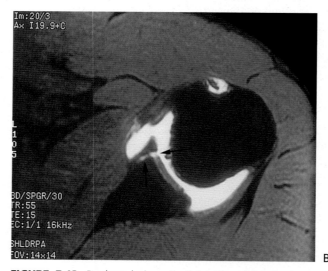

FIGURE 7.13. Bankart lesion. **A:** Axial T2-weighted sequence, TR/TE 2500/70. The absence of a joint effusion, the lack of fat suppression or improved contrast resolution of a T2* gradient echo sequence, limits visualization of the injury to the inferior labroligamentous complex (*arrow*). **B:** Axial T1-weighted MRI arthrogram in the same patient, TR/TE (800/20), reveals clear evidence of detachment of the anterior inferior labroligamentous complex from the glenoid margin (true "Bankart" lesion) (*arrows*).

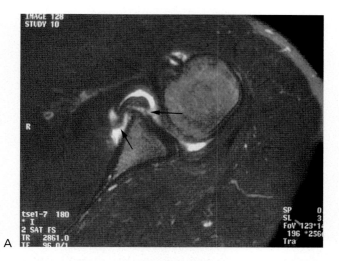

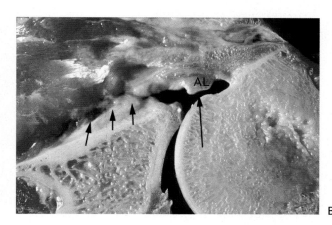

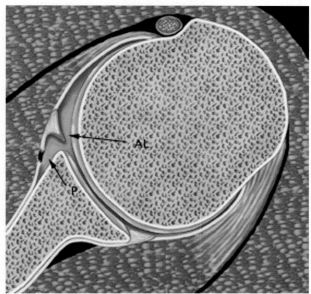

FIGURE 7.14. Bankart lesion. **A:** Axial fast spin echo T2-weighted image with fat suppression, TR/TE 2861/96. There is again evidence of detachment of the anterior inferior labroligamentous complex from the glenoid margin (true "Bankart" lesion) (*arrows*). **B:** Axial cadaver section from a specimen subjected to simulated dislocations in the laboratory. Tear and detachment of the anterior labrum are seen (*long arrow*), with disruption of the capsule and scapular periosteum (*arrows*). AL, anterior labrum. **C:** Artist's rendering of a Bankart lesion depicting the anterior labroligamentous tear and detachment with disruption of the scapular periosteum. AL, anterior labrum. P, scapular periosteum.

graphic MR examination on fast spin echo proton density, intermediate, or T2-weighted images with fat suppression, or with T2*-weighted 2D gradient echo techniques, particularly when there is a significant effusion. In the absence of an effusion, MR arthrography is very useful especially to identify clearly the anterior inferior labrum and inferior glenohumeral ligament (Fig. 7.13). With injury to this region, fluid or contrast may also be seen to extend beneath the soft-tissue mantle. In a typical Bankart lesion, the labrum will be torn or detached with the capsular structures, and fluid signal or contrast may extend within or beneath the labrum as well (Figs. 7.13, 7.14). The assessment of the capsule should be at the midglenoid or below, since on the more superior images, a distended subscapularis bursa or medial capsular insertion may mimic capsular stripping (64). Evaluation of

capsular stripping may then better reflect disruption of the anterior inferior labral ligamentous complex (67).

BANKART LESION VARIANTS

The discussion so far has focused on the typical lesion of anterior instability, which is the Bankart lesion (23), indicating an avulsion of the anterior inferior labrum, capsule, and inferior glenohumeral ligament complex, with an associated disruption of the scapular periosteum (Figs. 7.12–7.15). As noted earlier, this may occur with or without an injury to the bony glenoid (bony Bankart). In many cases, the labral lesion may extend to involve the midanterior and superior anterior labrum as the tear dissects upward (Fig. 7.12). The extent

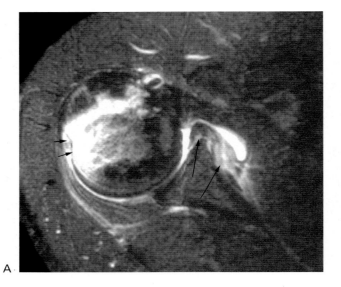

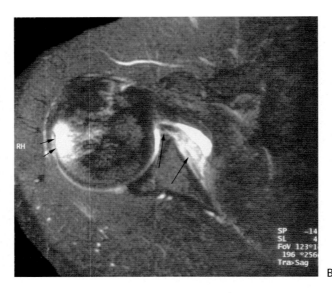

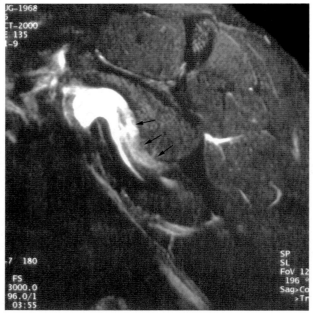

FIGURE 7.15. Bankart lesion. **A, B:** Axial fast spin echo T2-weighted image with fat suppression, TR/TE 3000/72. Note the injury to the anterior capsulolabroligamentous complex with disruption of the scapular periosteum (*longer arrows*). While the soft-tissue component of the lesion is nicely depicted with the use of fat-suppressed images and the presence of the effusion (contrast that with the image in Fig. 7.13A), the labral separation/detachment is not as well depicted as when the joint is distended with MR arthrography (see Fig. 7.13B) Also note the acute Hill-Sachs lesion (*shorter arrows*). **C:** Sagittal fast spin echo T2-weighted image with fat suppression, TR/TE 3000/72. Sagittal oblique images help reveal the extent of the injury, from superior to inferior (*arrows*) (see also Fig. 7.12D).

and nature are often best depicted with MR arthrography (53,55). There are, however, a number of variants of this typical lesion.

Perthes Lesion

This lesion was first described in the early 1900s by the German physician, Perthes (68). This lesion (68) is a labral ligamentous avulsion in which the scapular periosteum remains intact but is stripped medially (Fig. 7.16). The periosteum may then become redundant, and recurrent instability may occur as the humeral head moves forward into this region of acquired laxity (pseudojoint). The labrum may then lay back

down into a relatively normal position on the glenoid and resynovialize (heal back). It may then be very difficult to diagnose because the detachment may not be easily identified on conventional MRI or even on MR arthrography (Fig. 7.17) or at arthroscopy, unless specialized imaging positions, such as ABER, are employed (Fig. 7.17) (69,70, 159). With distension from MR arthrography and when needed with ABER positioning, only subtle displacement of the labral tissue may be seen (Fig. 7.17).

Wischer and coworkers (70) evaluated the use of MR imaging in the characterization of the Perthes lesion by correlating MR findings with findings at arthroscopy. They found that the use of a combination of axial and abduction-

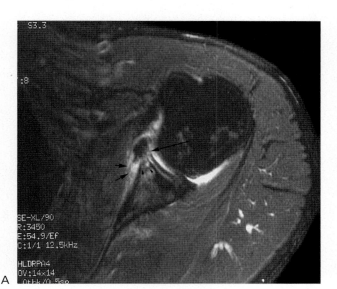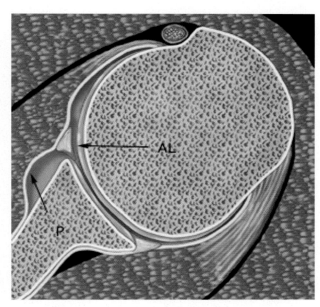

FIGURE 7.16. Bankart lesion variant: Perthes lesion. **A:** Axial fast spin echo T2-weighted image with fat suppression, TR/TE 3450/55. The labrum has healed back in near-normal position (*arrow*). The scapular periosteum is intact (*smaller arrows*) but mildly redundant. The edema and cystic alterations in the anterior inferior bony glenoid (*arrowheads*) help confirm the clinical diagnosis of anterior instability and point out the subtle soft-tissue MRI findings. MRI arthrography with ABER positioning as seen in Figure 7.17 may have been of benefit in this patient. **B:** Artist's depiction of a Perthes lesion. Note the detachment of the labroligamentous complex with the labrum resting in a relatively normal position on the glenoid margin (*AL*). There is an intact scapular periosteum that may become redundant (*P*).

external rotation position sequences on MR images (Fig. 7.17) can be helpful in the diagnosis of a Perthes lesion. A fluid-filled joint with capsular distension, caused by either a large amount of effusion or MR arthrography, was found to be helpful in outlining Perthes lesions. Adding the abduction-external rotation position to the protocol in patients in whom Perthes lesion was suspected increased the diagnostic accuracy and may reveal a Perthes lesion not visible on axial images, as was the case in 50% of the patients in their series.

Anterior Labroligamentous Periosteal Sleeve Avulsion

The ALPSA lesion (71) is anterior labroligamentous sleeve avulsion. In these cases, the scapular periosteum does not rupture, resulting in a medial displacement and inferior rotation of labroligamentous structures as they are stripped down to the scapular neck (peel-back lesion, which has been described as being similar to the rolling up of a shirt sleeve) (Figs. 7.18–7.20). The ALPSA lesion may then heal in this displaced position. This has also been termed a *medialized Bankart lesion*. A small cleft or separation can be seen between the glenoid margin and the labrum. With a chronic ALPSA lesion, fibrous tissue is deposited on the medially displaced labral ligamentous complex, and the entire lesion

then resynovializes along the articular surface (Figs. 7.18, 7.19). This lesion is associated with recurrent anterior dislocation of the glenohumeral joint owing to the resultant incompetence of the anterior portion of the inferior glenohumeral ligament. This may leave a deformed and redundant labrum.

This lesion may require a different repair than the typical Bankart lesion and therefore is important to recognize (71). In the chronic situation, the lesion may be difficult for the arthroscopist to find because it can be difficult to make the distinction as to whether the heaped-up region medially that is covered by synovium is labrum or synovial-lined fibrous tissue deposited on a medially displaced labrum. MRI may help in making this distinction (72), especially if there is an effusion present; however, since MR arthrography delineates the anterior inferior region of the labrum and capsule best, this approach is valuable in diagnosing such lesions (Figs. 7.19, 7.20) (55,58,69). MR arthrography in the ABER position may be valuable as well (Fig. 7.19), as the medial displacement can be visualized at the insertion point of the inferior glenohumeral ligament into the underlying glenoid. In the absence of an effusion, the ALPSA lesion may be missed on conventional MRI if the lesion does not extend to the midanterior labrum, as the fibrous medialized resynovialized mass can appear strikingly normal on MRI imaging (Fig. 7.19) in a patient with a paucity of joint fluid and magic angle artifact (67).

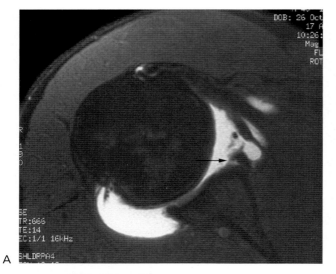

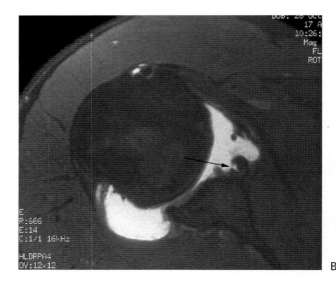

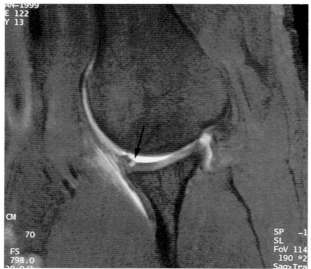

FIGURE 7.17. Bankart lesion variant: Perthes lesion. **A, B:** Axial T1-weighted MRI arthrogram images, TR/TE (666/14). The anterior labroligamentous complex has healed back in a near-normal position. The MR arthrogram images outline only subtle displacement of the labral tissue (*arrows*). **C:** Axial oblique (ABER) T1-weighted MRI arthrogram image, TR/TE (798/20), in another patient. Again only subtle displacement of the labral tissue is seen (*arrow*), in this case made visible only by carrying out imaging in this position.

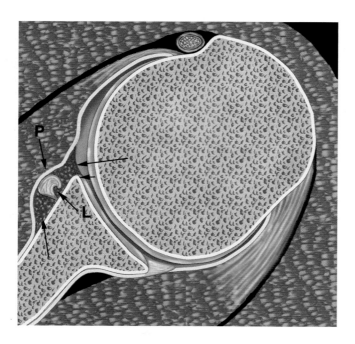

FIGURE 7.18. Bankart lesion variant: ALPSA lesion. Artist's depiction of a chronic lesion. The scapular periosteum remains intact. The labroligamentous complex is rolled up and displaced medially (*L*). Thick fibrous tissue surrounds this complex (*long arrows*) and separates the labrum from its expected location on the glenoid margin (*short arrow*). *P*, intact scapular periosteum.

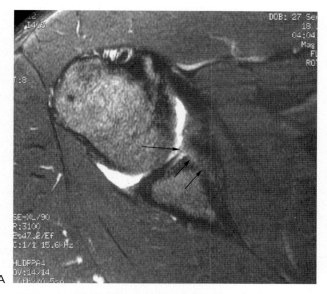

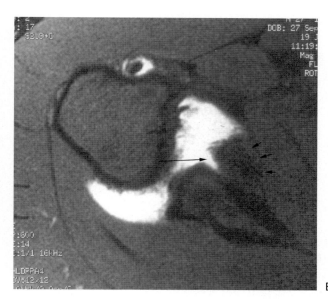

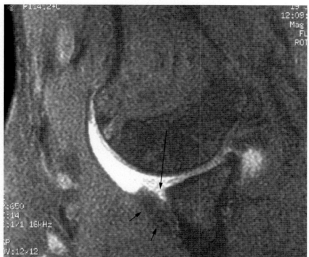

FIGURE 7.19. Bankart lesion variant: chronic ALPSA lesion. **A:** Axial fast spin echo T2-weighted image with fat suppression. Even though there is a small effusion, the fibrous medialized resynovialized mass of intermediate signal intensity is difficult to discern on conventional MRI images (*arrows*). **B:** Axial T1-weighted MRI arthrogram images, TR/TE (600/14). A cleft of contrast material (*long arrow*) outlines the anteromedially displaced healed over mass of labroligamentous tissue (*short arrows*). **C:** Axial oblique T1-weighted images taken in the ABER position; TR/TE 650/14 reveals the cleft of contrast (*long arrow*) and the thickened, anteromedially displaced mass of labroligamentous tissue to good advantage (*arrows*).

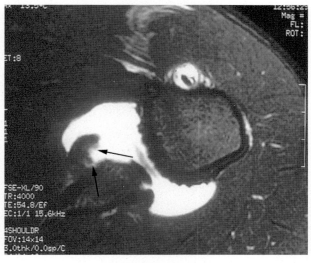

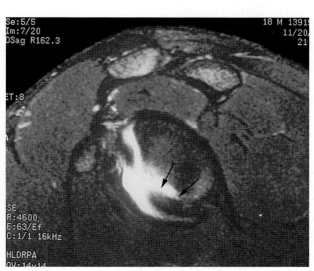

FIGURE 7.20. Bankart lesion variant: ALPSA lesion. Axial **(A)** and sagittal oblique **(B)** fast spin echo MR arthrogram images with fat suppression; TR/TE 4000/54 **(A)** and 4600/64 **(B)**. The thickened, anteriorly and medially displaced labroligamentous tissue, with intact scapular periosteum (*arrows*), is identified, after distension with intraarticular fluid.

Capsular and Intraligamentous Tears

These lesions may occur with anterior dislocation of the glenohumeral joint. In this case, there may be a tear of the middle portion of the capsule in association with the anterior band of the inferior glenohumeral ligament (73). These lesions usually occur at the time of the initial dislocation. In the acute stage, contrast may extravasate through the defect at MR arthrography, and periosteal bone formation may occur along the scapula at the site of injury in the more chronic situation.

Humeral Avulsion of the Glenohumeral Ligament

The HAGL lesion refers to *humeral avulsion of the glenohumeral ligament* (74–76). This lesion more typically occurs in individuals older than 30 years (76). It may be seen in conjunction with tear of the rotator cuff or fracture of the greater tuberosity of the humerus. It is not uncommonly associated with a tear of the subscapularis tendon. This lesion can be seen on conventional MR imaging as well as with MR arthrography (Fig. 7.21) (58,74). On MRI examination, the torn glenohumeral ligament may appear thick, wavy, and irregular, with increased signal intensity (74). MR arthrography may also show contrast material extravasating from the joint through the capsular disruption, at its humeral insertion. It may be feasible to repair this lesion arthroscopically via reattachment to the humerus using sutures. Recently the HAGL lesion was also seen after successful Bankart repair (77).

When patients avulse their subscapularis from the lesser tuberosity, they also avulse the glenohumeral ligament and capsule in association (Fig. 7.22). The HAGL lesion, however, refers to the situation when the subscapularis is not involved.

The bony humeral avulsion of the glenohumeral ligaments (BHAGL) (78) is a rare lesion that may occur after anterior dislocation of the shoulder. There is a bone fragment that may appear similar to a bony glenoid avulsion. Computed tomography or MRI can show that the bone is attached to the glenohumeral ligaments and does not originate from the glenoid, but rather from the bone at the site of humeral attachment of the inferior glenohumeral ligament. Treatment is through open excision of the bony fragment and reattachment of the glenohumeral ligaments to their origin on the anterior aspect of the humerus.

Glenoid and Humeral Avulsion of the Inferior Glenohumeral Ligament Complex

Recurrent anterior unidirectional shoulder instability is most commonly associated with an avulsion of the glenoid attachment of the labroligamentous complex (Bankart lesion). However, additional capsular injury is often considered necessary to allow anterior dislocation. Field and coworkers (79) described five patients undergoing surgical stabilization for recurrent anterior instability who were noted to have not only a classic Bankart lesion but also a complete disruption of the lateral capsule from the humeral neck. Repair of this "floating" anterior inferior glenohumeral ligament (AIGHL) (Fig. 7.8E) was accomplished by reattachment of the medial

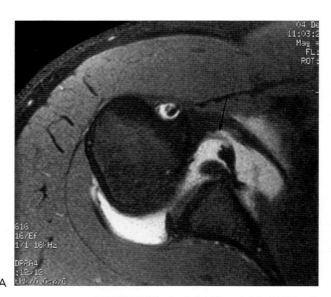 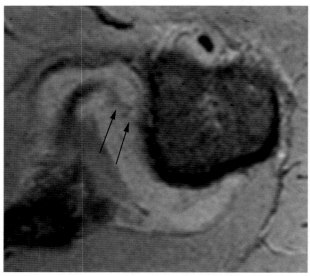

FIGURE 7.21. A: Axial T1-weighted MRI arthrogram image, TR/TE (616/16). The humeral attachment of the glenohumeral ligament is considerably attenuated (*arrow*). **B:** Axial fast spin echo proton density–weighted image, with fat suppression, TR/TE 2000/25, in a different patient than in A. A frayed, thinned, partly avulsed anterior band of the inferior glenohumeral ligament is seen (*arrows*). (Figure 7.21B courtesy of Javier Beltran MD, Brooklyn, NY.)

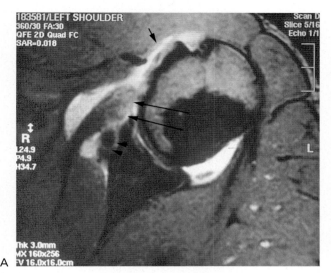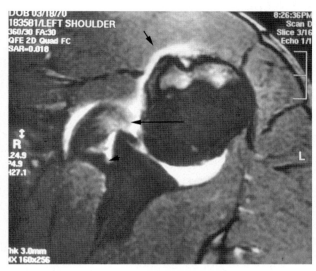

FIGURE 7.22. A, B: Axial 2D gradient echo images after the injection of intraarticular contrast, TR/TE 360/30 flip angle 30°. The subscapularis tendon is avulsed with the humeral attachments of the glenohumeral ligament and joint capsule (*long arrows*). Fluid and contrast extravasates out of the joint anteriorly and laterally (*short arrows*). Also note the medial and anterior displacement of the glenoid attachments of the labroligamentous complex (*arrowheads*).

and lateral capsular disruptions and has led to excellent postoperative function in these patients. A similar lesion was described by Warner and Beim (80), who also attained good results with treatment of both these lesions.

POSTERIOR INSTABILITY

Posterior instability of the shoulder is not well understood, in part because it is uncommon but also because of the confusion in terminology differentiating posterior subluxations and dislocations (81). Additionally, posterior labral tears may be less diagnostic of posterior instability than anterior labral lesions are for anterior instability (82–84). Posterior labral tears and capsular lesions may be found in patients with predominantly anterior instability, perhaps as a secondary phenomenon.

Isolated posterior instability is uncommon and accounts for only 5% of instability. Acute posterior dislocations of the glenohumeral joint are rare. They represent approximately 2% to 4% of all dislocations of the shoulder (85), and nearly all bilateral posterior dislocations are caused by epileptic convulsions. They may occur following trauma but are commonly associated with electric shock or seizures. They are managed with reduction and conservative measures. Recurrence is not common in this situation.

Recurrence is very common with atraumatic posterior dislocations and in patients with a history of a traumatic dislocation when large bony defects of the humerus and glenoid occur (86). The clinical situation of recurrent posterior subluxation rather than dislocation is, however, the more common lesion (87,88). Overuse, as in athletics (88), is usu-

ally involved in this circumstance rather than this circumstance developing after a traumatic dislocation. Abduction, flexion, and internal rotation are the mechanisms involved (swimming, throwing, and punching). This is a situation of repeated microtrauma. These patients, often young athletes, may present with pain rather than signs of instability. There may be some association with posterior laxity (89).

The posterior band of the inferior glenohumeral ligament is a primary static stabilizer of the glenohumeral joint with respect to translation posteriorly of the humeral head. Injury sufficient to cause posterior instability, however, requires injury to the posterior inferior labroligamentous complex as well as the posterior capsule. Pathologic findings in patients with prior posterior dislocations and resultant instability may be the reverse of those for recurrent anterior dislocations and include posterior labral and capsular detachments and tears, as well as posterior capsular laxity (82,90,91). An impaction type defect on the anteromedial aspect of the humeral head is known as a reverse Hill-Sachs lesion (notch sign or trough lesion). It is produced on the humeral head by the posterior cortical rim of the glenoid. It becomes larger with multiple posterior dislocations. Fractures off the posterior glenoid margin may also occur, not only from direct forces from an anterior direction, which push the humeral head out posteriorly, but also with dislocations due to indirect types of forces, such as those that occur during seizures or accidental electric shock. Deficiency of the posterior glenoid rim may also be a factor in patients with posterior instability, especially those with an atraumatic origin (92). Fractures of the lesser tuberosity may also develop during the process of a posterior dislocation. This is the result of considerable tension on the insertion of the subscapularis tendon.

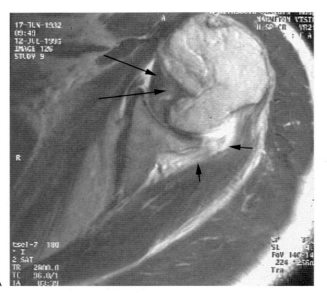

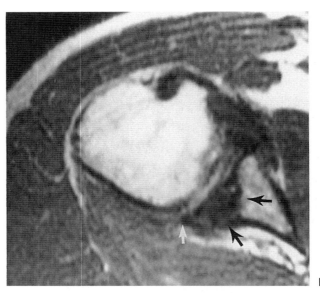

FIGURE 7.23. Posterior instability, bone lesions. **A:** Axial T2-weighted fast spin echo image, TR/TE 2800/96. There is a large bony defect on the anteromedial aspect of the humeral head consistent with a "reverse Hill-Sachs deformity" (*long arrows*). The posterior labrum and capsule are disrupted as well in this patient subsequent to a posterior dislocation (*short arrows*). **B:** Axial T1-weighted MR scan, TR/TE 800/20. Decreased signal intensity is present in the marrow of the mid- and posterior glenoid (*black arrows*) in this patient with a clinical history of posterior instability. The posterior labrum is also blunted (*white arrow*).

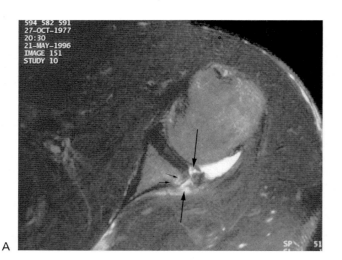

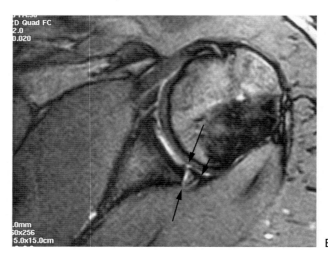

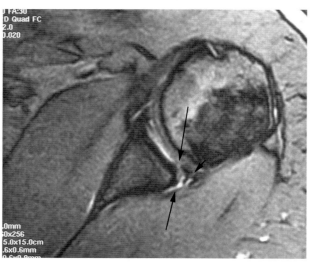

FIGURE 7.24. Posterior instability, posterior labroligamentous lesions. **A:** Axial T2-weighted fast spin echo image, TR/TE 2800/96. There is detachment of the posterior labroligamentous structures along the posterior inferior glenoid (reverse Bankart lesion) (*long arrows*). Note the edema in the posterior glenoid margin (*short arrows*). **B, C:** Axial 2D gradient echo images, TR/TE 360/30 flip angle 30°. There is evidence of both posterior labroligamentous detachment from the bony glenoid margin (*long arrows*) and a tear in the posterior labral substance (*short arrows*).

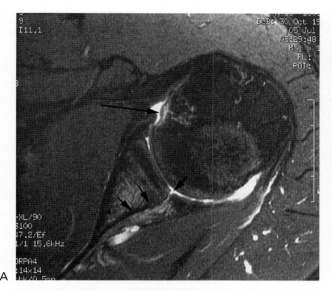

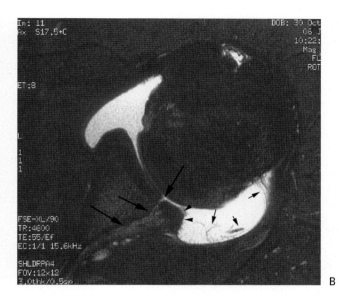

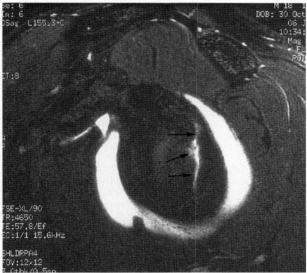

FIGURE 7.25. Posterior instability, posterior labroligamentous lesions, and MRI arthrography. **A:** Axial T2-weighted fast spin echo image with fat suppression, TR/TE 3100/47. The posterior glenoid labrum and capsule are torn along the posterior glenoid margin (*short arrows*). There is a bony defect on the anteromedial aspect of the humeral head consistent with a "reverse Hill-Sachs deformity." It is associated with marrow edema (*long arrow*). **B:** Axial T2-weighted fast spin echo image with fat suppression, TR/TE 4600/55, carried out after intraarticular fluid injection. With the joint distended, the capsulolabroligamentous tear is again noted (*larger arrows*). The posterior margin of the labrum is seen to be blunted (*arrowhead*), and there are some thickened synovial folds seen in the distended joint capsule now evident (*small arrows*). **C:** Sagittal oblique T2-weighted fast spin echo image with fat suppression, TR/TE 4650/57, carried out after intraarticular fluid injection. The superior inferior extent of the labral tear/detachment is seen best in this projection, outlined by the fluid signal and joint distension in this study (*arrows*).

The subscapularis tendon may be stretched or detached, and tears of the teres minor tendon my occur.

Posterior labrocapsular periosteal sleeve avulsion (POLPSA) has also been described. Due to the attachment of the posterior capsule to the posterior portion of the labrum, which in itself is attached to the posterior scapular periosteum, stripping of the labrum by the posterior capsule may result in a posterior labrocapsular periosteal sleeve avulsion (93).

The MR and MR arthrographic findings associated with patients with posterior instability mirror those described for anterior instability, except they involve the posterior capsule and labrum. The impaction-type defect on the anteromedial aspect of the humeral head, known as a *reverse Hill-Sachs lesion* (notch sign or trough lesion), is well seen on MRI images (Fig. 7.23). MRI and MR arthrography may be used to identify the presence and extent of a tear and detachment of the posterior labroligamentous complex (Figs. 7.24, 7.25).

Although the posterior capsule is injured, the capsular abnormalities may be less prominent than in anterior instability (94). MR-evident abnormalities that involve the bony glenoid include findings of marrow edema or sclerosis and cystic lesions, the nature of which often depends on the chronicity of the lesion (Figs. 7.23, 7.24). This is due to recurrent impaction or contusion of the bony glenoid by the humeral head with recurrent subluxations or dislocations. In patients with atraumatic recurrent posterior subluxation, joint laxity with redundancy of the posterior capsule may be the most prominent finding, and a posterior labral tear may not be found (95–97). This may also be associated with inferior redundancy (81,98,99), in which case multidirectional instability may result.

MR arthrography may be the only means of revealing this laxity (Fig. 7.25). Another clinical situation that may develop is in patients with chronic anterior instability, in

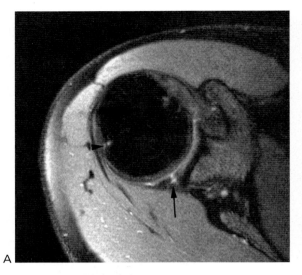

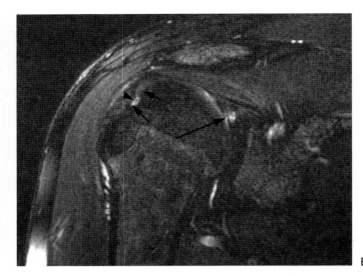

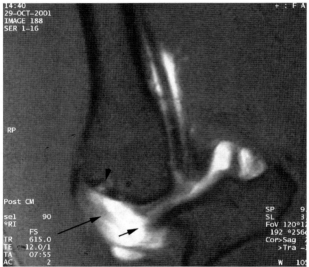

FIGURE 7.26. Posterior superior subglenoid impingement. **A, B:** Axial proton density–weighted fast spin echo image with fat suppression, TR/TE 3100/30, and coronal oblique T2-weighted fast spin echo image with fat suppression **(A)**, TR/TE 3100/55 **(B)**. A tear in the posterior superior labrum is seen (*longer arrow*), There is tendinosis and undersurface fraying of the infraspinatus tendon in B (*small arrows*) and a small posterior superior humeral head cyst (*arrowhead*). **C:** Axial oblique images T1-weighted images taken in the ABER position, TR/TE 615/12, in another patient. The posterior labrum is frayed and irregular (*short arrow*), there is some flaplike undersurface tearing of the posterior rotator cuff (*longer arrow*), and there is some cystic change in the posterior superior aspect of the humeral head (*arrowhead*). This constitutes the triad of changes seen in posterior superior subglenoid impingement.

whom secondary posterior abnormalities may develop (Figs. 7.8E, 7.10B). The outcome of this may be a situation of combined or bidirectional instability. MR and MR arthrography may demonstrate many or all the pathologic lesions recorded for recurrent anterior and posterior subluxations and dislocations that have been described previously (69). Treatment of posterior instability initially consists of conservative measures with exercise programs for the posterior musculature. Surgery may then be employed only if the disability and pain persist.

Isolated posterior labral tears are uncommon. They may occur due to direct trauma. They can also be seen in patients with anterior, posterior, bidirectional, or multidirectional instability. MRI will reveal high signal outlining of such lesions with brightening on images with T2 contrast, more conspicuous with fat suppression. Contrast will extravasate within or beneath such lesions at MR arthrography. Patients with posterosubglenoid impingement may develop posterior

labral fraying or attenuation, or even frank tears (100) (Fig. 7.26). Posterior labral tears, of course, may also be a component of tears of the superior labrum, anterior, and posterior (SLAP) (101) lesions, as discussed in more detail later. Certain contact athletes may develop posterior labral detachment (Fig. 7.27). In one series, this lesion was specific to contact athletes who engage their opponents with arms in front of the body, such as offensive lineman in football (102).

Bennett Lesion

The Bennett lesion is specific injury of the posterior labrum that occurs in overhead throwers such as baseball pitchers (103). It is associated with a posterior undersurface rotator cuff injury and ossification in the soft tissues adjacent to the posteroinferior glenoid (Fig. 7.28). Although originally thought by Bennett to be related to traction by the tendon

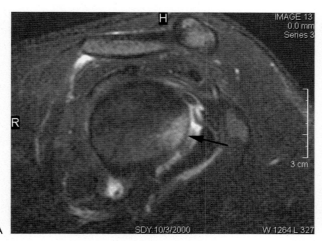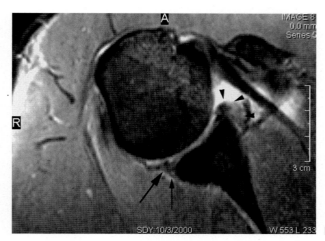

FIGURE 7.27. Posterior labral tear from contact sports: 18-year-old high school football player injured while blocking. **A:** Sagittal oblique fast spin echo T2-weighted image, TR/TE 2500/55. Edema is seen in the anteromedial aspect of the humeral head, indicating an acute reverse Hill-Sachs-like injury (*arrow*). **B:** Axial proton density–weighted fast spin echo image with fat suppression, TR/TE 3100/30. The posterior labrum is torn in its substance and irregular (*arrows*). Note the anterior labroligamentous tissues also appear blunted and irregular (*arrowheads*).

of the long head of the triceps muscle, it is now felt to be related to a posterior capsular avulsive injury related to traction by the posterior band of the inferior glenohumeral ligament, due either to posterior subluxation of the humeral head during the cocking motion of pitching or to posterior deceleration forces in follow-through (103). Recently, this lesion has also been discussed as an indicator of posterosuperior glenoid impingement (104).

The characteristic bone lesion can be seen on plain films, on CT scanning, and with conventional MRI as a crescent-shaped region of mineralization at the posteroinferior aspect of the glenoid rim, consistent with a Bennett lesion, arising

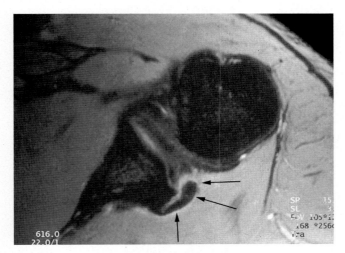

FIGURE 7.28. Bennett lesion, axial 2D gradient echo image, TR/TE 616/22, flip angle 25°. Note the large low signal focus of ossification in the soft tissues posterior to the posteroinferior glenoid (*arrows*).

at the insertion of the posterior joint capsule (104,105). The soft-tissue lesions in the rotator cuff, labrum, and capsule may be identified with conventional MRI (104,105), but they are perhaps best identified with MR arthrography.

MULTIDIRECTIONAL INSTABILITY

The concept of multidirectional instability (MDI) is a symptomatic glenohumeral subluxation or dislocation occurring in more than one direction (106). It is extremely relevant for the surgeon, in patients with unstable shoulders, to identify patients who are unstable in multiple directions, as they represent a separate subgroup in whom the history and physical exam can be confusing. In some of these patients, there may be a psychological component to the problem; in these cases, surgery may not be helpful. This is particularly true for patients who are voluntary dislocators. The direction of instability may be anterior or posterior and include an inferior component, or it may exist in all three directions. The basic causative factor is an abnormality of the soft-tissue elements that renders the joint hypermobile. This may be due to various degrees of inherent ligamentous laxity. Multidirectional instability is most often due to atraumatic factors.

Multidirectional instability may also occur following one or more episodes of significant trauma in contact sports or repetitive minor injury and stress on the capsule (microtrauma), as in gymnastics or overhead manual labor (106–108). An enlarged redundant joint capsule may be observed. Labral and capsular abnormalities similar to those in anterior and posterior instabilities may be seen, but less commonly (106–109) (Fig. 7.29). Not infrequently, the MRI exam may be completely normal, or the labrum may just appear small

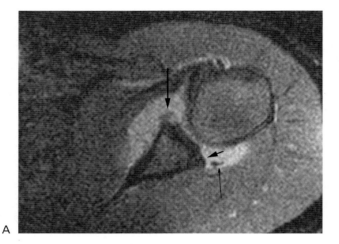
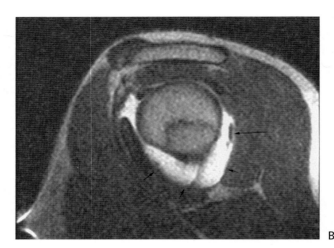

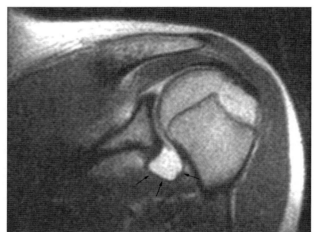

FIGURE 7.29. Multidirectional instability: 14-year-old female basketball player with atraumatic subluxations. **A:** Axial short tau inversion recovery weighted (STIR) image. The anterior labrum is blunted (*larger arrow*) and irregular; the posterior labrum is small (*smaller arrow*). There is a broad, medial capsular insertion along the anterior glenoid, outlined by the large effusion. The low signal focus in the posterior aspect of the joint is seen to be a thickened adherent area of capsular thickening on the sagittal image in B (*long thin arrows*). **B:** Sagittal oblique fast spin echo T2-weighted image, TR/TE 2550/80. Note the broad redundant joint capsule, anteriorly, posteriorly, and inferiorly (*shorter arrows*). There is an adherent fold of thickened capsular tissue seen posteriorly (*long thin arrow*). **C:** Coronal oblique fast spin echo T2-weighted image, TR/TE 2500/80. Note the prominent axillary recess, posteriorly, outlined by the joint effusion (*arrows*).

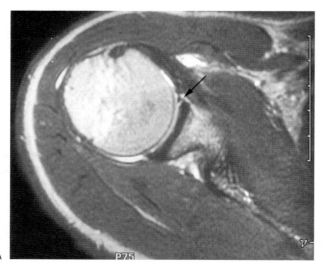
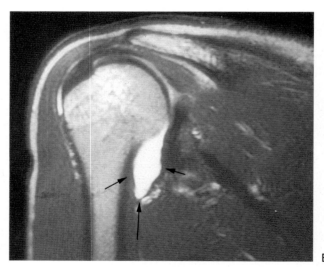

FIGURE 7.30. Multidirectional instability: 19-year-old female with involuntary dislocations. **A:** Axial T2-weighted image, TR/TE 2500/80. The anterior labrum is small and blunted, with a small area of separation at the glenoid attachment (*arrow*). **B:** Coronal oblique T2-weighted image, TR/TE 2500/55. There is a prominent axillary recess (*arrows*).

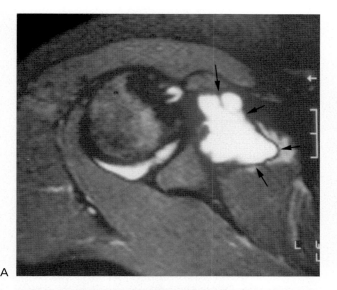

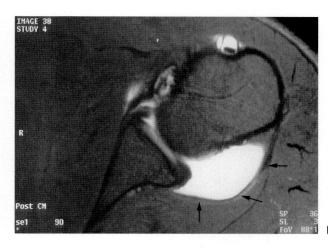

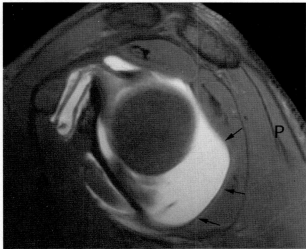

FIGURE 7.31. Multidirectional instability, MRI arthrography. **A:** Axial T1-weighted MRI arthrogram image, TR/TE (800/20). There is a broad, distended anterior inferior capsule identified (*arrows*). **B, C:** Axial (B) and sagittal oblique (C) T1-weighted MRI arthrogram images, TR/TE (616/16), in another patient. There is posterior and inferior capsular redundancy outlined by the intraarticular injection (*arrows*).

or have a degenerative appearance, especially in cases of atraumatic multidirectional instability (Fig. 7.30). Although difficult to quantify objectively, intraarticular injection of fluid and contrast may be the only way to assess the degree of redundancy of the capsule and ligaments (Fig. 7.31). It should be noted, again (this point has been discussed in the section on anterior instability), that patients with primarily anterior instability clinically, with evidence of a Bankart lesion, may occasionally have a posterior labral tear visualized. This is likely due to traction force applied to the posterior capsulolabral complex, in anterior subluxation or dislocation (94).

Therapy in these patients is usually initially conservative. Most patients with MDI can be treated successfully by conservative methods, such as patient education, a shoulder girdle–strengthening program, or modification of the patient's routine activity. There may be a high incidence of failures following operative treatment. If conservative therapy fails,

treatment may be some variation of the inferior capsular shift (107,108,110) or some other form of capsular shrinkage or ablation, which may be thermal and done arthroscopically (111,112).

CHRONIC DISLOCATIONS

Chronic dislocations are primarily found in the elderly. Although there is no strict rule as to when a dislocation is considered chronic, 3 weeks is an acceptable period to define them (113). Chronic anterior dislocations are more common than posterior (76% vs. 24%) (114), although the relative incidence of posterior dislocations that are chronic is higher than their proportionate number of dislocations overall (2%–4%). This implies that while posterior dislocations are infrequently encountered, they are more commonly

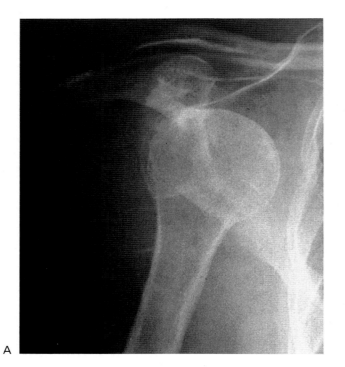

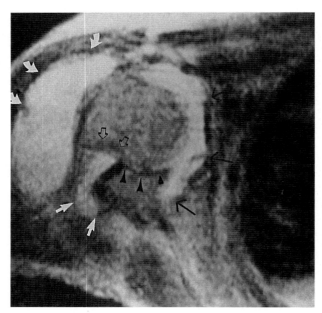

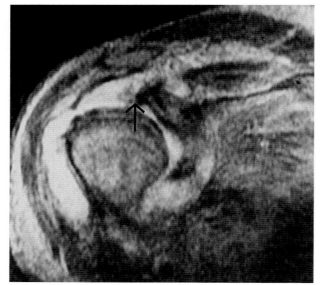

FIGURE 7.32. Chronic anterior dislocation: 77-year-old female with history of falls and recent stroke. **A:** Plain radiographs reveal an anterior dislocation. **B, C:** Axial MRI scan, TR/TE 2500/80, confirm the anterior dislocation. The anterior capsule is markedly redundant and bowed anteriorly by fluid (*black arrows*). Similar changes are present in the posterior capsule (*white arrows*). The glenoid labrum is completely effaced. The anterior glenoid margin is markedly resorbed with the humeral head is resting in this region of bone resorption (*arrowheads*). A small Hill-Sachs deformity is present (*open black arrows*). There is a massive amount of fluid present in the subdeltoid bursa (*curved white arrows*), due to a large rotator cuff tear. The cuff tear is seen in the coronal oblique images in **C** (*black arrow*).

missed (114,115). Chronic dislocations usually occur in elderly people and in people with impaired mental status, as these situations may prevent them from seeking help at the time of diagnosis. In elderly patients, the dislocation may be produced by a trivial injury, since with increasing age the soft-tissue supports become weaker and degenerated (116,117). The patient's history in relation to the time of injury and subsequent disability may be confusing and quite inadequate. The usual complaint is loss of motion and pain in the shoulder. In younger patients, the late diagnosis of an

old unreduced dislocation may arise when the patient is unconscious for some time at the time of initial injury and has multiple other injuries.

The usual soft-tissue and osseous pathology of traumatic dislocation is present in these patients. However, now reparative processes and degenerative changes in both the osseous and soft-tissue elements of the joint are superimposed, thereby compounding the magnitude of the pathology (Figs. 7.18, 7.19).

The usual modes of treatment in patients with chronic dislocations include (a) the decision to leave the shoulder

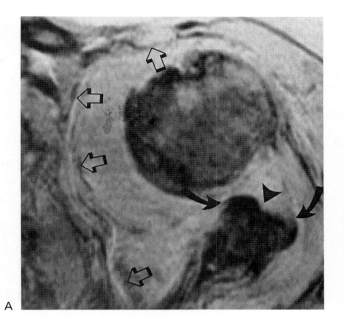

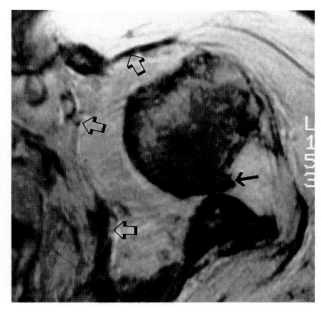

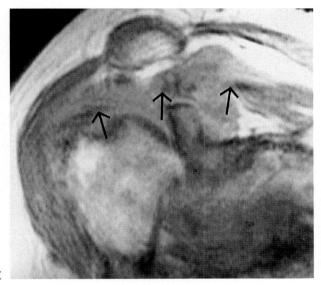

FIGURE 7.33. Chronic anterior dislocation. **A–C:** Axial 2D gradient echo images, TR/TE 400/13, flip angle 70° **(A, B)**. Coronal oblique image, proton density–weighted image, TR/TE 2500/25 **(C)**. Similar changes to those in Figure 7.32 are present in this older female patient. The humeral head is anteriorly dislocated in **A** and **B**. The capsule is markedly redundant and distended by fluid (*open black arrows in A and B*). The anterior and posterior labrum is absent (*curved black arrows in A*). An osteophyte is present on the humeral head in **B** (*black arrow*), and there is irregularity of the glenoid articular surface seen in A (*arrowhead*), indicating secondary degenerative arthritis. A large rotator cuff tear is also present (*black arrows in C*).

dislocated and attempt to regain as much motion as possible with physical therapy, (b) closed reduction, (c) open reduction, (d) insertion of a shoulder prosthesis, and (e) shoulder fusion. The prognosis is often not good with any of these methods. Although MRI is not commonly employed in these patients, it can be of value to help establish the chronicity of the lesion, if this is not clear. In addition, it is very effective in determining the extent of the bone and soft-tissue lesions that are present, in order to help decide the best mode of therapy in the individual patients. In the small number of patients whom my colleagues and I have imaged with chronic anterior dislocations, we have observed exten-

sive injury to the anterior and posterior capsular structures, the rotator cuff, as well as acute and chronic changes to the glenoid and humeral head (Figs. 7.32, 7.33).

Another difficult clinical problem is the locked posterior dislocation (115). In these patients, the diagnosis is often missed, and the dislocations then become chronic; therefore, early diagnosis is important. These cases may frequently be associated with fracture of the tuberosities or humeral neck. Cross-sectional imaging including both CT and MRI can be helpful in establishing a diagnosis in these cases. They can also be useful in assessing the extent of bone and soft-tissue injury and can therefore help guide treatment (Fig. 7.34).

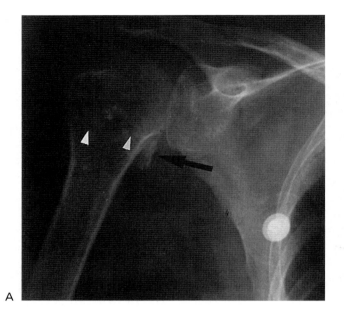

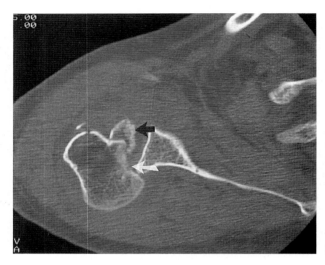

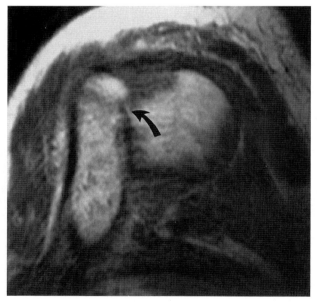

FIGURE 7.34. Locked posterior dislocation. **A:** Plain radiographic exam reveals a posterior dislocation, with a medial fracture fragment (*black arrow*). There is a suggestion of a nondisplaced fracture of the humeral neck (*white arrowheads*). **B:** Axial CT scan after an attempted reduction. This confirms the persistent posterior dislocation. The fracture fragment has arisen just medial to the lesser tuberosity and is blocking reduction. **C:** Sagittal T1-weighted MR scan, TR/TE 600/20, also after the attempted reduction, in addition now reveals an angulated fracture of the humeral neck (*black arrow*).

ISOLATED LABRAL TEARS INCLUDING SLAP LESIONS

The labrum can tear in the absence of demonstrable subluxation or dislocation. Some have termed this clinical situation as *functional instability* of the shoulder. The tears that have been described in this circumstance include flap or bucket handle tears, and at arthroscopy, these lesions may be present in the anterior superior portion of the labrum. They may respond to arthroscopic excision. Isolated glenoid labrum lesions may also occur in the throwing athlete, as fraying or separation in the superior quadrant of the labrum, adjacent to the origin of the long head of biceps. These patients present with a painful catching or snapping sensation, during throwing. This is related to overloading of the biceps tendon and subsequent avulsion of the superior part of the labrum during the follow-through, when the muscle eccentrically contracts to decelerate the elbow and to provide compressive force to the glenohumeral joint. The tearing of the labrum may be caused by the biceps tendon actually detaching portions of the glenoid labrum. In the throwing athlete, these lesions in the labrum may be associated with pathology in the rotator cuff (Fig. 7.35). Injuries that are seen in the rotator cuff, often partial tears of the rotator cuff undersurface more posteriorly, when associated with lesions in the posterior glenoid labrum, have been described as the "kissing le-

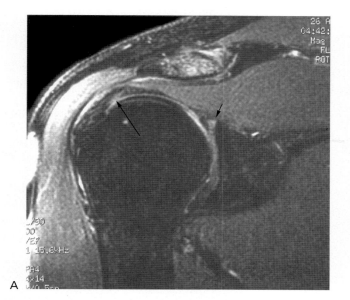

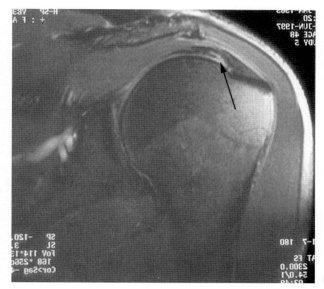

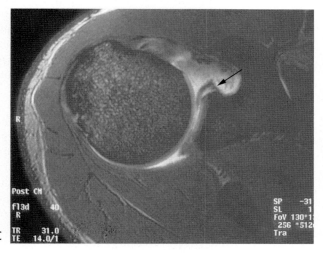

FIGURE 7.35. Superior labrum, rotator cuff lesions. **A:** Coronal oblique T2-weighted fast spin echo image, with fat suppression, TR/TE 3200/55. A tear in the superior labrum (*short arrow*) is accompanied by a small low-grade partial tear of the supraspinatus tendon undersurface (*long arrow*). **B, C:** Coronal oblique T2-weighted fast spin echo image, with fat suppression, TR/TE 2300/54 (**B**), reveals a flaplike partial tear of the posterior supraspinatus undersurface (*arrow*). Axial 3D gradient echo MRI arthrogram image (**C**) demonstrates contrast extending into a tear of the anterior superior labrum (*arrow*).

sion" (117). This lesion occurs in extreme external rotation, with the humeral head abutting against the labrum during the cocking phase of throwing. These labral lesions, as well as the accompanying cuff abnormalities, are often difficult to depict with conventional MRI. They are often subtle in nature, and there is often little or no associated fluid in the joint to outline their presence. MR arthrography (Fig. 7.35) is extremely useful in such cases, as these are often patients who are athletes with high demands for the shoulder, and the need is high for a precise diagnosis. Again, MR arthrography will leak into labral tears, imbibe into areas of labral fraying, detects areas of separation or detachment, and leak or imbibe into undersurface cuff injuries.

A similar situation is now more commonly described as *posterosuperior subglenoid impingement*, discussed more fully in Chapter 6 on the rotator cuff (118–124). This lesion is also known as *internal impingement* (125). This lesion occurs during the late cocking phase of throwing with abnormal contact between the posterosuperior portion of the glenoid rim and the undersurface of the rotator cuff, and it is thought to occur at the extremes of abduction and external rotation. A triad of findings have been described in association with this lesion (Figs. 7.5, 7.26), including injury to the rotator cuff undersurface at the junction of the infraspinatus and supraspinatus tendons, degenerative tearing of the posterosuperior glenoid labrum, as well as subcortical cysts and chondral lesions in the posterosuperior glenoid and humerus due to repetitive impaction. The lesion on the humerus may at times simulate a Hill-Sachs lesion (Fig. 7.5). There may in addition be an injury to the inferior glenohumeral ligament and anterior inferior labrum. The inferior glenohumeral ligament may be injured because it limits abduction in external rotation of the glenohumeral joint and is therefore under tension in this position.

SLAP Lesions

Snyder introduced the term for defining injuries to the superior portion of the labrum and adjacent biceps tendon (126, 127). A superior quadrant labral tear with anterior and posterior components of the tear is labeled a *SLAP lesion* (superior labrum anterior posterior) (128) (Fig. 7.14). This lesion may be more common than originally thought; however, a recent study by Handelburg and coworkers (129) found a similar incidence of such lesions as in Snyder and coworkers' (127) original series. These lesions may be acute or chronic, and, when acute, they may result from a fall on the outstretched arm, with the shoulder in abduction and forward flexion. Patients complain of pain, greater with overhead activity, and a painful popping or catching in the shoulder. It also may occur in athletes requiring repetitive overuse of the arm (130), including baseball, tennis, or volleyball. The injury to the superior portion of the glenoid labrum may result from sudden forced abduction of the arm. It results from excessive traction related to sudden pull from the long head of the biceps tendon. The lesion may typically begin posteriorly and then extends anteriorly, and it terminates at or before the midglenoid notch. It includes the biceps labral anchor.

SLAP tears were categorized into four basic types by Snyder and coworkers (127) (Fig. 7.36). Type 1 reveals superior labral roughening and degeneration. The labrum remains firmly attached to the glenoid. These represent 10% of SLAP lesions. This lesion is quite common in elderly persons and may represent a degenerative tear of the labrum. In younger, more athletic individuals, it may represent a traumatic injury. Type 2 is the most common lesion, representing 40% of all SLAP lesions. Type 2 represents a detachment of this roughened superior portion of the labrum and its biceps tendon anchor. As noted later, these lesions may be further subclassified based on their extension either anteriorly or posteriorly. Type 3 represents 30% of SLAP lesions. It is a bucket handle tear of the superior portion of the labrum. It does not involve the biceps labral anchor. The superior portion of the labrum is detached from both the glenoid and the biceps tendon and may be displaced into the joint space. The appearance is similar to that of a bucket handle tear of the knee meniscus (131). Type 4 represents 15% of SLAP lesions. It has, in addition to the bucket handle tear, a split tear of the biceps tendon.

Burkhart (130) describes three distinct categories of type 2 SLAP lesions: (a) anterior, (b) posterior, and (c) combined anteroposterior. Posterior type 2 SLAP lesions have distinct clinical and anatomical features that distinguish them from anterior type 2 SLAP lesions. Posterior and combined type 2 SLAP lesions can be disabling to overhead-throwing athletes apparently because of resultant posterosuperior instability and anteroinferior pseudolaxity that are present in these patients. Rotator cuff tears are frequently associated with posterior or combined anterior posterior SLAP lesions, and typically they begin as undersurface tears. Repair of posterior SLAP lesions can return overhead-throwing athletes to full overhead athletic functioning. The peel-back mechanism is a likely cause of posterior type 2 SLAP lesions.

Additional types of SLAP lesions have been described (132) (Fig. 7.37). Type 5 is a Bankart lesion of the anterior inferior labrum that then extends superiorly to include separation of the biceps tendon anchor. Type 6 lesions are unstable radial or flap tears that also involve separation of the biceps anchor. A type 7 lesion consists of anterior extension of the SLAP lesion to involve the middle glenohumeral ligament. Additional lesions that have been added to the list now include a type 8 lesion, which extends posteroinferiorly, with extensive detachment of the posterior labrum; and a type 9 lesion, which is complete concentric avulsion of the labrum circumferentially around the entire glenoid rim (127,133).

The pathogenesis of SLAP lesions may vary depending on the type of lesion present. Type 1 and 2 lesions may be related to athletes engaged in overhead activity and patients with atraumatic instability. Type 5 and 7 lesions may be seen in patients with shoulder instability after an acute traumatic episode. Type 2 lesions are associated with acute traction injuries. As noted earlier, a peel-back mechanism may be implicated in the posterior type 2 lesion. A fall on the outstretched hand may produce a type 3, 4, or 5 lesion.

MRI and MR arthography may be used in the detection of SLAP lesions (101,134–137) (Figs. 7.38–7.43). In the study by Cartland and coworkers (102), on MRI exam, type 1 lesions exhibit irregularity of the labral contour with mildly increased signal intensity. Type 2 lesions may reveal a globular region of increased signal interposed between the superior labrum and glenoid margin. Type 3 shows typical linear increased signal extending to the labral surface. Type 4 lesions show high signal within the superior labrum, extending into the proximal biceps tendon.

SLAP lesions may be difficult to detect on conventional MR imaging. The more superior portions of the tear can be difficult to visualize on axial images. External rotation as well as coronal oblique images help define these lesions. In the study by Monu and colleagues (138) using conventional MRI, all eight patients in their study showed an abnormal labrum on the coronal MR images, on 88% of the axial images, and on 50% of the sagittal images. Fifty percent of their cases also showed an intraarticular body, presumably representing the displaced fragment of a bucket handle tear, on all imaging planes (the MR "Cheerio" sign).

MR arthrography can be very helpful in detecting SLAP lesions, including the use of traction in some select situations (134–137). It will distend out buckle handle–type tears, outline morphological alterations, and imbibe into areas of degeneration and fraying of the labrum and biceps tendon. In Hodler et al.'s study of nine patients with SLAP lesions (139), differentiation between complete and partial labral detachments was not possible even with MR arthrog-

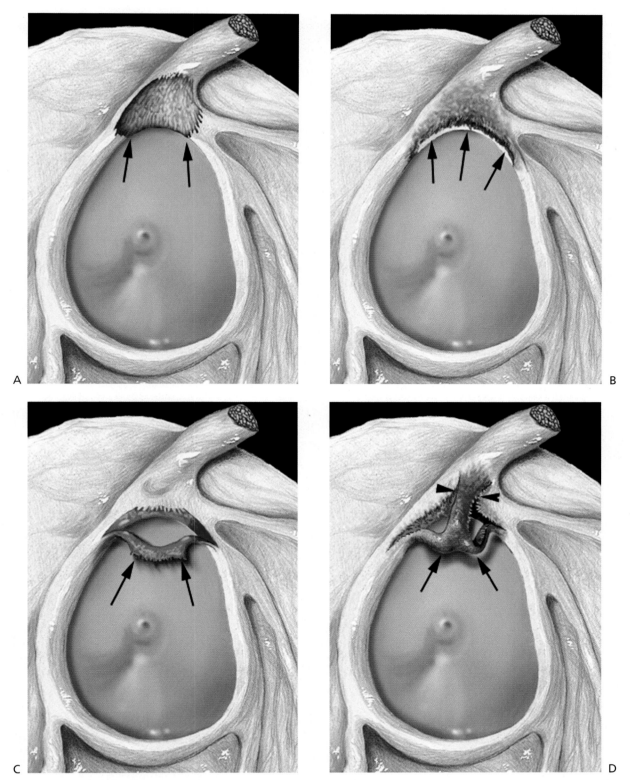

FIGURE 7.36. Artist's depiction of superior labrum, anterior and posterior (SLAP) lesions, types 1–4, lateral view. **A:** SLAP 1 lesion. The superior labrum is frayed, roughened, and degenerated (*arrows*). **B:** SLAP 2 lesion. The roughened superior labrum is detached with the biceps tendon anchor (*arrows*). **C:** SLAP 3 lesion. There is a bucket handle tear of the superior portion of the labrum. It does not involve the biceps labral anchor. The superior portion of the labrum is detached from both the glenoid and the biceps tendon and may be displaced into the joint space (*arrows*). **D:** In addition to the bucket handle tear (*arrows*), there is extension into the biceps, labral anchor in a longitudinal or split manner (*arrowheads*).

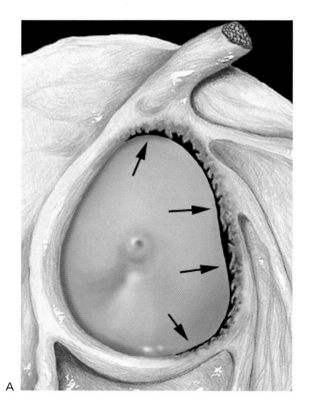

A

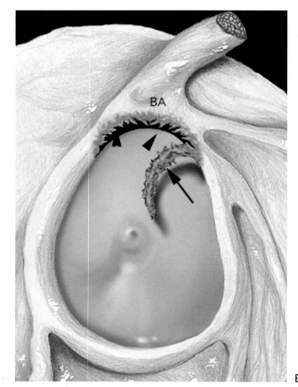

B

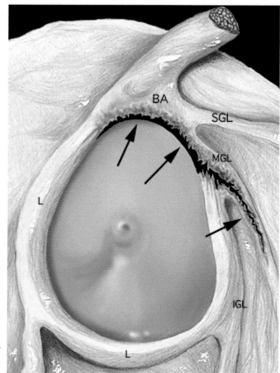

C

FIGURE 7.37. Artist's depiction of superior labrum, anterior and posterior (SLAP) lesions, types 5–9, lateral view. **A:** SLAP 5 lesion. This is a Bankart lesion of the anterior inferior labrum that then extends superiorly to include separation of the biceps tendon anchor (*arrows*). **B:** SLAP 6 lesion. This is an unstable radial or flap tear (*arrow*) that also involves separation of the biceps anchor (*arrowheads*). **C:** SLAP 7 lesion. This lesion consists of anterior extension of the SLAP (2) lesion (*arrows*) to involve the middle glenohumeral ligament (*shorter arrow*).

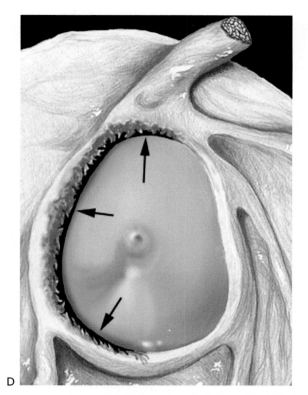
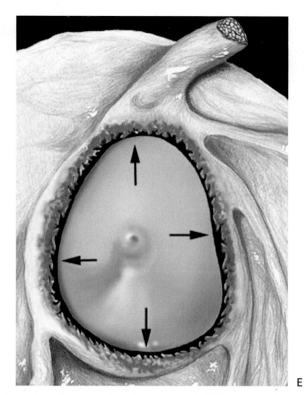

FIGURE 7.37 (continued). D: Type 8 SLAP lesion that extends posteroinferiorly (*arrows*). **E:** Type 9. There is complete concentric avulsion of the labrum (*arrows*). BA, biceps anchor; L, labrum; SGL, superior glenohumeral ligament; MGL, middle glenohumeral ligament; IGL, anterior band inferior glenohumeral ligament.

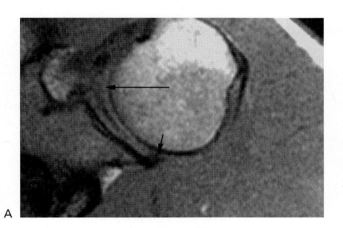
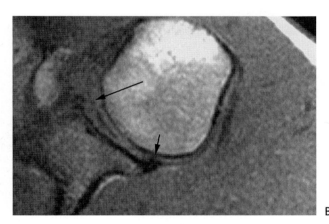
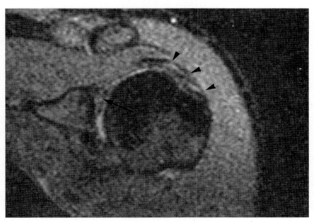

FIGURE 7.38. Type 1 SLAP lesion. Axial T1-weighted images **(A, B)** and coronal oblique STIR images **(C)**. There is irregularity of the labral contour, which is frayed, blunted, and irregular, with increased signal intensity in its substance more evident anteriorly (*longer arrow*) than posteriorly (*shorter arrow*), and identified superiorly in C (*arrow*). There is evidence of moderate rotator cuff tendinosis on the coronal oblique images in C (*arrowheads*).

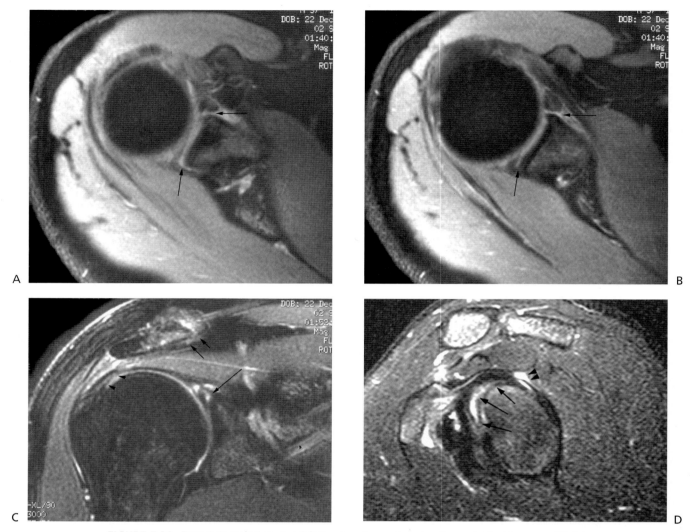

FIGURE 7.39. Type 2 SLAP lesion. Axial fast spin echo proton density–weighted images with fat suppression, TR/TE 2400/25 (**A, B**) and coronal oblique fast spin echo T2-weighted images (**C**), TR/TE 3000/55. The images reveal a globular region of fluidlike signal interposed between the superior labrum anterior and posterior and the glenoid margin (*arrows*). The tear extends into the posterior labrum beyond the biceps labral anchor. Note also the AC joint changes (*small arrows*) and the rotator cuff tendinosis and thinning (*arrowheads*) in this patient. Many patients with SLAP lesions may have concomitant rotator cuff alterations. **D:** Sagittal oblique fast spin echo T2-weighted sequence with fat suppression, TR/TE300/55. The superior labrum is separated from the superior glenoid by fluid signal (*arrows*). The sagittal images outline the more anteriorly predominant nature, but there is also a small posterior superior paralabral cyst (*arrowheads*).

raphy. Detection of abnormalities required the use of both the axial and coronal images. In addition, the authors emphasized the difficulty in separating SLAP lesions from both age-related labral separation and normal variants of labral attachment. They also expressed their difficulty identifying surface fraying and degeneration of the labrum even with the use of MR arthrography.

The use of traction with MR arthrography is helpful in the diagnosis of SLAP lesions as it apparently places tension on the biceps tendon and at its site of labral attachment and results in larger contrast-filled gaps between the labrum and the glenoid margin in cases of SLAP 2 lesions (137). This

helps to differentiate them from a sublabral recess or foramen. It also accentuates the abnormal intrabral collections of contrast material that characterize a SLAP 3 lesion. MR arthrography demonstrates the following signs in SLAP lesions (89): (a) contrast material possibly extended superiorly into the glenoid attachment of the long head of the biceps tendon (LHBT) on oblique coronal images, (b) irregularity of the insertion of the LHBT on oblique coronal and sagittal images, (c) accumulation of contrast material between the labrum and glenoid fossa on axial images, (d) detachment and displacement of the superior labrum on oblique sagittal and coronal images, and (e) a fragment of the labrum displayed

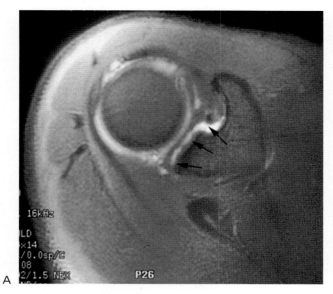

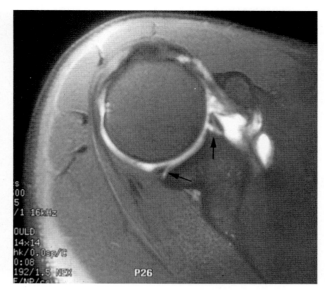

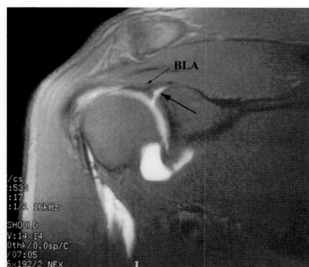

FIGURE 7.40. Type 2 SLAP lesion, MRI arthrography. Axial **(A, B)** and coronal **(C)** T1-weighted MRI arthrogram images, TR/TE 600/20. Contrast outlines separation of the anterior superior, superior, and posterior superior labrum and attached biceps labral anchor (*BLA*) from the glenoid margin (*arrows*).

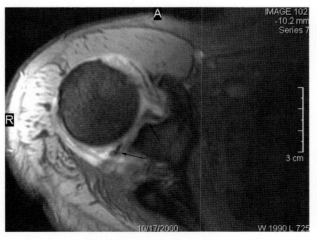

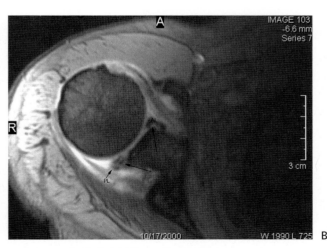

FIGURE 7.41. Type 2 SLAP lesion with posterior complex tear. **A, B:** Axial 2D gradient echo images, TR/TE 400/22, flip angle 25°. There is a tear and separation of the superior labrum, anterior and posterior (*larger arrows*). The posterior portion tear is more advanced and shows some fragmentation in B. Type 2 SLAP lesions can be anterior- or posterior-predominant, and if they extend and detach more posteroinferiorly, they may be considered a type 8 lesion. AL, anterior superior labrum; PL (*small arrow*), posterior superior labrum.

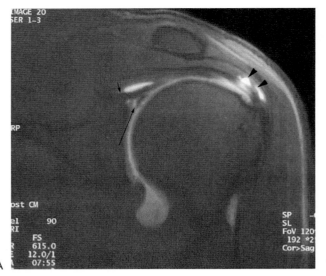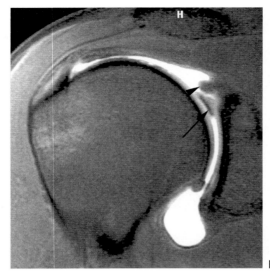

FIGURE 7.42. Type 3 SLAP lesion, MR arthrography. **A:** Coronal oblique T1-weighted MRI arthrogram image, TR/TE 615/12. Contrast extension reveals detachment and mild displacement of the superior labrum from the glenoid rim (*longer arrow*). The biceps tendon insertion remains intact (*shorter arrow*). Also note the small complete tear in the supraspinatus tendon (*arrowheads*). **B:** Coronal oblique T1-weighted MRI arthrogram image, TR/TE 600/15, in a patient different from that in **A**. Contrast outlines a detachment and inferior displacement of the superior labrum (*arrow*), consistent with a bucket handle tear. The biceps tendon insertion again is seen to be intact (*arrowhead*). (Figure **B**, courtesy of Javier Beltran MD, Brooklyn, NY.)

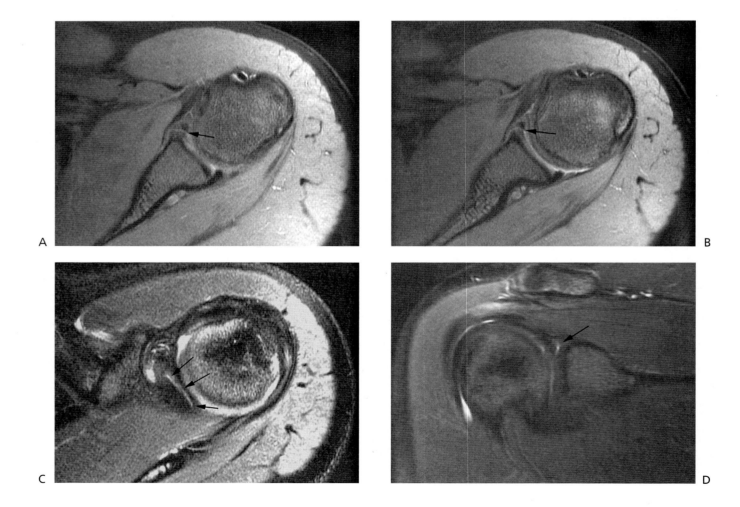

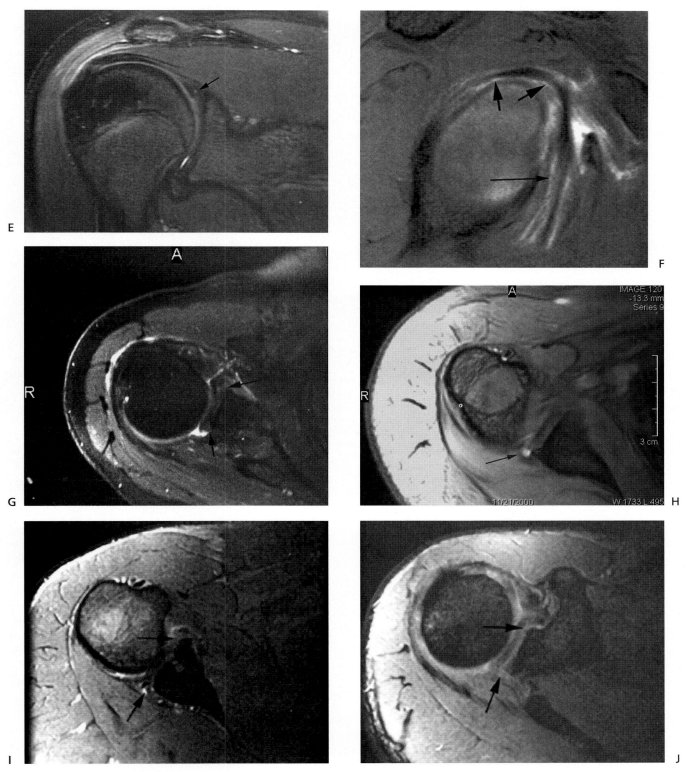

FIGURE 7.43. Other SLAP lesions. Type 5 lesion: axial **(A–C)** and coronal oblique fast spin echo images **(D, E)**, with fat suppression; TR/TE 3000/25 **(A, B, D, E)**, 3000/55 **(C)**. A tear of the anterior inferior labrum that then extends superiorly to include separation of the biceps tendon anchor is identified (*arrows*). Type 7 lesion: coronal oblique T1-weighted MRI arthrogram image **(F)**, TR/TE 600/15. Contrast extends into an irregular, frayed middle glenohumeral ligament (*long thin arrow*), representing extension of the SLAP lesion (*shorter thicker arrows*) into this structure. (Figure F, courtesy of Javier Beltran MD, Brooklyn, NY.) Type 8 lesion: axial fast spin echo T2-weighted image **(G)**, with fat suppression, TR/TE 3000/55, and 2D gradient echo image, TR/TE 400/22, flip angle 25° **(H)**. There is a tear of the superior labrum that extends posteroinferiorly (*arrows*). Type 9 lesion: axial 2D gradient echo images, TR/TE 616/22, flip angle 25° **(I, J)**. *(continued)*

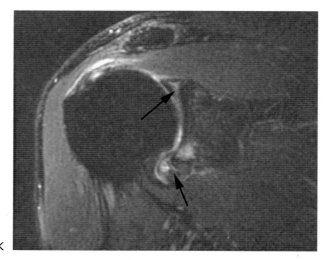
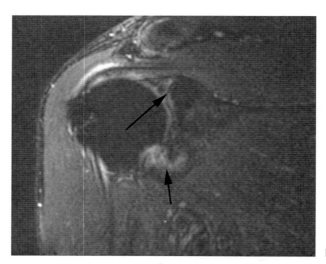

FIGURE 7.43 *(continued)*. Coronal oblique fast spin echo images, with fat suppression, TR/TE 3000/45 **(K, L)**. There is extensive circumferential tear and detachment of the labrum (*arrows*).

inferiorly between the glenoid fossa and the humeral head. In addition, paralabral cyst may be frequently associated with these lesions.

With respect to the diagnostic performance of MR arthrography in the diagnosis of SLAP lesions, Bencardino and coworkers studied (135) 52 patients who underwent arthroscopy or open surgery. Diagnostic criteria for SLAP lesions in this study included marked fraying of the articular aspect of the labrum, biceps anchor avulsion, an inferiorly displaced bucket handle fragment, and extension of the tear into the biceps tendon fibers. SLAP injuries were diagnosed at surgery in 19 of the 52 patients (37%). Six of the 19 lesions (32%) were classified as type 1, nine (47%) as type 2, one (5%) as type 3, and three (16%) as type 4. MR arthrography had a sensitivity of 89%, a specificity of 91%, and an accuracy of 90%. The MR arthrographic classification showed correlation with the arthroscopic or surgical classification in 13 of 17 patients (76%) in whom SLAP lesions were diagnosed at MR arthrography. Jee and coworkers (134) evaluated the MR arthrograms in 80 patients who underwent arthroscopy and MR arthrography. Type 1 SLAP lesions were regarded as negative as the authors felt that they are often not clinically relevant. There were 25 SLAP tears: type 2 (*n* = 22), type 3 (*n* = 2), and type 4 (*n* = 1). There were three different readers in this study. Sensitivity, specificity, and accuracy of each reader were 92%, 84%, and 86%; 92%, 82%, and 85%; and 84%, 69%, and 74%, for three different readers, respectively. Interobserver agreement for SLAP tears was substantial, and MR arthrography of the shoulder was felt to be a reliable and accurate method for detection of SLAP tears.

Tears of the superior portion of the labrum must be distinguished from the normal variants of the labrum and its attachments in this region, including the sublabral recess

which occurs at the 12 o'clock, the sublabral foramen that occurs more anteriorly at 2 o'clock, as well as the Buford complex (absent anterior superior labrum associated with a cordlike middle glenohumeral ligament), the latter of which is less common than the sublabral foramen (136). These normal anatomic variants are not uncommon and have been described and discussed in some detail in the chapter on shoulder anatomy (140–142). Among the criteria for distinguishing these lesions from SLAP tears are that these lesions do not extend to involve the superior or posterior labrum beyond the level of the biceps labral anchor; there should be no associated morphological alterations. In addition, they should not extend below the level of the equator of the glenoid, which may be marked by the coracoid process. Increased distance between the labrum and the glenoid, an irregular appearance of the labral margin, or lateral extension of the separation may suggest a SLAP lesion rather than a normal anatomic variant (136). However, differentiation between normal variants and pathologic conditions and among various types of SLAP lesions remains difficult. MR arthrography is helpful in the differentiation of SLAP tears from normal anatomical variants because it can help identify a cordlike middle glenohumeral ligament to good advantage, especially in the sagittal oblique plane (140–142). It can also reveal the smooth nature of the labrum and establish the location and extent of these normal variants and help to separate them from true SLAP tears.

SLAP lesions may be treated with arthroscopic debridement, excision of a portion of the labrum, or labral repair. Labral repair will usually be carried out with the use of suture anchors (143,144). The surgical treatment may be based on whether there is compromise of the biceps labral anchor; therefore, special attention must be paid to the integrity of this region in preoperative planning (129,133).

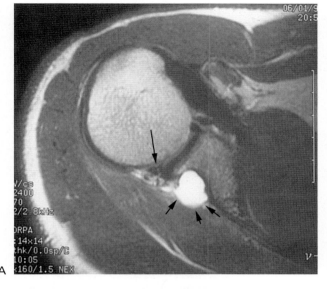

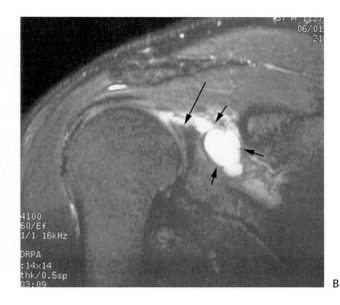

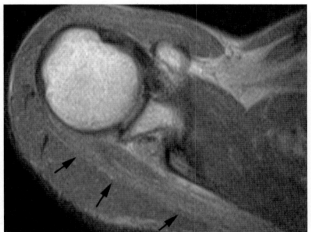

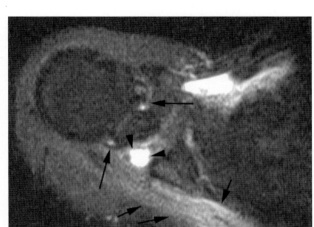

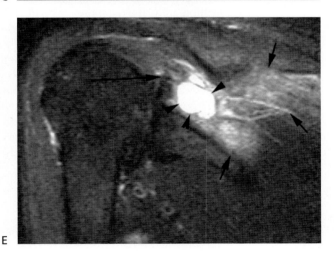

FIGURE 7.44. Paralabral cyst. **A, B:** Axial T2-weighted image, TR/TE 2500/70, and coronal oblique fast spin echo T2-weighted sequence with fat suppression. A large paralabral cyst is identified (*shorter arrows*). It is arising in relation to a posterosuperior labral tear (*longer arrows*) and extends into the spinoglenoid notch region. Axial T1-weighted image **(C)**, axial and coronal oblique STIR images **(D, E)**. A type 2 SLAP lesion is seen (*longer arrows*). A paralabral cyst is arising from the posterior superior portion (*arrowheads*). There is denervation edema/atrophy in the infraspinatus muscle (*shorter arrows*).

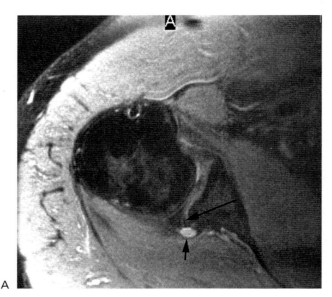
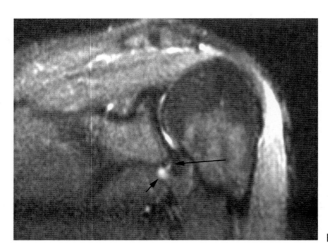

FIGURE 7.45. Posterior inferior labral tear, small paralabral cyst. **A:** Axial fast spin echo proton density–weighted sequence with fat suppression, TR/TE 2600/12. A small postinferior labral tear is seen (*longer arrow*), communicating with a small paralabral cyst (*shorter arrow*). **B:** Coronal oblique STIR image. A tear in the inferior labrum (*longer arrow*) is associated with a small paralabral cyst (*shorter arrow*).

Results of arthroscopic treatment of SLAP lesions have been variable. This may in part be related to the difficulty in diagnosis and particularly the difficulty in distinguishing these lesions from the age-related labral separation that also occurs superiorly and from the normal variation in anatomy that occurs in the superior portion of the labrum (145), alluded to earlier and elsewhere in the text.

As with other tears of the superior labrum, SLAP lesions are frequently associated with rotator cuff lesions, particularly partial tears (Figs. 7.35, 7.42). One study found such lesions in 42% of cases (135). Other associated lesions that may be seen less commonly include a frayed or lax inferior glenohumeral ligament, chondral lesions, loose bodies, Bankart or Hill-Sachs lesions, complete rotator tear, and posterior labral tear (135,146).

Paralabral Ganglion Cysts

These types of cysts are discussed elsewhere in the text; however, these are ganglion cysts arising adjacent to the glenoid labrum (121,147) and most commonly associated with a labral tear (Figs. 7.44–7.46). This labral tear is often a SLAP lesion, and the paralabral cyst most commonly arises in relation to the posterosuperior component (Figs. 7.44, 7.46). They may, however, occur anywhere in the glenohumeral joint (Fig. 7.45). Pathophysiologically, they may be similar to cysts of this nature elsewhere in the body, such as meniscal cysts, or cysts associated with tears of the acetabular labrum. In this situation, fluid arising from the joint extends through the labral tear into the surrounding soft tissues and

leads to ganglion cyst formation. When large, these cysts extend into the spinoglenoid notch, the suprascapular notch, or both notches.

Tung and coworkers studied 46 patients with paralabral cysts with MRI, MR arthrography, and arthroscopy (148). They found that most paralabral cysts are associated with labral tears. On MR imaging and arthroscopy, a labral tear was identified in 27 (53%) and 15 (88%) patients, respectively. They stated that paralabral cysts may be difficult to identify on MR arthrography unless some form of T2-weighted sequence is performed, since direct communication between a cyst and the joint space rarely occurs (Fig. 7.46). A posterior or inferior cyst may cause compression neuropathy of the suprascapular or axillary nerve, respectively. Compression of the suprascapular nerve is usually with extension of the posterior cyst into the spinoglenoid notch. Cysts that cause nerve compression are usually large (mean size 3.1 cm). Cyst aspiration may result in temporary relief of symptoms, but an untreated labral tear should be suspected if the cyst recurs.

Glenoid Labrum Articular Disruption

Another recently described lesion occurs in athletes and has been described at arthroscopy (150). This refers to tears of the superficial anterior inferior labrum and also involves articular cartilage (Fig. 7.47). This is the *GLAD lesion* (glenoid labrum articular disruption). This occurs from a forced adduction across the chest from an abducted and externally rotated position. The GLAD lesion is identified by

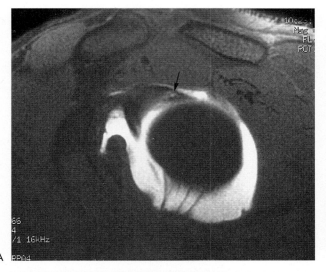

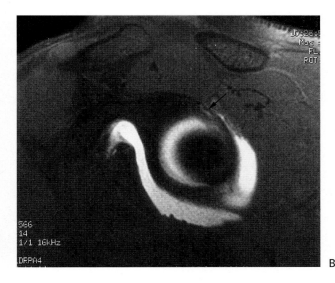

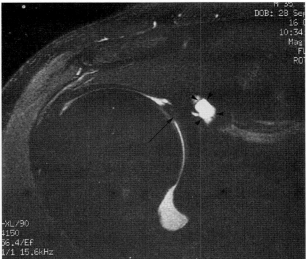

FIGURE 7.46. Paralabral cyst and MR arthrography. **A, B:** Sagittal oblique T1-weighted MR arthrogram images with fat suppression, TR/TE 566/14. Contrast outlines a small posterior superior labral tear (*arrows and larger arrow in* **C**). **C:** Coronal oblique fast spin echo T2-weighted MR arthrogram images with fat suppression. The small posterior paralabral cyst is seen with the T2-weighted images (*arrowheads*).

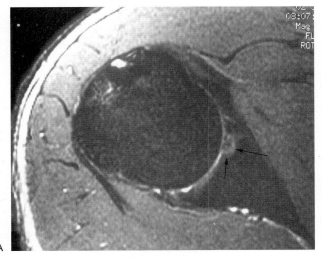

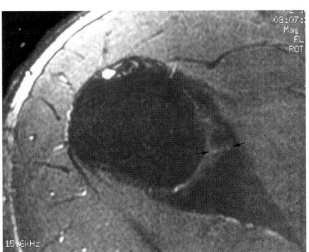

FIGURE 7.47. Glenoid labrum articular disruption (GLAD) lesion. This refers to tears of the superficial anterior inferior labrum and also involves articular cartilage. **A, B:** Axial 2D gradient echo images. There is a tear of the anterior inferior labrum in B (*smaller arrows*). It is associated with an osteochondral lesion of the inferior anterior margin of the glenoid articular surface seen in A (*arrows*). There is no demonstrable disruption of the capsuloligamentous structures. *(continued)*

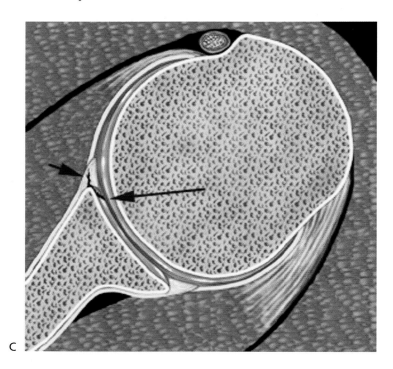

C

FIGURE 7.47 *(continued)*. C: Artist's depiction of a GLAD lesion. There is a flap tear of the anterior labrum (*shorter arrow*), with a defect of the adjacent articular cartilage (*longer arrow*).

an inferior flap-type tear. It is not associated with any glenohumeral instability, and the deep fibers of the inferior glenohumeral ligament remain strongly attached to the labrum and glenoid rim. In addition, there is fibrillation and erosion of the articular cartilage in the anteroinferior quadrant of the glenoid fossa. Experience with these lesions is limited. MR arthrography may improve the sensitivity to these lesions (69,150,151). In some cases, a depressed osteochondral lesion is also seen, thus suggesting an overlap of this condition and osteochondiritis dissecans.

REFERENCES

1. Obrien SJ, Neves MC, Arnoczcky SP, et al. The anatomy and histology of the inferior glenohumeral ligament complex of the shoulder. *Am J Sports Med* 1990;18:449–456.
2. Resnick D. Internal derangement of joints. In: *Diagnosis of bone and joint disorders,* 4th ed. Philadelphia: WB Saunders, 2002: chap. 65.
3. Obrien SJ, Warren RF, Schwartz E. Anterior shoulder instability. *Orthop Clin North Am* 1987;18:395–408.
4. Matsen FA III, Thomas SC, Rockwood CA, Wirth MA. Glenohumeral instability. In: Rockwood CA, Matsen FA III, eds. *The shoulder.* Philadelphia: WB Saunders, 1998:611–755.
5. Zarins B, Rowe CR. Current concepts in the diagnosis and treatment of shoulder instability in athletes. *Med Sci Sports Exerc* 1984; 16:444–448.
6. Pappas AM, Goss TP, Kleinman PK. Symptomatic shoulder instability due to lesions of the glenoid labrum. *Am J Sports Med* 1983;11:279–288.
7. Sperling JW, Anderson K, McCarty EC, Warren RF. Complications of thermal capsulorrhaphy. *Instr Course Lect* 2001;50:37–41.
8. Matsen FA, Harryman DT, Sidles JA. Mechanics of glenohumeral stability. *Clin Sports Med* 1991;10:783–791.
9. Symeonides PP, Hatzokos I, Christoforides J, Pournaras J. Humeral head torsion in recurrent anterior dislocation of the shoulder. *J Bone Joint Surg Br* 1995;77:687–690.
10. Brewer BJ, Wubben RC, Carrera GF. Excessive retroversion of the glenoid cavity: a cause of non-traumatic posterior instability of the shoulder. *J Bone Joint Surg Am* 1986;68:724–731.
11. *The genuine works of Hippocrates.* Translated by Francis Adams. London: Sydenham Society, 1849;vol. 2:553–654.
12. Goss TP. Anterior glenohumeral instability. *Orthopedics* 1988;2: 87–95.
13. Rowe CR. Acute and recurrent anterior dislocations of the shoulder. *Orthop Clin North Am* 1980;11:253–270.
14. Hovelius L. Anterior dislocation of the shoulder in teenagers and young adults. *J Bone Joint Surg Am* 1987;69:393–399.
15. Henry JH, Genung JA. Natural history of glenohumeral dislocation-revisited. *Am J Sports Med* 1982;10:135–141.
16. Rowe CR. Prognosis in dislocations of the shoulder. *J Bone Joint Surg* 1956;38A:957–977.
17. Rowe CR. Acute and recurrent anterior dislocations of the shoulder. *Orthop Clin North Am* 1980;11: 253–270.
18. Cofield RH, Kavanagh BF, Frassica FJ. Anterior shoulder instability. *Instr Course Lect* 1985;34:210–227.
19. Kinnett JG, Warren RF, Jacobs B. Recurrent dislocation of the shoulder after age fifty. *Clin Orthop Rel Res* 1980;149:164–168.
20. Kinnett JG, Warren RF, Jacobs B. Recurrent dislocation of the shoulder after age fifty. *Clin Orthop Rel Res* 1980;149: 164–168.
21. Neviaser RJ, Neviaser TJ, Neviaser JS. Current rupture of the rotator cuff and anterior dislocation of the shoulder in the older patient. *J Bone Joint Surg Am* 1988;70:1308–1311.
22. Morton KS. The unstable shoulder: recurring subluxation. *Injury* 1979;10:304–306.
23. Bankart ASB. The pathology and treatment of recurrent dislocation of the shoulder joint. *Br J Surg* 1938;26:23–29.

24. DeAnquin CE. Recurrent dislocation of the shoulder roentgenographic study. *J Bone Joint Surg Am* 1965; 47:1085–1088.
25. Saha AK. Dynamic stability of the glenohumeral joint. *Acta Orthop Scand* 1971;42:491–505.
26. McGlynn FJ, Caspari RB. Arthroscopic findings in the subluxating shoulder. *Clin Orthop Rel Res* 1984;183:173–178.
27. Rowe CR. Anterior glenohumeral subluxation/dislocation: the Bankart procedure. In: Torg JS, Welsh RP, Sheperd RJ, eds. *Current therapy in sports medicine—2* (EDS) Toronto: BC Decker, 399–404.
28. Caspari R, Savoir B. Arthroscopic reconstruction of the shoulder: the Bankart repair. In: Pariesien JS, ed. *Operative arthroscopy.* New York, Raven Press, 1990:65–74.
29. McGlynn FJ, Caspari RB. Arthroscopic findings in the subluxating shoulder. *Clin Orthop Rel Res* 1984;183:173–178.
30. Palmer WE, Brown JH, Rosenthal DI. Labral ligamentous complex of the shoulder: evaluation with MR arthrography. *Radiology* 1994;190:645–651.
31. Hill HA, Sachs MD. The grooved defect of the humeral head: a frequently unrecognized complication of dislocation of the shoulder joint. *Radiology* 1940;65:690–700.
32. Pavlov H, Warren RF, Weiss CB, Dines DW. The roentgenographic evaluation of anterior shoulder instability. *Clin Orthop* 1985;194:153–158.
33. Obrien SJ, Warren RF, Schwartz E. Anterior shoulder instability. *Orthop Clin North Am* 1987;18:395–408.
34. Danzig LA, Greenway G, Resnick D. The Hill Sachs lesion: an experimental study. *Am J Sports Med* 1980;8:328–332.
35. Pavlov H, Warren RF, Weiss CB, Dines DW. The roentgenographic evaluation of anterior shoulder instability. *Clin Orthop* 1985;194:153–158.
36. Zlatkin MB, Iannotti JP, Esterhai JL, Dalinka MK, Kressel HY, Spindler K. Evaluation of rotator cuff disease and glenohumeral instability with MR imaging: correlation with arthroscopy and arthrotomy in a large population of patients. *Magn Reson Imaging* 1990;8(suppl 1):78(abstr).
37. Iannotti JP, Zlatkin MB, Esterhai JL, Dalinka MK, Kressel HY, Spindler K. Magnetic resonance imaging of the shoulder: sensitivity, specificity and predictive value. *J Bone Joint Surg Am* 1991; 73:17–29.
38. Zlatkin MB, Dalinka MK, Kressel HY. Magnetic resonance imaging of the shoulder. *Magn Reson Q* 1989;5:3–22.
39. Seeger LL. Magnetic resonance imaging of the shoulder. *Clin Orthop* 1989;244:48–59.
40. Altchek DW, Skyhar MJ, Warren RF. Shoulder arthroscopy for shoulder instability. *Instr Course Lect* 1989;38:187–198.
41. Mclaughlin HL. Recurrent anterior dislocations of the shoulder. *Am J Surg* 1956;99:628–632.
42. Workman TL, Burkhard TK, Resnick D, et al. Hill-Sachs lesion: comparison of detection with MR imaging. *Radiology* 1992;185: 847–852.
43. Itoi E, Lee SB, Berglund LJ, Berge LL, An KN. The effect of a glenoid defect on anteroinferior stability of the shoulder after Bankart repair: a cadaveric study. *J Bone Joint Surg Am* 2000;82:35–46.
44. Singson R, Feldman F, Bigliani L. CT arthrographic patterns in recurrent glenohumeral instability. *AJR* 1987;149:749–753.
45. Tullos HS, Bennett JB, Braly WJ. Acute shoulder dislocations: factors influencing diagnosis and treatment. *Instr Course Lect* 1984; 33:364–385.
46. Rowe CO, Patel D, Southnayd WW. The Bankart procedure. *J Bone Joint Surg Am* 1978;60A:1–16.
47. Massengill AD, Seeger LL, Yao L, Gentili A, Shnier RC, Shapiro MS, Gold RH. Labrocapsular ligamentous complex of the shoulder: normal anatomy, anatomic variation, and pitfalls of MR imaging and MR arthrography. *RadioGraphics* 1994;14:1211–1223.
48. Cole BJ, Warner JJ. Arthroscopic versus open Bankart repair for traumatic anterior shoulder instability. *Clin Sports Med* 2000;19:19–48.
49. Steinbeck J, Liljenqvist U, Jerosch J. The anatomy of the glenohumeral ligamentous complex and its contribution to anterior shoulder stability. *J Shoulder Elbow Surg* 1998;7:122–126.
50. Loredo R, Longo C, Salonen D, Yu J, Haghighi P, Trudell D, Clopton P, Resnick D. Glenoid labrum: MR imaging with histologic correlation. *Radiology* 1995;196:33–41.
51. Legan JM, Burkhead TK, Goff WB, et al. Tears of the glenoid labrum: MR imaging of 88 arthroscopically confirmed cases. *Radiology* 1991;179:241–246.
52. Iannotti JP, Zlatkin MB, Esterhai JL, Kressel HY, Dalinka MK, Spindler KP. Magnetic resonance imaging of the shoulder. *J Bone Joint Surg Am* 1991;73:17–29.
52a. Garneau RA, Renfrew DL, Moore TE, et al. Glenoid lebrum: evaluation with MR imaging. *Radiology* 1991;179:519–522.
53. Chandnani VP, Yeager TD, DeBerardino T, et al. Glenoid labral tears: prospective evaluation with MR imaging, MR arthrography and CT arthrography. *AJR* 1993;161:1229.
54. Karzel RP, Snyder SJ. Magnetic resonance arthrography of the shoulder. *Clin Sports Med* 1993,12:123.
55. Palmer WE, Caslowitz PL. Anterior shoulder instability: diagnostic criteria determined from prospective analysis of 121 MR arthrograms. *Radiology* 1995;197:819–825.
56. Tirman PFJ, Stauffer AE, Crues JV, et al. Saline magnetic resonance arthrography in the evaluation of glenohumeral instability. *Arthroscopy* 1993;9:550–559.
57. Gusmer PJ, Potter HG, Schatz JA, et al. Labral injuries: accuracy of detection with unenhanced MR imaging of the shoulder. *Radiology* 1996;200:519–524.
58. Stoller DW. MR Arthrography of the glenohumeral joint. *Radiologic Clin North Am* 1997;35:97–116.
59. Cvitanic O, Tirman PFJ, Feller JF, et al. Using abduction and external rotation of the shoulder to increase the sensitivity of MR arthrography in revealing tears of the anterior glenoid labrum. *AJR* 1997;169:837.
60. Coumas JM, Waite RJ, Goss TP, et al. CT and MR evaluation of the labral capsular ligamentous complex of the shoulder. *AJR* 1992;158:591–597.
61. Chandnani VP, Gagliardi JA, Murnane TG, Bradley YC, DeBerardino TA, Spaeth J, Hansen MF. Glenohumeral ligaments and shoulder capsular mechanism: evaluation with MR arthrography. *Radiology* 1995;196:27–32.
62. Zlatkin MB, Bjorkengren AG, Gylys-Morin V, Resnik D, Sartoris DJ. Cross-sectional imaging of the capsular mechanism of the glenohumeral joint. *AJR* 1988;150:151–158.
63. Mendoza FX, Nicholas JA, Reilly J. Anatomic patterns of glenoid labrum tears. *Orthop Trans* 1987;11:246.
64. Rafii M, Firooznia H, Golimbu C, Weinreb J. Magnetic resonance imaging of glenohumeral instability. *MRI Clin North Am* 1993;1:87–104.
65. Warner JJ, McMahon PJ. The role of the long head of the biceps brachii in superior stability of the glenohumeral joint. *J Bone Joint Surg Am* 1995;77:366–372.
66. Rothman RH, Marvel JP, Heppenstall RB. Anatomic considerations in the glenohumeral joint. *Orthop Clin North Am* 1975;6:341–352.
67. Tirman PFJ. Glenohumeral instability. In: Steinbach LS, Tirman PFJ, Peterfy CG, Feller JF. *Shoulder magnetic resonance imaging.* Philadelphia: Lippincott-Raven, 1998:135–167.
68. Perthes G. Uber Operationen bei habitaller Schulterluxationen. *Deutsch Z Chir* 1906;85:199–227.
69. Tirman PFJ, Palmer WE, Feller JF. MR arthrography of the shoulder. *MRI Clin North Am* 1997;5:811–839.
70. Wischer TK, Bredella MA, Genant HK, Stoller DW, Bost FW, Tirman PF. Perthes lesion (a variant of the Bankart lesion): MR

imaging and MR arthrographic findings with surgical correlation. *AJR* 2002;178:233–237.

71. Neviaser TJ. The anterior labroligamentous periosteal sleeve avulsion injury: a cause of anterior instability of the shoulder. *Arthroscopy* 1993;9:17–21.

72. Connell DA, Potter HG. Magnetic resonance evaluation of the labral capsular ligamentous complex: a pictorial review. *Australas Radiol* 1999;43:419–426.

73. Ogawa K, Yoshida A. Extensive shoulder capsule tearing as a main cause of recurrent anterior shoulder dislocation. *J Shoulder Elbow Surg* 1997;6:1–5.

74. Tirman PFJ, Steinbach LS, Feller JF, et al. Humeral avulsion of the anterior shoulder stabilizers after anterior shoulder dislocation: demonstration by MR and MR arthrography. *Skeletal Radiol* 1996;25:743–748.

75. Wolf EM, Cheng JC, Dickson K. Humeral avulsion of glenohumeral ligaments as a cause of anterior shoulder instability. *Arthroscopy* 1995;11:600–607.

76. Bokor DJ, Conboy VB, Olson C. Anterior instability of the glenohumeral joint with humeral avulsion of the glenohumeral ligament: a review of 41 cases. *J Bone Joint Surg Br* 1999;Jan;81(1):93–96.

77. Schippinger G, Vasiu PS, Fankhauser F, Clement HG. HAGL lesion occurring after successful arthroscopic Bankart repair. *Arthroscopy* 2001;Feb;17(2):206–208.

78. Oberlander MA, Morgan BE, Visotsky JL. The BHAGL lesion: a new variant of anterior shoulder instability. *Arthroscopy* 1996;12:627–633.

79. Field LD, Bokor DJ, Savoie FH III. Humeral and glenoid detachment of the anterior inferior glenohumeral ligament: a cause of anterior shoulder instability. *J Shoulder Elbow Surg* 1997;Jan–Feb; 6(1):6–10.

80. Warner JJ, Beim GM. Combined Bankart and HAGL lesion associated with anterior shoulder instability. *Arthroscopy* 1997;13:749–752.

81. Hawkins RJ, Koppert G, Johnston G. Recurrent posterior instability (subluxation) of the shoulder. *J Bone Joint Surg* 1984;66A:169–174.

82. Petersen SA. Posterior shoulder instability. *Orthop Clin North Am* 2000;31:263–274.

83. Bigliani LU, Kelkar R, Flatow EL, Pollock RG, Mow VC. Glenohumeral stability: biomechanical properties of passive and active stabilizers. *Clin Orthop* 1996;330:13–30.

84. Weber SC, Caspari RB. A biochemical evaluation of the restraints to posterior shoulder dislocation. *Arthroscopy* 1989;5:115–121.

85. Pavlov M, Freiberger RH. Fractures and dislocations about the shoulders. *Semin Roentgenol* 1978;13:85–96.

86. Matsen FA III, Thomas SC, Rockwood CA. Anterior glenohumeral instability. In: Rockwood CA, Matsen FA III, eds. *The shoulder*. Philadelphia: WB Saunders, 1990.

87. Hawkins RJ, Belle RM. Posterior instability of the shoulder. *Instr Course Lect* 1989;38:211–215.

88. Norwood LA, Terry GC. Shoulder posterior subluxation. *Am J Sports Med* 1984;12:25–30.

89. Shankman S, Bencardino J, Beltran J. Glenohumeral instability: evaluation using MR arthrography of the shoulder. *Skeletal Radiol* 1999;28:365–382.

90. Hawkins RJ, Janda DH. Posterior instability of the glenohumeral joint: a technique of repair. *Am J Sports Med* 1996;24(3):275–278.

91. Murrell GA, Warren RF. The surgical treatment of posterior shoulder instability. *Clin Sports Med* 1995;14:903–915.

92. Weishaupt D, Zanetti M, Nyffeler RW, Gerber C, Hodler J. Posterior glenoid rim deficiency in recurrent (atraumatic) posterior shoulder instability. *Skeletal Radiol* 2000;29:204–210.

93. Simons P, Joekes E, Nelissen RG, Bloem JL. Posterior labrocapsular periosteal sleeve avulsion complicating locked posterior shoulder dislocation. *Skeletal Radiol* 1998;27:588–590.

94. Rafii M, Firooznia H, Golimbu C. MR Imaging of the glenohumeral instability. *MRI Clin North Am* 1997;5:787–809.

95. Bell RH, Nobel JS. An appreciation of posterior instability of the shoulder. *Clin Sports Med* 1991;10:887–893.

96. Pollock RG, Bigliani LU. Recurrent posterior shoulder instability: diagnosis and treatment. *Clin Orthop* 1993;291:85–96.

97. Tibone JE, Bradley JP. The treatment of posterior subluxation in athletes. *Clin Orthop* 1993;291:124–137.

98. Hawkins RJ, Belle RM. Posterior instability of the shoulder. *Instr Course Lect* 1989;38:211–215.

99. Hawkins RJ, McCormack RG. Posterior shoulder instability. *Orthopedics* 1988;11:101–107.

100. Halbrecht JL, Tirman P, Atkin D. Internal impingement of the shoulder: comparison of findings between the throwing and nonthrowing shoulders of college baseball players. *Arthroscopy* 1999;Apr;15(3):253–258.

101. Cartland JP, Crues JV II, Stauffer A, et al. MR imaging in the evaluation of SLAP injuries of the shoulder: findings in 10 patients. *AJR* 1992;159:787–792.

102. Mair SD, Zarzour RH, Speer KP. Posterior labral injury in contact athletes. *Am J Sports Med* 1998;26:753–758.

103. Ferrari JD, Ferrari DA, Coumas J, et al. Posterior ossification of the shoulder: the Bennett lesion. Etiology, diagnosis and treatment. *Am J Sports Med* 1994;22:171–176.

104. Miniaci A, Mascia AT, Salonen DC, Becker EJ. Magnetic resonance imaging of the shoulder in asymptomatic professional baseball pitchers. *Am J Sports Med* 2002;30:66–73.

105. De Maeseneer M, Jaovisidha S, Jacobson JA, Tam W, Schils JP, Sartoris DJ, Fronek J, Resnick D. The Bennett lesion of the shoulder. *J Comput Assist Tomogr* 1998;22:31–34.

106. An YH, Friedman RJ. Multidirectional instability of the glenohumeral joint. *Orthop Clin North Am* 2000;31:275–285.

107. Neer CS, Foster CR. Inferior capsular shift for involuntary inferior and multidirectional instability of the shoulder. *J Bone Joint Surg* 1980;62A:897–908.

108. Neer CS. Involuntary inferior and multidirectional instability of the shoulder: etiology, recognition and treatment. *Instr Course Lect* 1985;34:232–238.

109. Arendt EA. Multidirectional shoulder instability. *Orthopedics* 1988;11:113–120.

110. Bak K, Spring BJ, Henderson JP. Inferior capsular shift procedure in athletes with multidirectional instability based on isolated capsular and ligamentous redundancy. *Am J Sports Med* 2000;28:466–471.

111. Gartsman GM, Roddey TS, Hammerman SM. Arthroscopic treatment of multidirectional glenohumeral instability: 2- to 5-year follow-up. *Arthroscopy* 2001;17:236–243.

112. Lyons TR, Griffith PL, Savoie FH III, Field LD. Laser-assisted capsulorrhaphy for multidirectional instability of the shoulder. *Arthroscopy* 2001;17:25–30.

113. Rowe CR, Zarins B. Chronic unreduced dislocations of the shoulder. *J Bone Joint Surg* 1982;64A:494–505.

114. Shultz TJ, Jacobs B, Patterson RL. Unrecognized dislocations of the shoulder. *J Trauma* 1969;9:1009–1023.

115. Perrenoud A, Imhoff AB. Locked posterior dislocation of the shoulder. *Bull Hosp Joint Dis* 1996;54(3):165–168.

116. Neer CS III, Rockwood CA Jr. Fractures and dislocations of the shoulder. In: Rockwood CA Jr., Green GP, eds. *Fractures*. Philadelphia: JB Lippincott, 1975;585–815.

117. Shuman WP, Kilcoyne RF, Matsen FA, Rogers JV, Mack LA. Double contrast computed tomography of the glenoid labrum. *AJR* 1983;141:581–584.

118. Giombini A, Rossi F, Pettrone FA, Dragoni S. Posterosuperior glenoid rim impingement as a cause of shoulder pain in top level waterpolo players. *J Sports Med Phys Fitness* 1997;37:273–278.

119. Davidson PA, Elattrache NS, Jobe CM, et al. Rotator cuff and posterosuperior glenoid labrum injury associated with increased glenohumeral motion: a new site of impingement. *J Shoulder Elbow Surg* 1995;4:384–390.

120. Jobe CM. Posterior superior glenoid impingement: expanded spectrum. *Arthroscopy* 1995;11:530–536.

121. Tirman TFJ, Bost FW, Steinbach LS, et al. MR arthrographic depiction of tears of the rotator cuff: benefit of abduction and external rotation of the arm. *Radiology* 1994;192:851–856.

122. Halbrecht JL, Tirman P, Atkin D. Internal impingement of the shoulder: comparison of findings between the throwing and nonthrowing shoulders of college baseball players. *Arthroscopy* 1999;15:253–258.

123. Walch G, Boileau P, Noel E, et al. Impingement of the deep surface of the supraspinatus tendon on the posterior superior glenoid rim: an arthroscopic study. *J Shoulder Elbow Surg* 1992;1:238–245.

124. Liu SH, Boynton E. Posterior superior impingement of the rotator cuff on the glenoid rim as a cause of shoulder pain in the overhead athlete. *Arthroscopy* 1993;9:697–701.

125. Edelson G, Teitz C. Internal impingement in the shoulder. *J Shoulder Elbow Surg* 2000;9:308–315.

126. Esch JC, Baker CL. *Arthroscopic surgery: the shoulder and elbow.* Philadelphia: JB Lippincott, 1993:133–142.

127. Snyder SJ, Karzel RP, Delpizzo W, Ferkel RD, Friedman MJ. SLAP lesions of the shoulder. *Arthroscopy* 1990;6:274–279.

128. Musgrave DS, Rodosky MW. SLAP lesions: current concepts. *Am J Orthop* 2001;30:29–38.

129. Handelberg F, Willems S, Shahabpour M, Huskin JP, Kuta J. SLAP lesions: a retrospective multicenter study. *Arthroscopy* 1998;14:856–862.

130. Burkhart SS, Morgan CD, Kibler WB. Shoulder injuries in overhead athletes. The "dead arm" revisited. *Clin Sports Med* 2000;19:125–158.

131. Bresler F, Blum A, Braun M, Simon JM, Cossin M, Regent D, Mole D. Assessment of the superior labrum of the shoulder joint with CT-arthrography and MR-arthrography: correlation with anatomical dissection. *Surg Radiol Anat* 1998;20:57–62.

132. Maffet MW, Gartsman GM, Moseley B. Superior labrum-biceps tendon complex lesions of the shoulder. *Am J Sports Med* 1995;23:93–98.

133. Mileski RA, Snyder SJ. Superior labral lesions in the shoulder: pathoanatomy and surgical management. *J Am Acad Orthop Surg* 1998;6:121–131.

134. Jee WH, McCauley TR, Katz LD, Matheny JM, Ruwe PA, Daigneault JP. Superior labral anterior posterior (SLAP) lesions of the glenoid labrum: reliability and accuracy of MR arthrography for diagnosis. *Radiology* 2001;218:127–132.

135. Bencardino JT, Beltran J, Rosenberg ZS, Rokito A, Schmahmann S, Mota J, Mellado JM, Zuckerman J, Cuomo F, Rose D. Superior labrum anterior-posterior lesions: diagnosis with MR arthrography of the shoulder. *Radiology* 2000;214:267–271.

136. De Maeseneer M, Van Roy F, Lenchik L, Shahabpour M, Jacobson J, Ryu KN, Handelberg F, Osteaux M. CT and MR arthrography of the normal and pathologic anterosuperior labrum and labral-bicipital complex. *Radiographics* 2000;20 Spec No:S67–S81.

137. Chan KK, Muldoon KA, Yeh L, Boutin R, Pedowitz R, Skaf A, Trudell DJ, Resnick D. Superior labral anteroposterior lesions: MR arthrography with arm traction. *AJR* 1999;173:1117–1122.

138. Monu JU, Pope TL Jr., Chabon SJ, Vanarthos WJ. MR diagnosis of superior labral anterior posterior (SLAP) injuries of the glenoid labrum: value of routine imaging without intraarticular injection of contrast material. *AJR* 1994;163:1425–1429.

139. Hodler J, Kursunoglu-Brahme S, Flannigan B, Snyder SJ, Karzel RP, Resnick D. Injuries of the superior portion of the glenoid labrum involving the insertion of the biceps tendon: MR imaging findings in nine cases. *AJR* 1992;159:565–568.

140. Beltran J, Bencardino J, Mellado J, Rosenberg ZS, Irish RD. MR Arthrography of the shoulder: variants and pitfalls. *Radiographics* 1997;17:1403–1412.

141. Tirman PFJ, Feller JF, Palmer WE, Carroll KW, Steinbach LS, Cox I. The Buford complex: a variation of normal shoulder anatomy: MR arthrographic imaging features. *AJR* 1996;166:869–873.

142. Tuite MJ, Orwin JF. Anterosuperior labral variants of the shoulder: appearance on gradient-recalled-echo and fast spin-echo MR images. *Radiology* 1996;199:537–540.

143. Resch H, Gosler K, Thoem H, Sperner G. Arthroscopic repair of superior glenoid labral detachment (the SLAP lesion). *J Shoulder Elbow Surg* 1993;2:147–155.

144. Gartsman GM, Hammerman SM. Superior labrum, anterior and posterior lesions: when and how to treat them. *Clin Sports Med* 2000;19:115–124.

145. Cooper DE, Arnoczky SP, O'Brien SJ, Warren RF, DiCarlo E, Allen AA. Anatomy, histology, and vascularity of the glenoid labrum: an anatomical study. *J Bone Joint Surg Am* 1992;74:46–52.

146. Warner JJ, Kann S, Marks P. Arthroscopic repair of combined Bankart and superior labral detachment anterior and posterior lesions: technique and preliminary results. *Arthroscopy* 1994;10:383–391.

147. Chochole MH, Senker W, Meznik C, Breitenseher MJ. Glenoid-labral cyst entrapping the suprascapular nerve: dissolution after arthroscopic debridement of an extended SLAP lesion. *Arthroscopy* 1997;13:753–755.

148. Tung GA, Entzian D, Stern JB, Green A. MR imaging and MR arthrography of paraglenoid labral cysts. *AJR* 2000;174:1707–1715.

149. Neviaser TJ. The GLAD lesion: another cause of anterior shoulder pain. *Arthroscopy* 1993;9:22–25.

150. Uri DS, Kneeland BJ, Dalinka MKD. Update in shoulder magnetic resonance imaging. *Magn Reson Q* 1995;11:21–44.

151. Sanders TG, Tirman PF, Linares R, Feller JF, Richardson R. The glenolabral articular disruption lesion: MR arthrography with arthroscopic correlation. *AJR* 1999;172:171–175.

BICEPS TENDON AND MISCELLANEOUS SHOULDER LESIONS

JAVIER BELTRAN
JENNY BENCARDINO

BICIPITAL TENDON LESIONS

Normal Anatomy

The biceps muscle has two muscle bellies, each one of them terminating in a corresponding tendon (1). The short bicipital tendon inserts onto the coracoid process, along with the tendons of the pectoralis minor and coracobrachialis muscles. A subcoracoid bursa is located between the coracoid process, the subscapularis, and the short head of the biceps and coracobrachialis tendons (2). This bursa alleviates friction between these tendinous structures during the arc of rotation of the humeral head. Distended subcoracoid bursa can be diagnosed using MR imaging (Fig. 8.1).

The long bicipital tendon (LBT) inserts onto the supraglenoid tubercle and/or the superior aspect of the glenoid labrum after arching over the humeral head (3). This tendon enters the joint capsule through the bicipital groove, formed between the lesser and greater humeral tuberosities (Fig. 8.2). The LBT is maintained within the bicipital groove by the transverse humeral ligament and more distally it is roofed by the tendinous insertions of the pectoralis major (4). Proximal to the transverse humeral ligament, the LBT is roofed by the coracohumeral ligament, which also contributes to the stability of the tendon within the groove as it enters the joint capsule. The coracohumeral ligament extends from the base of the coracoid process to the bicipital groove, with attachments at both sides of the groove (Fig. 8.3). The coracohumeral ligament fills a natural gap existing between the supraspinatus and subscapularis muscles, the rotator interval (Fig. 8.4) (1).

The joint capsule inserts onto the surgical neck of the humerus and glenoid margin. A bicipital recess of the synovial capsule accompanies the LBT for a short segment, to a level just distal to the transverse humeral ligament. The medial fibers of the transverse humeral ligament are intimately related to the insertional fibers of the subscapularis tendon (5). Within the joint capsule, the LBT is covered anteriorly by the superior glenohumeral ligament and the edges of the supraspinatus and infraspinatus tendons.

The structures described are well depicted with conventional MR imaging and MR arthrography (6). Axial images obtained at the level of the uppermost portion of the humeral head often demonstrate the LBT as it curves around the anterior portion of the humeral head (Fig. 8.5) (1). The curved orientation of the tendon, with the concavity directed posteriorly and concentrically with the anterior cortex of the humeral head, is related to the fact that the axial images are obtained in most cases with the arm in neutral or slight internal rotation. This brings the bicipital groove anteriorly, in the 12 o'clock position. With the arm in external rotation, the portion of the bicipital tendon adjacent to the humeral head is difficult to visualize since it becomes aligned on top of the humeral head.

Axial images obtained slightly inferiorly depict the LBT as a low signal intensity (SI) round structure that can be followed to the bicipital groove (Fig. 8.2). Anteriorly, the superior glenohumeral ligament is identified as a low SI band concentrically aligned with the lateral cortex of the coracoid process.

On sections obtained more distally with the arm in moderate internal rotation, the LBT can be seen adjacent to the medial aspect of the groove, covered by the transverse humeral ligament and more distally by the pectoralis major tendon. Not infrequently, a small amount of fluid distending the synovial sheath can be seen at this level. Fluid in the synovial sheath should not be confused with the high SI of the anterior circumflex humeral vessels. These vessels are located within the bicipital groove, anterior to the tendon and extrasynovial in position (7).

Oblique coronal images obtained at the anterior portion of the humeral head often reveal the extracapsular portion of the LBT and occasionally the intracapsular portion, as the tendon turns over the head of the humerus to insert in the superior labrum (Fig. 8.6). At this point a small sulcus or recess oriented toward the midline can be observed between

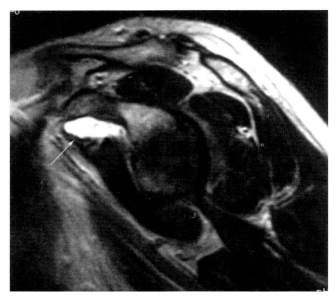

FIGURE 8.1. A well-defined fluid collection (*arrow*) extending beneath the coracoid process consistent with subcoracoid bursitis is noted on this oblique sagittal T2-weighted MR image.

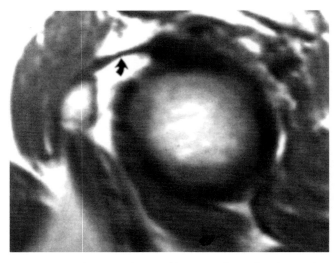

FIGURE 8.3. The coracohumeral ligament (*arrow*) is depicted as a low-signal structure extending from the coracoid process to the proximal humerus on this oblique sagittal T1-weighted MR arthrogram.

the superior labrum and the articular cartilage covering the glenoid (Fig. 8.7) (3). This bicipitolabral sulcus or sublabral recess can be filled with contrast material when performing an MR arthrogram and should not be more than a few millimeters deep.

Oblique sagittal images obtained at the level of the glenoid fossa reveal the insertion of the LBT in the superior aspect of the glenoid labrum, between the coracohumeral ligament and the superior glenohumeral ligament (Fig. 8.8). Sections obtained more laterally demonstrate the LBT as a low SI rounded structure over the head of the humerus (Fig. 8.9). Using high-resolution MR arthrogram, the coraco-

humeral ligament can be seen covering the tendon at the level of the bicipital groove. Oblique sagittal sections obtained at the plane of the coracoid process also demonstrate the insertion of the short bicipital tendon (Fig. 8.9). More laterally, the extracapsular portion of the tendon is observed as a low SI band extending distally.

It is important to remember that the portion of the LBT located over the lateral aspect of the humeral head is oriented about 55 degrees in relationship with the main magnetic field. This orientation creates a magic angle effect when using pulse sequences with TE of 20 ms or less, rendering the tendon as a high SI structure, easily misinterpreted as abnormal. This artifact can be seen on T1- and proton den-

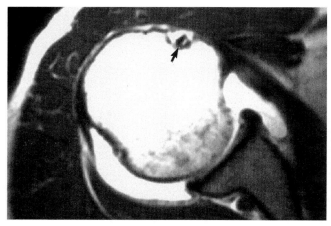

FIGURE 8.2. Axial T1-weighted MR arthrogram shows the long bicipital tendon (LBT) (*arrow*) as a low-signal round structure within the groove formed by the lesser and greater humeral tuberosities.

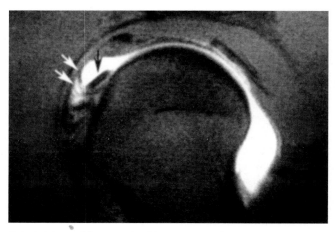

FIGURE 8.4. Oblique sagittal fat-suppressed T1-weighted (900/20) MR arthrogram demonstrates the coracohumeral ligament (*white arrows*) covering the rotator interval underneath which the LBT (*black arrow*) enters the joint capsule.

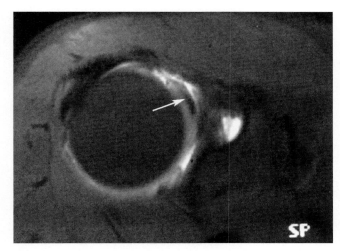

FIGURE 8.5. Axial fat-suppressed T1-weighted MR arthrogram shows the intracapsular LBT (*arrow*) as it curves around the anteromedial humeral head.

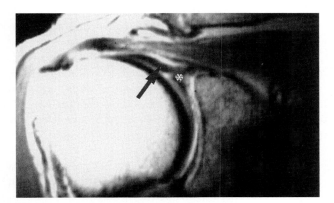

FIGURE 8.6. The intracapsular LBT (*arrow*) and its insertion onto the superior glenoid labrum (*white asterisk*) are depicted on this oblique coronal T1-weighted MR arthrogram.

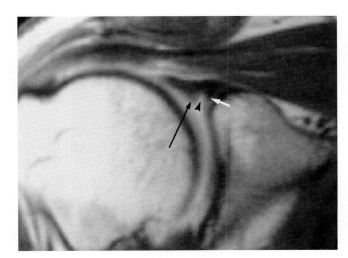

FIGURE 8.7. Pseudo-SLAP lesion. Oblique coronal T1-weighted MR arthrogram shows a medially oriented linear deposit of contrast (*arrowhead*) between the superior labrum (*black arrow*) and the glenoid rim (*white arrow*) consistent with a synovial recess.

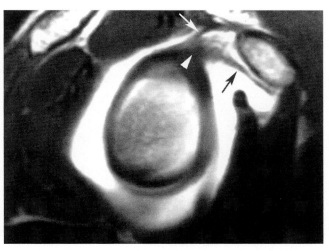

FIGURE 8.8. The LBT insertion (*arrowhead*) onto the superior glenoid is shown between the superior glenohumeral ligament (*black arrow*) and coracohumeral ligament (*white arrow*) on this sagittal T1-weighted MR arthrogram.

sity–weighted images and also using GRE sequences with a short TE (Fig. 8.10) (8).

Biceps Tenosynovitis, Tendinosis, and Tears

Tendinosis or tenosynovitis of the LBT has been classified into two types: impingement tendinosis and attrition tendinosis (9). The first type occurs in association with shoulder impingement syndrome and rotator cuff tears, where the intracapsular portion of the LBT is compressed between the humeral head, the acromion, and the coracoacromial ligament during abduction and rotation of the arm. Attritional

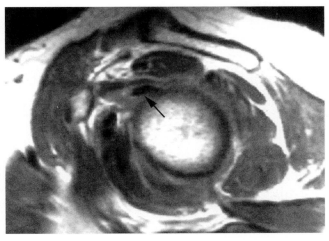

FIGURE 8.9. Sagittal T1-weighted MR image demonstrates the intracapsular portion of the LBT (*arrow*) as a low signal somewhat elongated structure over the humeral head.

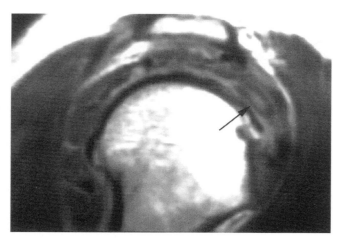

FIGURE 8.10. Spurious increased signal intensity (*arrow*) is noted involving the LBT on this sagittal T1-weighted MR image related to magic angle effect.

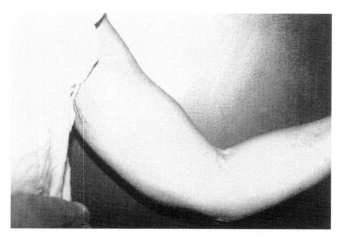

FIGURE 8.12. Complete extracapsular tear of LBT associated with inferior displacement of the biceps muscle belly resulted in "Popeye arm" deformity.

tendinosis is said to be associated to a narrow bicipital groove; hence, it affects the extracapsular portion of the tendon.

Clinically, patients present with anterior shoulder pain extending down to the arm, commonly unilateral. It is more often seen during the fifth or sixth decade of life (9, 10). Predisposing factors include inflammatory disease or

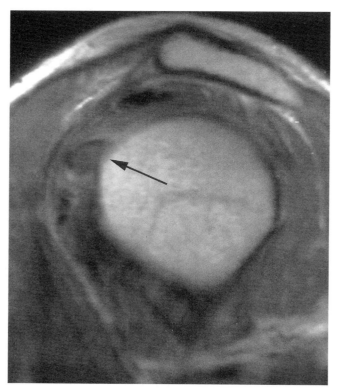

FIGURE 8.11. Marked thickening and increased signal intensity of the LBT (*arrow*) consistent with tendinosis is evident on this sagittal proton density–weighted MR image.

chronic repetitive stress of the glenohumeral joint. On physical examination, there is tenderness on palpation of the bicipital groove.

MR imaging may demonstrate fluid in the joint extending into the bicipital groove, although this is a nonspecific sign. Kaplan et al. (7) studied 30 shoulder MR examinations in asymptomatic volunteers, concluding that fluid in the tendon sheath of the LBT is abnormal if it completely surrounds the tendon, in the absence of a joint effusion.

Trauma and degeneration may involve the LBT, producing swelling and increased SI on T2 and T2* pulse sequences (Fig. 8.11) (11). This finding is particularly evident on oblique sagittal sections obtained at the level of the intracapsular portion of the LBT. In these cases, the term tendinosis is preferred to tendinitis, since inflammatory cells are not found upon histological examination.

Complete rupture of the LBT more often occurs proximally, at the level of the proximal portion of the extracapsular segment, within the groove (11). Neer classified ruptures of the long head of the biceps tendon into three types. Type 1 is tendon rupture without retraction. Type 2 is tendon rupture with partial recession, and type 3 is a self-attaching rupture without retraction (12). Clinically, complete extracapsular tears present with an audible pop and deformity of the arm secondary to the distal displacement of the belly of the biceps muscle ("Popeye arm") (Fig. 8.12). MR imaging demonstrates the absence of the LBT in the groove and its distal displacement (Fig. 8.13).

Attritional tendinosis affecting the intertubercular portion of the LBT can progress to longitudinal splits within the tendon resulting in thickening of the LBT with increased intrasubstance signal intensity on T2-weighted images. As the lesion progresses, attenuation and stretching of the torn tendon fibers will occur (Fig. 8.14). Fluid in the tendon sheath that is out of proportion of that in the joint space is another ancillary finding. A bifid LBT (normal vari-

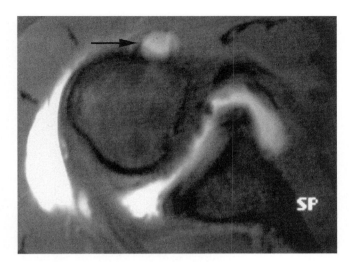

FIGURE 8.13. Axial fat-suppressed T1-weighted MR arthrogram demonstrates absent LBT within this contrast-filled bicipital groove (*arrow*).

ant) should not be confused with a partial longitudinal tear (Fig. 8.15) (12).

Intracapsular tears of the LBT are seen more often in patients with rotator cuff tears. MRI reveals absence of the in-

tracapsular portion of the tendon and the associated rotator cuff lesion (Fig. 8.16) (11).

Biceps Tendon Dislocation

As indicated earlier, the major restrains preventing dislocation of the biceps tendon are the subscapularis tendon and coracohumeral ligament (13). Disruption of these structures predisposes to dislocation or subluxation of the LBT. The transverse ligament is the least important structure in keeping the LBT within the groove (14). It is considered that the broad insertion of the subscapularis tendon plays a significant role in preventing medial slippage of the LBT (13,15). Another factor predisposing to dislocation of the LBT is hypoplasia of the bicipital groove.

Meyer described this abnormality in 1926 (14). In a series of 286 anatomic dissections, medial dislocation of the LBT was found in four instances, all of them associated with destruction of the articular surface and occasionally with rupture of the supraspinatus tendon.

According to Chan et al. (13), clinical symptoms of tendon dislocation are nonspecific and are often masked by associated rotator cuff tears. Preoperative diagnosis of this entity is important since repair of the rotator cuff without biceps tenodesis may not restore full range of motion or may

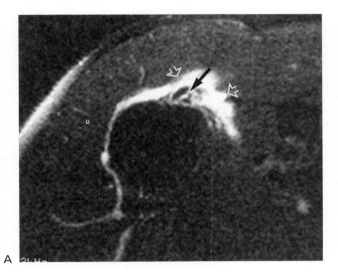

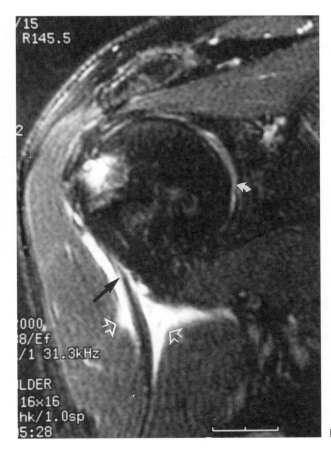

FIGURE 8.14. Partial extracapsular tear of the LBT. Longitudinal splits of the LBT (*arrow*) and fluid within the bicipital tendon sheath (*open arrows*) that is out of proportion to that seen in the joint space (*curved arrow*) are noted on these axial and coronal fat-suppressed T2-weighted MR images **(A, B)**.

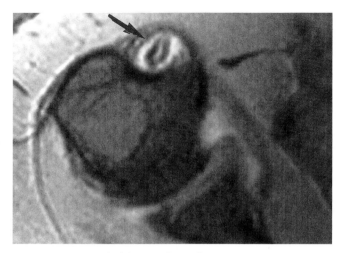

FIGURE 8.15. A bifid LBT (*arrow*) representing a normal anatomic variant is demonstrated on this axial fat-suppressed T1-weighted MR arthrogram.

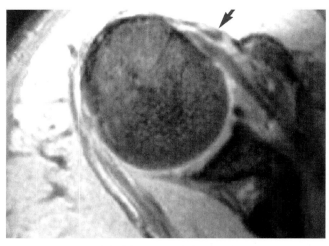

FIGURE 8.17. Medial dislocation of the LBT (*arrow*) over the intact attachment fibers of the subscapularis tendon is demonstrated on this axial T2*-weighted image.

not alleviate the clinical symptoms (10). Intermittent dislocation of the LBT is thought to be rare because once dislocation has occurred, scar tissue within the groove will prevent reduction (9).

Two types or dislocation of the LBT have been described, depending on whether the tendon is located in front or behind the subscapularis tendon (5,16,17). In the first type, the insertional fibers of the subscapularis tendon are intact (Fig. 8.17). In the second type, the subscapularis tendon is detached, and the LBT is medially displaced, becoming entrapped intrarticularly (15). Cervilla et al. (5) were able to diagnose coracohumeral ligament tear in one of six cases as well as rotator cuff tears in all of them. At surgery, flattening, fraying, and degenerative changes of the LBT were found. Slätis and Aalto (18) reported medial dislocation of the LBT over the subscapularis tendon in six cases and subluxation in

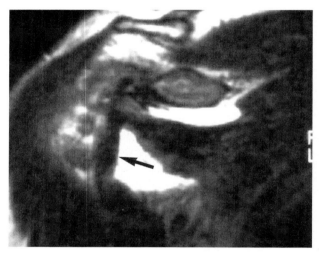

A

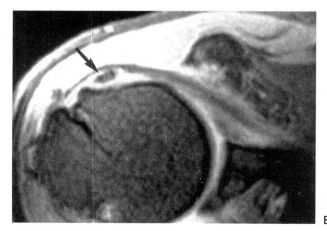

B

FIGURE 8.18. Dislocation of the LBT medial to the bicipital groove (*arrow*) is shown on these oblique coronal T2-weighted **(A)** and axial T2*-weighted images **(B)**. Although the superficial fibers of the subscapularis tendon are still intact, the deeper fibers have detached from the medial margin of the bicipital groove allowing the LBT to dislocate under the subscapularis tendon.

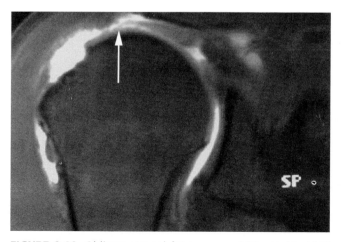

FIGURE 8.16. Oblique coronal fat-suppressed T1-weighted MR arthrogram shows complete intracapsular tear of the LBT (*arrow*) associated with complete tear of the rotator cuff.

four cases, in a series of 45 patients. These authors also stressed the significance of proper intraoperative assessment of the biceps tendon during reconstructive procedures of the shoulder capsule.

Dislocation of the LBT under the subscapularis tendon was described by Peterson (Fig. 8.18) (15). This author indicated that in some instances, the external fibers of the subscapularis muscle appear intact at visual inspection, although the deep fibers are detached from the medial margin of the bicipital groove.

MR imaging provides valuable information about the intra- or extraarticular location of the LBT tear and the integrity of the rotator cuff, specifically of the subscapularis tendon. Kynematic magnetic resonance imaging may be useful to demonstrate a dislocating biceps tendon during maximal external rotation of the shoulder (19,20).

Surgical treatment of biceps tendon dislocation includes arthroscopic debridement of partial subscapularis tendon tears, repair of subscapularis full-thickness tears, and tenodesis of the LBT to the intertubercular groove (21). Opening of the rotator cuff interval is an essential component of rotator cuff repair in order to avoid overlooking associated medial dislocation of LBT.

COMPRESSIVE AND ENTRAPMENT NEUROPATHIES

Compressive and entrapment neuropathy (CEN) refers to an alteration of nerve function due to compression by a mechanical or dynamic force. Anatomically narrow passages predispose individual nerves to these neuropathies. The compression can be acute, continuous, or intermittent. In general, CENs are produced by tumors, cysts, inflammatory processes (rheumatoid arthritis, tuberculosis), or trauma (hematoma, myositis ossificans, and callous formation). In some instances, minor changes of the surrounding soft tissues, such as a slight thickening of connective tissue, can produce signs and symptoms of CEN. Edema caused by hormonal changes associated with pregnancy, use of oral contraceptives, menopause, and hypothyroidism are also known causes. Dynamic changes within a narrow space or "tunnel" during repetitive daily activity can create compression of a nerve with only minimal anatomic variations (22,23,24,25).

Most commonly, CENs are manifested by nonspecific signs and symptoms, such as muscle weakness, with or without associated sensory loss over a localized skin area. Sharp burning pain and paresthesia may be present. In advanced cases, muscle atrophy and vegetative disturbances can occur. Electromyography and nerve conduction studies may show abnormal response to nerve stimulation.

In most cases, conservative treatment (immobilization heat, anti-inflammatory medications) of CENs is successful. Other cases may require injection of steroids or even surgery to remove the cause of the compression.

Imaging techniques other than MR imaging are extremely useful in detecting CENs. Plain film radiography and CT may show bony changes—such as exostosis, osteophytes, fracture callus, and anatomic bone variants—that may produce a CEN (26). None of these techniques, however, except occasionally CT, can show the nerves directly; the specific diagnosis of a CEN can therefore only be inferred.

Because of its exquisite spatial resolution and multiplanar capabilities, MR imaging has been used to evaluate CENs. Normal peripheral nerves are seen on MR images as structures with low to intermediate signal intensity surrounded by fat, in specific anatomic locations. Changes in signal intensity, size, and position of the involved peripheral nerve are valuable MR findings suggestive of a CEN. Osseous and soft-tissue lesions can also be well depicted with MR imaging. In acute stage of muscle denervation, MR imaging typically shows increased T2 signal of the corresponding muscle group. On advanced cases produced by a long-standing CEN, muscle atrophy with fatty infiltration will take place (27,28,29).

The diagnosis of a CEN should be established first by using clinical findings, electromyography, and possibly conventional radiographs. CT can also be used to exclude an osseous cause of the symptoms. Probably the most important roles of MR imaging in CEN are to (1) confirm the presence of nerve compression or entrapment, (2) determine whether the syndrome is produced by mechanical compression (e.g., soft-tissue mass), (3) determine the nature and extent of the lesion and the site of nerve compression, and (4) exclude other lesions that can cause similar signs and symptoms (e.g., rotator cuff tear).

Recent developments in pulse sequences and surface coils will further enhance the usefulness of MR imaging in depicting normal and abnormal peripheral nerves. Small flexible surface coils, circularly polarized coils, and phase array coils designed for imaging the different joints of the upper extremity are being tested. Increased contrast-to-noise and signal-to-noise ratios at very small fields of view that are achievable with these techniques will probably allow detection of subtle changes in size and abnormal signal intensity of the peripheral nerves.

The use of IV paramagnetic contrast agents might also prove to be valuable in assessing CENs. Sugimoto et al. (30), using dynamic MR imaging, have suggested that symptoms of carpal tunnel syndrome are produced by circulatory disturbances in the median nerve with chronic hypoxia rather than by compression alone. In their experience, dynamic MR imaging could be used to distinguish normal from abnormal nerves by their different patterns of enhancement.

Suprascapular Nerve Syndrome

The suprascapular nerve originates from the brachial plexus, traverses the supraclavicular fossa, and enters the supraspinatus fossa through the scapular notch, making a sharp turn around the scapular spine. The transverse scapular ligament bridges the scapular notch or incisura superiorly, creating a fibro osseous tunnel. At the scapular incisura, the suprascapular nerve branches into the supraspinatus and infraspinatuous nerves. In about 50% of the population, a second ligament, the spinoglenoid ligament, produces a second tunnel traversed by the infraspinatus nerve (22,31). Therefore, proximal entrapment at the scapular incisura may result in supra and infraspinatus muscle denervation syndrome while distal entrapment at the spinoglenoid notch may be manifested as isolated compromise of the infraspinatus muscle.

The suprascapular nerve or its branches can become compressed or entrapped by stretching due to repetitive scapular motion or can be damaged by scapular fractures or other direct trauma. In a recent anatomic and morphological study in 23 shoulder specimens, adduction and internal rotation were noted to cause stretching of the suprascapular nerve underneath the spinoglenoid ligament (32). Overhead activities (e.g., as done by painters, electricians, volleyball and tennis players) may also result in chronic mechanical stretching and irritation of the suprascapular nerve. In these patients, T2-weighted MR images can show hyperintense signal of the involved muscle. Nerve thickening and muscle atrophy due to denervation may be noted in advanced cases.

Soft-tissue masses, osseous tumors, and vascular malformations can also compress the nerve along its course. Ganglion cysts at the scapular incisura typically associated with posterior labral tears can be easily detected on MR images of the shoulder (31,33).

Quadrilateral Space Syndrome

The quadrilateral space syndrome is caused by compression of the axillary nerve at the quadrilateral space. This space is bounded by the long head of the triceps brachii muscle medially, the teres minor muscle superiorly, the teres major muscle inferiorly, and the medial aspect of the humerus laterally. The axillary nerve originates from the brachial plexus and passes through the quadrilateral space together with the posterior circumflex artery. The teres minor and deltoid muscles and the posterolateral cutaneous region of the shoulder and upper arm are innervated by the axillary nerve (22,29).

Proximal humeral and scapular fractures or axillary mass lesions can result in damage or compression of the axillary nerve. Entrapment of this nerve can also be produced by extreme abduction of the arm during sleep, hypertrophy of teres minor muscle in paraplegic patients, or by a fibrous band within the quadrilateral space (34). Patients may have shoulder pain and paresthesia. In advanced cases, atrophy of the deltoid and teres minor muscles can occur.

The normal axillary nerve is easily visualized on routine oblique sagittal MR images. Osseous lesions involving the axillary nerve, such as fracture callus or bone tumors, can be

assessed with plain film radiography or CT. Soft-tissue lesions can be detected with MR imaging. Selective atrophy of the teres minor muscle caused by axillary nerve compression has been reported (29).

Parsonage-Turner Syndrome

Parsonage-Turner syndrome, also referred to as *acute brachial neuritis*, is clinically characterized by sudden onset of severe atraumatic pain in the shoulder girdle (35). The pain typically decreases spontaneously in 1 to 3 weeks and is followed by weakness of at least one of the muscles about the shoulder. The exact etiology has not been established, but viral and immunological causes have been considered (36). The age-range at presentation is quite wide. There is typically male predominance for this disorder (male : female = 2–11.5 : 1) (35,37,38).

In the description by Parsonage and Turner (35), the long thoracic nerve was thought to be most frequently compromised. However, later reports have shown higher rate of isolated suprascapular nerve disease (37,38). The axillary, radial, and phrenic nerves may also be affected (39) as well as the entire brachial plexus (40). Bilateral involvement is found in as many as one-third of the patients (38). Abnormal electromyographic pattern with fibrillation potentials and positive waves is characteristically encountered in this condition (40).

MR imaging findings in acute stage include diffuse increased signal intensity on T2-weighted images consistent

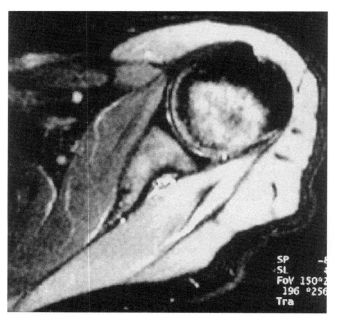

FIGURE 8.19. Parsonage-Turner syndrome. Axial T2*-weighted MR image demonstrates diffuse increased T2* signal intensity involving the infraspinatous and deltoid muscles. The increased signal intensity is not related to coil-proximity artifact since the signal intensity of subcutaneous fat is low.

with interstitial muscle edema associated with denervation (Fig. 8.19) (28). The most commonly affected muscles are those innervated by the suprascapular nerve, including the supra and infraspinatus. The deltoid muscle can also be compromised in cases of axillary nerve involvement. Later in the course of the disease, muscle atrophy manifested by decreased muscle bulk may be visualized (41).

This disorder can resemble a variety of other clinical diagnosis, including rotator cuff pathology, cervical radiculopathy, spinal cord tumor, and peripheral nerve compression. The most confusing differential diagnosis is probably that of compressive neuropathy of the suprascapular nerve (40). The more insidious onset of pain and lack of spontaneous resolution of symptoms can help to distinguish compressive neuropathy from Parsonage-Turner syndrome. MR imaging is the diagnostic technique of choice to solve this diagnostic dilemma by excluding suprascapular nerve entrapment related to paralabral ganglions or other impinging mass lesions (41). Rotator cuff pathology can also be readily excluded using MR imaging.

PECTORALIS AND DELTOID MUSCULOTENDINOUS LESIONS

Pectoralis Tendon Lesions

Pectoralis major musculotendinous injuries are relatively uncommon but have become more prevalent due to increased popularity of recreational sport activities. Weightlifting, wrestling, football, and water skiing have been associated with these lesions. Skeletally mature men are more commonly affected than women (42). However, complete bony avulsions of the pectoralis major have also been reported in skeletally immature individuals (43).

The pectoralis major muscle is composed by two major heads, clavicular and sternal, and a smaller abdominal head. The upper abdominal/sternal and lower clavicular insertional fibers are distributed along the lateral lip of the bicipital tendon groove of the humerus.

Injuries to the pectoralis major musculotendinous unit can involve the humeral insertion, muscle belly, or myotendinous junction (4). The larger sternal head is more frequently injured than the smaller clavicular head (42). Clinical evaluation can be difficult in the acute setting due to the presence of pain, intramuscular hematoma, and spasm. MR imaging is then useful for distinguishing avulsive from myotendinous injuries (44). Partial tears are more frequent at the myotendinous junction, while complete tears are usually noted at the insertion site. This is of clinical importance since the former lesions are commonly treated conservatively as opposed to the latter ones that require surgical correction (4). Timely surgical reattachment of the pectoralis major muscle prevents the formation of scarring and tendon retraction (42) allowing earlier incorporation of the professional or recreational athlete in sports activities. In cases of

complete avulsion, MR imaging can demonstrate the degree of tendon retraction and scarring, which are important preoperative planning factors (4,45).

Deltoid Muscle Lesions

Lesions involving the deltoid muscle include chronic avulsion injury, muscle contracture, and muscle dehiscence following rotator cuff repair. Chronic avulsion injuries in general occur more frequently in adolescents and present radiographically as an area of cortical irregularity and periosteal reaction simulating a malignant process (44,46), occasionally leading to biopsy. Most frequently chronic avulsion injuries occur at the pelvis and proximal femora. Chronic avulsion at the humeral insertion of the deltoid muscle is relatively rare. Radiographic manifestations also include cortical thickening and irregularity. On MRI, these findings are associated with focal areas of increased T2 signal involving the soft tissues adjacent to the humerus (46). Bone scintigraphy may demonstrate a focal area of increased uptake in the region of the deltoid tubercle. The treatment is conservative.

Deltoid muscle contracture has been described as a complication of repeated intramuscular injections leading to fibrosis (47). Patients present with a characteristic deformity of the shoulder which includes anterolateral scapular rotation ("winging"), inferolateral rotation or lateral shift of the scapula, associated with flexion and abduction contracture of the glenohumeral joint. Patients complain of pain and decreased range of motion. Clinical history of repeated intramuscular injections is a clue to the diagnosis of this entity. Occasionally there is a family history of keloid formation and muscle contracture. This lesion involves more often the midportion of the deltoid. It is postulated that mechanical injury, drug toxicity muscle ischemia, and chemical myositis are potential etiologic factors. In addition to the abnormal position of the scapula, radiological examination may reveal soft-tissue calcifications, prominent deltoid tuberosity, lateral downsloping of the acromion due to scapular rotation, and enthesopathy of the superolateral of the acromion process, and distal deltoid insertion in the humerus.

MR findings include the abnormal scapular orientation and a hypointense cordlike structure within the deltoid representing the fibrotic bundle of muscle fibers. This finding is more conspicuous on gradient echo pulse sequences. Treatment is conservative, but surgery with distal release of the contracture has reported to give good results in 96% of cases in a series of 43 postoperated shoulders. Resolution of anterosuperior subluxation of the humeral head and rotation of the scapula were noted after surgical treatment in this recent report (48).

Temporal detachment of the deltoid tendon insertion from the anterolateral acromion is a frequent surgical practice that improves exposure during acromioplasty (49). Postoperative dehiscence of the deltoid is a potential complication after this procedure. MR imaging is a valuable tool in identifying this condition that can be repaired surgically if promptly identified. The prognosis worsens if deltoid atrophy ensues due to chronic detachment.

INFLAMMATORY AND INFECTIOUS CONDITIONS

Idiopathic Synovial Osteochondromatosis

Idiopathic synovial osteochondromatosis is a benign disorder characterized by cartilaginous metaplastic changes of synovium. These synovial cartilaginous nodules are often multiple and may undergo ossification. Idiopathic synovial chondromatosis often involves large, capacious joints including the knee, the hip, shoulder, and elbow.

The radiographic manifestations of idiopathic synovial osteochondromatosis include numerous ossified intraarticular nodules of approximately equal size without joint space narrowing (50). Nonossified cartilaginous nodules (synovial chondromatosis) will escape radiographic detection, requiring advanced imaging techniques such as arthrography, computed tomography, ultrasonography, or MRI (51,52, 53). Pressure erosions may be occasionally present, in which case the differential diagnosis with pigmented villonodular synovitis is difficult (54). These erosions are more frequent around the proximal humerus. Other radiographic manifestations of idiopathic synovial osteochondromatosis are subchondral cysts and joint subluxation, probably related to synovial nodular proliferation.

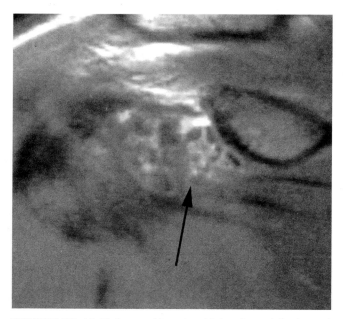

FIGURE 8.20. Multiple round low signal intensity nodules (*arrow*) are noted in the subscapularis recess on this oblique coronal fat-suppressed T1-weighted MR arthrogram consistent with synovial chondromatosis.

The MR manifestations of idiopathic synovial osteochondromatosis depend on the degree of calcification or ossification of the cartilaginous bodies (53). If no calcification is present, it may simulate a joint effusion, with low SI on T1-weighted images and high SI on T2-weighted images. However, high-resolution MR imaging may be able to demonstrate a signal more inhomogeneous than fluid. If calcifications are present, these will manifest themselves as multiple small foci of decreased SI on both T1- and T2-weighted pulse sequences (Fig. 8.20), surrounded by high SI haloes on T2-weighted images, representing the cartilaginous coverage. The presence of low SI material mixed with hyperintense cartilage may mimic pigmented villonodular synovitis, especially if bone erosions are present. Other differential diagnostic considerations include entities that can produce multiple intraarticular bodies, such as osteocartilaginous loose bodies related to osteoarthritis or osteochondral trauma and "rice bodies" such as those seen in rheumatoid arthritis and tuberculosis.

The intraarticular bodies have a tendency to lodge in the synovial recesses of the joint, including the subscapularis recess, the axillary recess, and the synovial sheath in the bicipital groove (Fig. 8.21).

Pigmented Villonodular Synovitis (PVNS)

Pigmented villonodular synovitis is a synovial disorder characterized by villous hyperplasia of the synovium and hemosiderin deposition (55). It is most often a monoarticular process that can be seen in any structure lined by synovium, such as bursae (56) and tendon sheaths (57). In the latter, the term *giant cell tumor of the tendon sheaths* is applied, indicating the same condition (58). The shoulder joint is not as frequently involved by PVNS as the knee, hip, elbow, and ankle. Articular involvement by PVNS can present as diffuse or localized forms.

PVNS occurs more often during the third or fourth decade of life, but it can also be seen in children and in the elderly. It involves males slightly more often than females, and a history of trauma can be found in about 50% of the cases (55). Occurrence of PVNS following anterior capsulolabral reconstruction of the shoulder was recently reported (59). Concomitant articular involvement by PVNS and rheumatoid arthritis has also been described (60).

Clinical manifestations include pain, swelling, tenderness, stiffness, and warmth in the diffuse form. In the localized form, signs of internal joint derangement are more frequent. Joint aspiration reveals brown fluid secondary to chronic hemorrhage or fresh blood.

The radiographic manifestations of PVNS include joint effusion, soft-tissue swelling, bone erosions, cystic lesions, absence of calcifications with diffuse increased opacity of the soft tissues around the affected joint due to hemosiderin deposition (61). Typically, the joint space is maintained as well as the overall bone density, but, occasionally, joint space

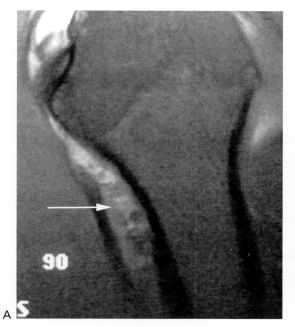 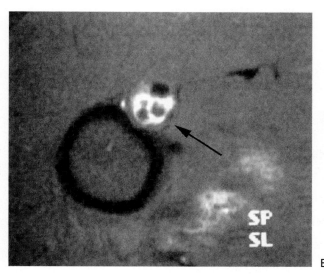

FIGURE 8.21. Oblique sagittal **(A)** and axial **(B)** fat-suppressed T1-weighted MR arthrograms demonstrate multiple intraarticular bodies (*arrows*) lodged in the bicipital tendon sheath in this patient with synovial chondromatosis.

narrowing and osteoporosis may be present late in the disease process (62). Not infrequently, the localized form of PVNS reveals no abnormalities on conventional radiographs except for a joint effusion. Diagnostic overlap between noncalcified synovial osteochondromatosis and PVNS has been stressed in the literature (63).

The MR findings of PVNS are quite distinct, due to the paramagnetic effect of the hemosiderin deposit that produces characteristic foci of low SI on T1- and T2-weighted sequences (64). Heterogeneous pattern is also frequently observed, due to the presence of areas of low hemosiderin deposition and associated joint effusion (Fig. 8.22) (65,66). The paramagnetic effect of hemosiderin is enhanced on gradient echo pulse sequences (66). Associated ancillary findings such as bone erosions and capsular distension are often seen in the diffuse form of PVNS. The differential diagnosis of this entity, based on MR findings, includes synovial chondromatosis, gout, amyloidosis, synovial hemangioma, and hemophilic arthropathy (Fig. 8.23) (63). All these entities can produce intraarticular masses with areas of low SI in all pulse sequences, very similar to PVNS. The presence of pressure erosions makes the differentiation between synovial osteochondromatosis and PVNS more difficult. Malignant transformation of PVNS to spindle-shaped cell sarcomas has been reported (67).

Crystal Deposition Diseases

Calcific deposits around the shoulder can be seen on conventional radiographs in a variety of conditions including calcific tendinitis and bursitis secondary to hydroxiapatite or pyrophosphate crystal deposits, renal osteodystrophy (Fig. 8.24), idiopathic tumoral calcinosis, collagen vascular disorders, milk alkali syndrome, and hypervitaminosis D.

Intraarticular deposition of hydroxiapatite crystal can trigger a series of events leading to the development of severe osteoarthritis and joint disintegration with associated rotator cuff tears (68,69). This condition has been termed "Milwaukee

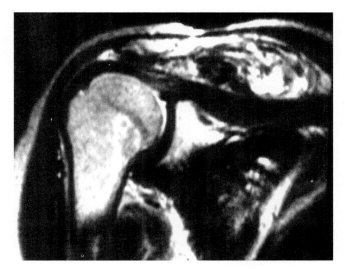

FIGURE 8.22. Pigmented villonodular synovitis involving the subacromial bursa characterized by heterogeneous T2 signal intensity related to areas of low hemosiderin deposition and associated hyperintense joint effusion.

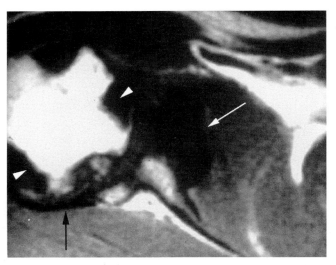

FIGURE 8.23. Hemophilic arthropathy. Axial T1-weighted MR image shows homogeneously hypointense hemarthrosis (*white arrow*) associated with humeral head erosions (*arrowheads*) and thickened low signal posterior capsule (*black arrow*).

shoulder." The radiographic manifestations of this entity include intraarticular calcifications, joint space narrowing, severe osteolysis, subchondral cysts, sclerosis and superior migration of the humeral head, related to advanced chronic rotator cuff tear (70) (Fig. 8.25). Osteophytes are not characteristic of this syndrome. Other conditions that can produce severe disintegration of the glenohumeral joint include

neuroarthropathy (Fig. 8.26), cuff-tear arthropathy, CPPD crystal deposition disease, alkaptonuria, septic arthritis, idiopathic chondrolysis, rheumatoid arthritis, ischemic necrosis, and senile hemorrhagic shoulder syndrome. It is accepted that hydroxiapatite crystal deposition disease may coexist with CPPD crystal deposition disease (mixed crystal deposition disease) (71).

The MRI manifestations of hydroxiapatite crystal deposition disease involving the shoulder include focal areas of low SI, often associated with edematous changes of the surrounding soft tissues. The most frequently involved structure is the distal portion of the supraspinatus tendon (70) (Fig. 8.27), but it may involve other tendons, including the bicipital tendon (Fig. 8.25).

Osteoarthritis

Primary osteoarthritis of the glenohumeral joint is not so common. Degenerative changes are often associated with a history of previous shoulder trauma or underlying conditions, including CPPD crystal deposition disease, hydroxyapatite crystal deposition disease, acromegaly, or hemophilia. The radiographic manifestations of osteoarthritis are well known and include joint space narrowing, subchondral cyst formation, loose bodies, and osteophytes. MRI may reveal in addition the presence of rotator cuff abnormalities, including tendinosis and rotator cuff tears, as well as degenerative changes of the labrum and glenoid margins. Large subchondral cyst of the greater tuberosity can be occasionally noted

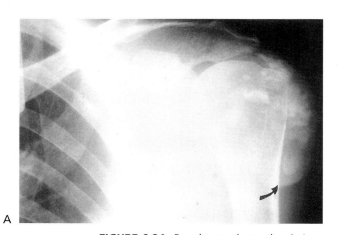
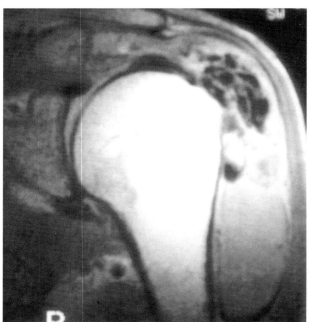

FIGURE 8.24. Renal osteodystrophy. **A:** Large saclike collections of calcification (*curved arrow*) about the shoulder are depicted on this conventional anteroposterior radiograph. **B:** Oblique coronal T2-weighted MR image shows extensive subacromial-subdeltoid bursitis with layering areas of low signal intensity corresponding to calcification in this end-stage renal disease patient.

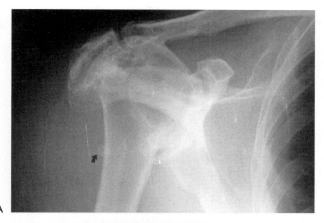

A

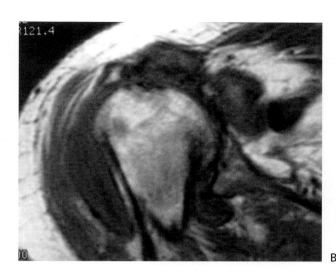

B

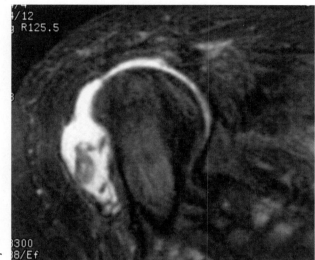

C

FIGURE 8.25. Milwaukee shoulder. **A:** Anteroposterior radiograph of the shoulder demonstrates advanced degenerative changes of the glenohumeral joint associated with superior migration of the humeral head related to rotator cuff tear, and long bicipital calcific tendinitis (*curved arrow*). Coronal T1-weighted **(B)** and fat-suppressed T2-weighted **(C)** MR images show extensive rotator cuff tear, subdeltoid bursitis, and intraarticular loose bodies in this patient with hydroxyapatite crystal deposition disease.

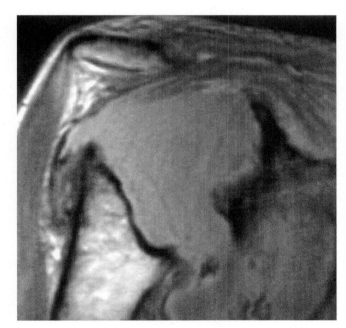

FIGURE 8.26. Neuroarthropathy. Oblique coronal proton density–weighted MR image shows severe desintegration of the humeral head and glenoid cavity associated with large joint effusion.

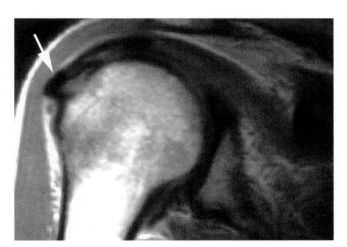

FIGURE 8.27. Calcific tendinitis involving the distal portion of the supraspinatous tendon (*arrow*) is demonstrated on this oblique coronal proton density–weighted MR image.

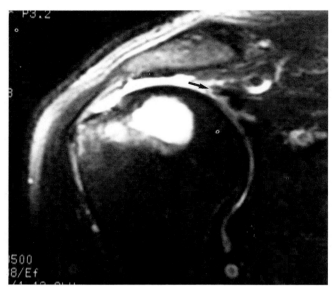

FIGURE 8.28. Oblique coronal fat-suppressed T2-weighted MR image demonstrates degenerative changes of the shoulder joint with large subchondral cyst or geode involving the humeral head. A complete tear of the supraspinatus tendon is also noted (*arrow*).

in association with degenerative osteoarthritis and rotator cuff tears (Fig. 8.28) (72).

Rheumatoid Arthritis

Shoulder involvement by rheumatoid arthritis is often seen. Its classic radiographic manifestations include uniform narrowing of the joint space, marginal erosions, erosions of the greater tuberosity, subchondral cystic lesions, osteophytes, bone reabsorption of the proximal humerus, flattening of the glenoid cavity, and sclerosis of apposing surfaces of the glenoid and humerus. Elevation of the humerus with respect to the glenoid cavity, due to rotator cuff atrophy or tear, is also a prominent finding. The acromioclavicular joint is also often affected in rheumatoid arthritis, with soft-tissue swelling and subchondral osteoporosis and erosions, predominating on the clavicle with extensive osteolysis and subluxation. Pseudowidening of the acromioclavicular joint space due to distal clavicle resorption is a common associated finding.

Additional features of rheumatoid arthritis revealed by MR imaging include joint effusion, subacromial-subdeltoid bursitis, rotator cuff tendinosis, and tears secondary to the effect of the inflamed synovium on the undersurface of the tendons and "rice bodies" (73,74,75,76). Chronic articular inflammation evolves into proliferation of elongated synovial villi (Fig. 8.29) that become fibrotic and eventually detach, producing grains similar to polished rice. On MRI, these "rice bodies" manifest themselves as numerous rounded nodules of intermediate SI occupying the joint

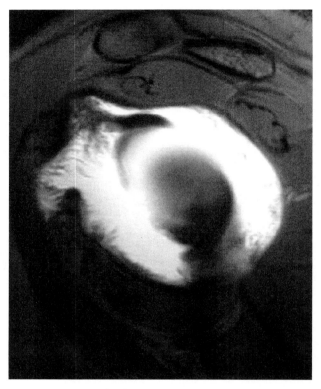

FIGURE 8.29. Multiple elongated synovial villi related to chronic articular inflammation are depicted on this oblique sagittal fat-suppressed T1-weighted MR arthrogram.

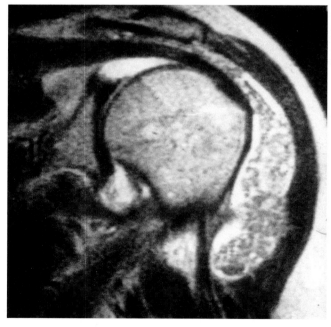

FIGURE 8.30. Tuberculosis. Oblique coronal T2-weighted MR image shows extensive subacromial subdeltoid bursitis with innumerable punctate foci of low signal intensity consistent with rice bodies.

space and/or the subacromial bursa. Similar findings can be seen in tuberculous arthritis (Fig. 8.30) and even synovial chondromatosis (Fig. 8.20).

Septic Arthritis

Septic arthritis of the shoulder has predilection for either the very young infant population or elderly patients with chronic debilitating diseases such as diabetes, malignancies, liver disease, and alcoholism (77,78). Septic arthritis is most likely to develop in a joint with preexisting chronic arthritis. Septic arthritis can manifest as a complication of rheumatoid arthritis, systemic lupus erythematosus, and mixed connective tissue disorder (79). Therefore, other signs of arthritis can be seen on MRI, such as bone erosions, bone resorption, and subchondral cysts.

Clinical diagnosis of shoulder septic arthritis requires a high index of suspicion (80). Aspiration of synovial fluid is necessary to make the diagnosis and identify the offending pathogen, although it is important to be aware of a high rate (90%) of false-negative gram stains in this condition. Conversely, synovial fluid cultures often reveal the pathogen (88%). Conventional radiographs are frequently unremarkable in early stages of the disease. Ultrasound may be useful in demonstrating joint effusion. Indium-labeled leucocytes may be helpful, specially if coexistent osteomyelitis is suspected (Fig. 8.31).

The MR manifestations of septic arthritis are not different from those seen in other joints—namely, joint effusion with associated soft-tissue pericapsular edema and occasionally bone marrow edema. Inferior subluxation of the glenohumeral joint, "drooping shoulder," is a manifestation of joint effusion that can be seen associated with septic arthritis (81). However, since the MR examination is performed with the patient in the supine position, this sign may not be as evident as it is on a conventional radiograph, obtained with the patient upright.

Tuberculosis

Tuberculosis of the shoulder is unusual as compared with tuberculous involvement of other joints (82,83). The classic triad of radiographic manifestations (Phemister triad) includes juxtaarticular osteoporosis, peripherally located osseous erosions (corner erosions), and gradual narrowing of the joint space (84). Loss of articular space is a late part of the radiographic picture, as opposed to rheumatoid arthritis in which joint narrowing occurs early in the process. Other manifestations include subchondral erosions, bone sclerosis (unusual), periostitis, bone sequestrate, and bony ankylosis as the end result of tuberculous arthritis (84).

MRI findings of tuberculous arthritis include the previously described bony changes in addition to soft-tissue manifestations of tuberculosis, such as large synovial cysts,

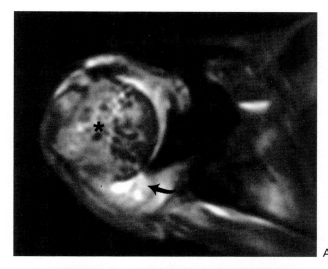

A

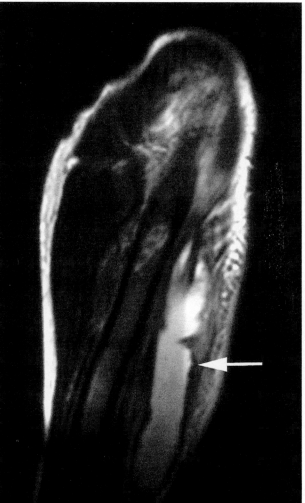

B

FIGURE 8.31. Humeral head osteomyelitis (*asterisk*) associated with septic shoulder effusion (*curved arrow*) and infectious bicipital bursitis (*arrow*) are noted on these axial **(A)** and sagittal **(B)** fat-suppressed T2-weighted MR images. Fluid/fluid level within the bicipital bursa is probably related to debris.

soft-tissue abscesses, and fistulous communication with internal organs (85). "Rice bodies" are also characteristic of tuberculous arthritis, with similar MRI findings as those seen in rheumatoid arthritis (Fig. 8.30). Areas of decreased signal intensity on T1- and T2-weighted images probably representing hemosiderin deposition in hemorrhagic synovium have been described (85).

FRACTURES AND OSTEOCHONDRAL LESIONS

Occult Fractures

Occult fractures of the proximal humerus often involve the greater tuberosity and occur as a result of injuries such as seizures, glenohumeral dislocations, and forced abduction. These fractures can be classified as one part fractures using the Neer classification of proximal humeral fractures (86). Mason et al. (87) described the MRI findings of occult greater tuberosity in 12 patients, in whom prospective review of the plain films failed to demonstrate minimally displaced fractures. All patients in this series had partial tears or tendinosis of the rotator cuff, but none had full-thickness tears. These authors postulate that the presence of a fracture precludes a full-thickness tear of the cuff. Conversely, Zanneti et al. found nondisplaced greater tuberosity fractures in 9 of 24 patients following acute substantial trauma to the shoulder associated with complete tears of the supraspinatus, infraspinatus, and subscapularis tendons (88). Management of acute traumatic tears of the rotator cuff is surgical, while nondisplaced fractures of the greater tuberosity require only conservative therapy. Awareness of the associated finding of

greater tuberosity fracture give reasons for persistence of pain after rotator cuff repair (89).

MR imaging demonstrates the fracture line as a low signal irregular area, surrounded by bone marrow edema (Fig. 8.32). Retrospective evaluation of the plain films in Mason et al. series revealed subtle findings such as irregularities and defects of the curved surface of the greater tuberosity in 8 of 11 patients, highlighting the need for careful inspection of this area to avoid unnecessary MRI studies. Clinically, these patients present with symptoms that simulate rotator cuff tears.

Osteochondral Lesions

Osteochondral lesions of the shoulder are rare. Different names and descriptions have been used by different authors

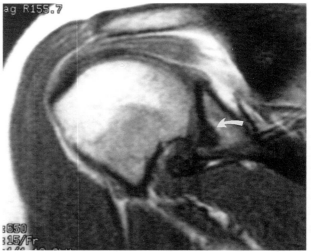

A

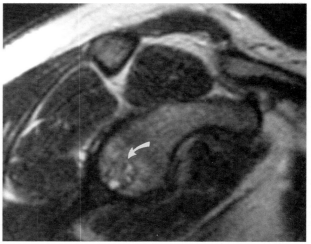

B

FIGURE 8.33. Oblique coronal T1-weighted **(A)** and oblique sagittal T2-weighted images demonstrate cystic changes in the subchondral bone of inferior glenoid fossa related to osteochondral lesion (*curved arrows*).

FIGURE 8.32. A nondisplaced, occult fracture of the greater tuberosity (*arrows*) associated with edema of adjacent bone marrow is depicted on this oblique coronal proton density–weighted MR image.

to describe a group of lesions that involve the articular surface of the glenoid fossa, including osteochondritis dissecans (OCD) (90), subchondral avascular necrosis (91), juxtaarticular bone cyst (92), posttraumatic subchondral cyst (92), and glenoid articular rim divot (GARD). Recently, Yu et al. (93) described the MRI findings of osteochondral defects of the glenoid fossa. Their results indicate that these lesions are related to acute trauma and are often associated with glenohumeral instability, labral tears, and intraarticular loose bodies. Cystic changes in the subchondral bone of the glenoid fossa are the most frequent radiographic feature. Similar findings are also seen using CT and MRI (Fig. 8.33). Another frequent radiographic manifestation is the presence of a radiolucent area in the subchondral bone surrounded by a rim of sclerosis. Occasionally loose bodies are found on plain radiographs, CT, or MRI. Careful attention to the articular surface of the glenoid may reveal the presence of a chondral or osteochondral defect.

Based on arthroscopic findings, Snyder et al. described a glenoid chondral defect called "GARD" for glenoid articular rim divot (94). MRI examination in these patients may reveal the chondral defect as well as a cartilaginous loose fragment in a joint recess. A similar entity was reported by Chan et al. (95) in which multiloculated subchondral cysts are present in the posterior superior quadrant of the glenoid fossa. These authors used the same acronym (GARD) to indicate glenoid articular rim disruption. They postulated that the specific location of these lesions is related to a developmentally weak area of the glenoid fossa related to an area of junction between the ossification centers of the glenoid. All these osteochondral lesions are often detected in the throwing athlete.

AVASCULAR NECROSIS

Avascular necrosis or osteonecrosis of the humeral head is not as frequent as osteonecrosis of other parts of the skeleton such as the femoral head (96). It is often seen associated with predisposing conditions like sickle-cell anemia, alcoholism, pancreatitis, steroid use, systemic lupus erythematosus, and trauma, among others. The radiographic manifestations and clinical staging are similar to osteonecrosis of the femoral head. In the early phases, no radiographic findings are detected (stage 1). Subchondral bone sclerosis and lucencies with preservation of the shape of the humeral head correspond to stage 2. In stage 3, there is subchondral fracture and collapse (Fig. 8.34) that evolves into incongruity of the glenohumeral joint and subsequent osteoarthritis (stage 4).

MRI manifestations of osteonecrosis of the humeral head are also similar to those seen in the femoral head (97). The more characteristic MR finding is the presence of the "double line" sign, with a band of low SI surrounding a band of higher SI on proton density– and T2-weighted images. Both

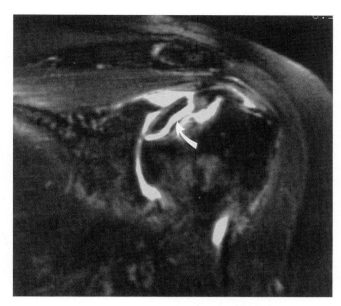

FIGURE 8.34. Oblique coronal fat-suppressed T2-weighted MR image shows subchondral fracture (*curved arrow*) with articular fluid interposed between the fragment and the donor site, findings in keeping with stage 3 avascular necrosis of the humeral head.

bands appear to correspond to the reactive interphase as described microscopically (97). The hypointense line or band correlates with the outer layer of osteoclastic proliferation and bone sclerosis and the hyperintense line corresponds to an area of hypervascularity and granulation tissue.

ACROMIOCLAVICULAR JOINT

The articular surfaces of the acromioclavicular joint are covered with fibrocartilage and confined by a fibrous capsule. There is a disc occupying the central portion of the joint. The distal end of the clavicle is stabilized to the scapula by the acromioclavicular and the coracoclavicular ligaments (Fig. 8.35). The coracoclavicular ligament has two components, trapezoid and conoid. These two components are separated by fatty tissue and occasionally a bursa. An articulation between the undersurface of the clavicle and the coracoid process can be found in less than 1% of the population. In these cases, a bony protuberance extends inferiorly from the clavicle toward the coracoid process. This joint is covered by a fibrous capsule, and it contains fibrocartilage and occasionally a fibrous disc.

The acromioclavicular joint may be involved in a variety of pathologic conditions, including osteoarthritis, inflammatory arthritis, trauma, metabolic diseases, crystal deposition diseases, and septic arthritis. Most of the findings caused by these entities are well identified with conventional radiographic techniques. However, from the MRI standpoint, it is important to be familiar with their manifestations

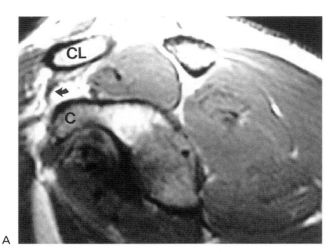
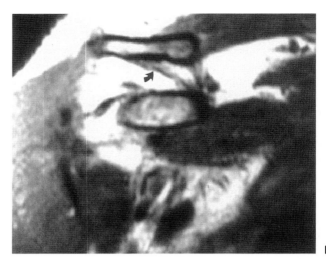

A   B

FIGURE 8.35. Oblique sagittal **(A)** and oblique coronal **(B)** T1-weighted images through the plane of the coracoid process demonstrate a low signal linear structure extending from the clavicle (CL) to the coracoid **(C)** consistent with the coracoclavicular ligament (*curved arrow*).

since the acromioclavicular joint is part of any shoulder MRI examination, and significant pathology of this area can be detected.

The classic radiographic signs of osteoarthritis, including subchondral cysts, osteophytes, joint space narrowing, and irregularity of the joint, can be observed also with MRI. Hypertrophy of the joint and osteophytes are particularly important to recognize since they can produce compression

of the rotator cuff and impingement syndrome, leading to rotator cuff tear (Fig. 8.36). Full-thickness rotator cuff tears allow communication between the glenohumeral joint and subacromial subdeltoid bursa. Occasionally, additional communication between the subacromial-subdeltoid bursa and the acromioclavicular joint can be found. This communication can be seen with arthrographic techniques (the geyser sign) (98,99) as well as MRI with fluid accumulating in the

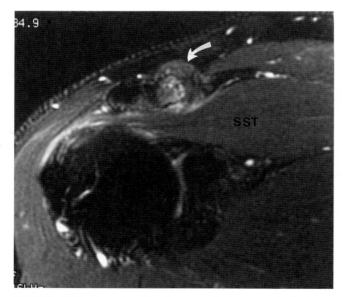

FIGURE 8.36. Hypertrophic changes of the acromioclavicular joint and acromial marrow edema (*curved arrow*) associated with impingement of the musculotendinous junction of supraspinatus tendon (SST) are seen on this oblique coronal fat-suppressed T2-weighted MR image.

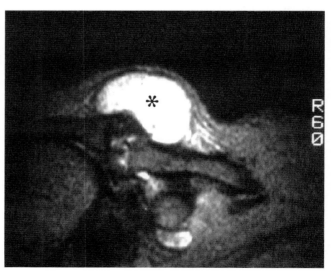

FIGURE 8.37. Acromioclavicular joint cyst. Oblique coronal T2-weighted MR image depicts a large fluid collection (*asterisk*) overlying the acromioclavicular joint related to leakage of synovial fluid from the glenohumeral joint space through a torn rotator cuff.

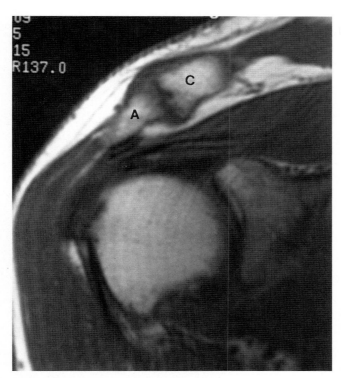

FIGURE 8.38. Oblique coronal T1-weighted MR image shows a bulbous appearance of the acromioclavicular joint related to volume averaging from the plane of scanning. A, acromion; C, clavicle.

acromioclavicular joint and occasionally producing distension of the capsule and a cyst-like fluid collection (Fig. 8.37) (100).

Hypertrophy of the acromioclavicular joint is often overdiagnosed with MRI because the normal joint can offer a bulbous appearance on oblique coronal and oblique sagittal images (Fig. 8.38). As indicated earlier the diagnosis of osteoarthritis requires the visualization of osteophytes, subchondral cysts, irregular and narrow articular surfaces, and subchondral sclerosis, manifested on MRI as areas of low SI on various pulse sequences.

Distal resorption of the clavicle is a classical radiographic finding in a number of conditions, including rheumatoid arthritis, ankylosing spondylitis, infection, other collagen vascular disorders, hyperparathyroidism, and following trauma (posttraumatic osteolysis) (101). MRI does not provide additional information, but it may be helpful to detect associated lesions in other areas of the shoulder (Fig. 8.39).

The presence of fluid within the acromioclavicular joint is nonspecific, and it can be related to a variety of conditions, including inflammatory, degenerative, posttraumatic, and infectious. Occasionally bone marrow edema of the distal end of the clavicle and the acromion process may be seen associated with any of these conditions.

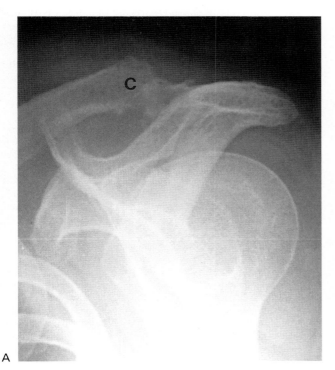

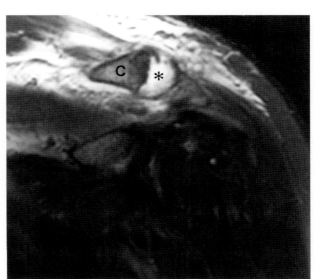

FIGURE 8.39. Septic acromioclavicular arthritis. Distal resorption of the clavicle (C) and periostitis are seen in this conventional scapular view **(A)**. Oblique coronal fat-suppressed T2-weighted MR image **(B)** in this same patient demonstrates erosion of distal clavicle **(C)** associated with acromioclavicular joint effusion (*asterisk*) and extensive edema of adjacent soft-tissue planes.

REFERENCES

1. Erickson SJ, Fitzgerald SW, Quinn SF, Carrera GF, Black KP, Lawson TL. Long bicipital tendon of the shoulder: normal anatomy and pathologic findings on MR imaging. *AJR* 1992;158:1091–1096.
2. Bureau NJ, Dussault RG, Keats TE. Imaging of bursae around the shoulder joint. *Skeletal Radiol* 1996;25:513–517.
3. Smith DK, Chopp TM, Aufdemorte TB, Witcowski EC, Jones RC. Sublabral recess of the superior glenoid labrum: study of cadavers with conventional nonenhanced MR imaging, MR arthrography, anatomic dissection and limited histologic examination. *Radiology* 1996;201:251–256.
4. Connell DA, Potter HG, Sherman MF, Wickiewicz TL. Injuries of the pectoralis major muscle: evaluation with MR imaging. *Radiology* 1999;210:785–791.
5. Cervilla V, Schweitzer ME, Ho C, Motta A, Kerr R, Resnick D. Medial dislocation of the biceps brachii tendon: appearance at MR imaging. *Radiology* 191;180(2):523–526.
6. Van Leersum M, Schweitzer ME. MRI of the biceps complex. *MRI Clin North Am* 1993;1:77–86.
7. Kaplan PA, Bryans KC, David JP, et al. MR imaging of the normal shoulder: variants and pitfalls. *Radiology* 1992;184:519–524.
8. Erickson SJ, Cox IH, Hyde JS, Carrera GF, Strandt JA, Estokowski LD. Effect of tendon orientation on MR. Signal intensity: a manifestation of the "magic angle" phenomenon. *Radiology* 181:389–392.
9. Burkhead WZ Jr. The biceps tendon. In: Rockwood CA Jr., Matsen II. FA, eds. *The shoulder.* Philadelphia: WB Saunders, 1990:791.
10. Hitchcock HH, Bechtol CO. Painful shoulder: observation on the role of the tendon of the long head of the biceps brachii in its causation. *J Bone Joint Surg Am* 1948;30:263.
11. Tuckman GA. Abnormalities of the long head of the biceps tendon of the shoulder: MR imaging findings. *AJR* 1994;163:1183–1188.
12. Stoller DW, Wolf EM. The shoulder. In: Stoller DW, ed. *Magnetic resonance imaging in orthopaedics and sports medicine*, 2nd ed. Philadelphia: Lippincott-Raven, 1997:728.
13. Chan TW, Dalinka MK, Kneeland JB, Chervrot A. Biceps tendon dislocation: evaluation with MR imaging. *Radiology* 1991;179: 649–652.
14. Meyer AW. Spontaneous dislocation of the tendon of the long head of the biceps brachii. *Arch Surg* 1926;13:109.
15. Petersson CJ. Spontaneous medial dislocation of the tendon of the long biceps brachii: an anatomic study of prevalence and pathomechanics. *Clin Orthop* 1994;211:224–227.
16. Rokito AS, Bilgen OF, Zuckerman JD, Cuomo F. Medial dislocation of the long head of the biceps tendon: magnetic resonance imaging evaluation. *Am J Orthop* 1996;25:314, 318–323.
17. Walch G, Nove-Josserand L, Boileau P, Levigne C. Subluxations and dislocations of the tendon of the long head of the biceps. *J Shoulder Elbow Surg* 1998;7:100–108.
18. Slätis P, Aalto K. Medial dislocation of the tendon of the long head of biceps brachii. *Acta Orthop Scand* 1979;50:71–77.
19. Boden BP, Hanks GA, Chesnick RM. Diagnosis of biceps tendon dislocation by kynematic magnetic resonance imaging. *Am J Orthop* 1996;25:709–711.
20. Farin PU, Jaroma H, Harju A, Soimakallio S. Medial displacement of the biceps brachii tendon: evaluation with dynamic sonography during maximal external shoulder rotation. *Radiology* 1995;195:845–848.
21. Deutsch A, Altchek DW, Veltri DM, Potter HG, Warren RF. Traumatic tears of the subscapularis tendon: clinical diagnosis, magnetic resonance imaging findings, and operative treatment. *Am J Sports Med* 1997;25:13–22.
22. Pecina MM, Krmpotic-Nemanic J, Markiewitz AD. Tunnel syndromes in the upper extremities. In: Pecina MM, Krmpotic-Nemanic J, Markiewitz AD, eds. *Tunnel syndromes.* New York: CR. Press, 1991:29–53.
23. Mulder DG, Lambert EH, Bastron J, Sprague RG. The neuropathies associated with diabetes mellitus: clinical and electromyographic study of 103 unselected diabetic patients. *Neurology* 1961;11:275–291.
24. Lambert EH, Mulder DW. Nerve function studies in experimental polyneuritis. *Electroencephalogr Clin Neurophysiol Suppl* 1964:22:29–33.
25. Gilliatt RW, Willison RG. Peripheral nerve conduction in diabetic neuropathies. *J Neurol Neurosurg Psychiatry* 1962;25:11–17.
26. Golimbu CN. Elbow. In: Firooznia H, Golimbu CN, Raffii M, Raushing W, Weinreb JC, eds. *MRI and CT of the musculoskeletal system.* St. Louis: Mosby 1991:564–593.
27. Uetani M, Kuniaki H, Matsunaga N, Imamura K, Ito N. Denervated skeletal muscle: MR imaging. *Radiology* 1983;189:511–515.
28. Fleckenstein JL, Watumull D, Conner KE, et al. Denervated human skeletal muscle: MR imaging evaluation. *Radiology* 1993;187:213–218.
29. Linker CS, Helms CA, Fritz RC. Quadrilateral space syndrome: evaluation of median nerve circulation with dynamic contrast-enhanced MR imaging. *Radiology* 1993;188:675–676.
30. Sugimoto H, Miyaji N, Ohsawa T. Carpal tunnel syndrome: evaluation of median nerve circulation with dynamic contrast-enhanced MR imaging. *Radiology* 1994;190:459–466.
31. Fritz RC, Helms CA, Steinbach LS, Genant HK. Suprascapular nerve entrapment: evaluation with MR imaging. *Radiology* 1992;182:437–444.
32. Demirhan M, Imhoff AB, Debski RE, Patel PR, Fu FH, et al. The spinoglenoid ligament and its relationship to the suprascapular nerve. *J Shoulder Elbow Surg* 1998;7:238–243.
33. Tirman PF, Feller JF, Janzen DL, Peterfy CG, Bergman AG. Association of glenoid labral cysts with labral tears and glenohumeral instability: radiologic findings and clinical significance. *Radiology* 1998;190:653–658.
34. Spinner M, Linschied RL. Nerve entrapment syndromes. In: Morrey BF, ed. *The elbow and its disorders.* Philadelphia: Saunders, 1985:691–712.
35. Parsonage MJ, Turner JWA. Neuralgic amyotrophy: the shoulder-girdle syndrome. *Lancet* 1948;1:973–978.
36. Pellas F, Olivares JP, Zandotti C, Delarque A. Neuralgic amyotrophy after parvovirus B19 infection. *Lancet* 1993;342:503–504.
37. Magee KR, DeJong RN. Paralytic brachial neuritis. *J Am Med Assn* 1960;174:1258–1262.
38. Tsairis P, Dyck P, Mulder DW. Natural history of brachial plexus neuropathy: report on 99 patients. *Arch Neurol* 1972;27:109–117.
39. Lahrmann H, Grisold W, Authier FJ, Zifko UA. Neuralgic amyotrophy with phrenic nerve involvement. *Muscle Nerve* 1999;22:437–442.
40. Misamore GW, Lehman DE. Parsonage-Turner syndrome (acute brachial neuritis). *J Bone Joint Surg Am* 1996;78A:1405–1408.
41. Helms CA, Martinez S, Speer KP. Acute brachial neuritis (Parsonage-Turner syndrome): MR imaging appearance-report of three cases. *Radiology* 1999;207:255–259.
42. Wold SW, Wickiewicz, TL Cavanaugh JT. Ruptures of the pectoralis major muscle: an anatomic and clinical analysis. *Am J Sports Med* 1992;20:587–593.
43. Simian PT, Morris ME. Pectoralis tendon avulsion in the skeletally immature. *Am J Orthop* 1996;25:563–564.
44. Stevens MA, El-Cheery GY, Kathol MH, Brandser EA, Chow S. Imaging features of avulsion injuries. *Radiographics* 1999;19:655–672.
45. Ohashi K, El-Khoury GY, Albright JP, Tearse DS. MRI of com-

plete rupture of the pectoralis major muscle. *Skeletal Radiol* 1996;25:625–628.

46. Donelly LF, Helms CA, Bisset II. GS. Chronic avulsive injury of the deltoid insertion in adolescents: imaging findings in three cases. *Radiology* 1999;211: 233–236.

47. Chen CK, Yeh L, Chen CT, Pan HB, Yang CF, et al. Contracture of the deltoid muscle: imaging findings in 17 patients. *AJR* 1998; 170:449–453.

48. Ko JY, An KN, Yamamoto R. Contracture of the deltoid muscle: results of distal release. *J Bone Joint Surg Am* 1998;80:229–238.

49. Oxner KG. Magnetic resonance imaging of the musculoskeletal system. Part 6. The shoulder. *Clin Orthop* 1997;334: 354–373.

50. Crotty JM, Monu JU, Pope TL Jr. Synovial osteochondromatosis. *Radiol Clin North Am* 1996;34: 327–342.

51. Campeau NG, Lewis BD. Ultrasound appearance of synovial osteochondromatosis of the shoulder. *Mayo Clin Proc* 1998;73: 1079–1081.

52. Blacksin MF, Ghelman B, Freiberger RH, Salvati E. Synovial chondromatosis of the hip: evaluation with air computed arthrotomography. *Clin Imaging* 1990;14:315–318.

53. Kramer J, Recht M, Deely DM, Schweitzer M, Pathria MN, et al. MR appearance of idiopathic synovial osteochondromatosis. *J Comput Assist Tomogr* 1993;17:772–776.

54. Goldberg RP, Weissman BNW, Naimark A, Braunstein EM. Femoral neck erosions: sign of hip joint synovial disease. *AJR* 1983;141: 107–111.

55. Granowitz SP, D'Antonio J, Mankin HL. The pathogenesis and long-term end results of pigmented villonodular synovitis. *Clin Orthop* 1976;114:335–351.

56. Konrath GA, Nahigian K, Kolowich P. Pigmented villonodular synovitis of the subacromial bursa. *J Shoulder Elbow Surg* 1997;6: 400–404.

57. Karasick D, Karasick S. Giant cell tumor of tendon sheath: spectrum of radiologic findings. *Skel Radiol* 1992;21:219–224.

58. Jaffe HL, Lichtenstein L, Sutro CJ. Pigmented villonodular synovitis, bursitis, and tenosynovitis: a discussion of the synovial and bursal equivalents of the tenosynovial lesion commonly denoted as xanthoma, xanthogranuloma, giant cell tumor, or myeloplaxoma of the tendon sheath and some consideration of this tendon sheath lesion itself. *Arch Pathol* 1941;31:731.

59. Vigorita VJ. Pigmented villonodular synovitis-like lesions in association with rare cases of rheumatoid arthritis, osteonecrosis, and advanced degenerative joint disease: report of five cases. *Clin Orthop* 1984;183:115–121.

60. Cheng JC, Wolf EM, Chapman JE, Johnston JO. Pigmented villonodular synovitis of the shoulder after anterior capsulolabral reconstuction. *Arthroscopy* 1997;13:257–261.

61. Flandry F, McCann SB, Hughston JC, et al. Roentgenographic findings in pigmented villonodular synovitis of the knee. *Clin Orthop* 1989247:208–219.

62. Rydholm U: Pigmented villonodular synovitis of the hip joint. *Intern Orthop (SICOT)* 1987;11:307–310.

63. Cardinal E, Dussault RG, Kaplan PA. Imaging and differential diagnosis of masses within a joint. *Can Assoc Radiol J* 1994;45:363–372.

64. Hughes TH, Sartoris DJ, Schweitzer ME, Resnick KL. Pigmented villonodular synovitis: MR characteristics. *Skel Radiol* 1995;24:7–12.

65. Jelinek JS, Krandsdorf MJ, Schmookler BM, Aboulafia AA, Malawer MM. Giant cell tumor of the tendon sheath: MR findings in nine cases. *AJR* 1995;162: 919–922.

66. Lin J, Jacobson JA, Jamadar DA, Ellis JH. Pigmented villonodular synovitis and related lesions: the spectrum of imaging findings. *AJR* 1999;172:191–197.

67. Kalil RK, Unni KK. Malignancy in pigmented villonodular synovitis. *Skel Rad* 1998;27:392–395.

68. McCarty DJ, Halverson PB, Carrera GF, et al. "Milwaukee shoulder"—association of microspheroids containing hydroxyapatite crystals, active collagenase, and neutral protease with rotator cuff defects. I. Clinical aspects. *Arthritis Rheum* 1981;24:464–473.

69. Halverson PB, Cheung HS, McCarty DJ, et al. "Milwaukee shoulder"—association of microspheroids containing hydroxyapatite crystals, active collagenase, and neutral protease with rotator cuff defects. II. Synovial fluid studies. *Arthritis Rheum* 1981;24: 474–483.

70. Halverson PB, Cheung HS, Carrera GF, et al. Rotator cuff tears associated with synovial fluid hydroxyapatite crystals and activated collagenase (abstr). *Arthritis Rheum* 1980;23:687.

71. Halverson PB, Cheung HS, Johnson R, Struve J. Simultaneous occurrence of calcium pyrophosphate dihydrate and basic calcium phosphate hydroxyapatite crystals in a knee. *Clin Orthop* 1990; 257:162–165.

72. Needell SD, Zlatkin MB, Sher JS, Murphy BJ, Uribe JW. MR imaging of the rotator cuff: peritendinous and bone abnormalities in an asymptomatic population. *AJR* 166:863–867.

73. Ostergaard M, Stoltenberg M, Lovgreen-Nielsen P, Volck B, Jensen CH. Magnetic resonance imaging-determine synovial membrane and joint effusion volumes in rheumatoid arthritis and osteoarthritis. *Arthritis Rheum* 1997;40:1856–1867.

74. McGonagle D, Conaghan PG, O'Connor P, Gibbon W, Green M, et al. The relationship between synovitis and bone changes in early untreated rheumatoid arthritis. *Arthritis Rheum* 1999;42:1706–1711.

75. Griffith JF, Peh WC, Evans NS, Smallman LA, Wong RW, et al. Multiple rice body formation in chronic subacromial/subdeltoid bursitis: MR appearances. *Clin Radiol* 1996;51:511–514.

76. Chung C, Coley BD, Martin LC. Rice bodies in juvenile rheumatoid arthritis. *AJR* 1998;170:698–700.

77. Lossos, IS, Yossepowitch, O, Kandel, L, Yardeni, D, Arber N. Septic arthritis of the glenohumeral joint: a report of 11 cases and review of the literature. *Medicine* 1998;77:177–187.

78. Chaudhuri K, Lonergan D, Portek I, et al. Septic arthritis of the shoulder after mastectomy and radiotherapy for breast carcinoma. *J Bone Joint Surg Br* 1993;75:318–321.

79. Gompels BM, Darlington LG. Septic arthritis in rheumatoid disease causing bilateral shoulder dislocation: diagnosis and treatment assisted by grey scale ultrasonography. *Ann Rheum Dis* 1981; 40:609–611.

80. Leslie BM, Harris JM III, Driscoll D. Septic arthritis of the shoulder in adults. *J Bone Joint Surg Am* 1981;71:1516–1522.

81. Resnik CS. Septic arthritis: a rare cause of drooping shoulder. *Skel Radiol* 1992;21:307–309.

82. Antti-Poika I, Vankka E, Santavirta S, et al. Two cases of shoulder joint tuberculosis. *Acta Orthop Scand* 1991;62–63:81–83.

83. Stecher DR, Gusis SE, Cocco JAM. Tuberculous arthritis in the course of connective tissue disease: report of 4 cases. *J Rheumatol* 1992;19:1418–1420.

84. Schultz E, Richterman I, Dorfman HD. Case report 739: tuberculous arthritis of the knee. *Skel Radiol* 1992;21:330–334.

85. Araki Y, Tsukaguchi I, Shinok. Tuberculous arthritis of the knee: MR. findings. *AJR* 1993;160:664.

86. Neer CS. Displaced proximal humeral fractures. I. Classification and evaluation. *J Bone Joint Surg Am* 1970;52:1077–1089.

87. Mason BJ, Kier R, Bindleglass DF. Occult fractures of the greater tuberosity of the humerus: radiographic and MR imaging findings. *AJR* 1999;172:469–473.

88. Zanetti M, Weishaupt D, Jost B, Gerber C, Hodler J. MR imaging for traumatic tears of the rotator cuff: high prevalence of greater tuberosity fractures and subscapularis tendon tears. *AJR* 1999;172:463–467.

89. Basset RW, Cofield RH. Acute tears of the rotator cuff: the timing of surgical repair. *Clin Orthop* 1983;175:18–24.

90. Dzioba RB, Quinlan WJ. Avascular necrosis of the glenoid. *J Trauma* 1984;24:448–451.
91. Shanley DJ, Mulligan ME. Osteochondrosis dissecans of the glenoid. *Skel Radiol* 1990;19:419–421.
92. Greenan TJ, Zlatkin MB, Dalinka MK, Estehai JL. Posttraumatic changes in the posterior glenoid and labrum in a handball player. *Am J Sports Med* 1993;21:153–156.
93. Yu JS, Greenway G, Resnick D. Osteochondral defect of the glenoid fossa: cross-sectional imaging features. *Radiology* 1998;206: 35–40.
94. Snyder SJ. *Shoulder arthroscopy*. New York: McGraw-Hill, 1994: 121–124.
95. Chan KK, Skaff A, Roger B, Resnick DL. Glenoid articular rim disruption (GARD) and its relationship to osteochondritis dissecans: routine radiography, standard arthrography, CT arthrography, and MR arthrography in eighteen patients. *Radiology* 1998; 209(P):236.

96. Loebengerg MI, Plate AM, Zuckerman JD. Osteonecrosis of the humeral head. *Instr Course Lect* 1999;48:349–357.
97. Mitchell DG, Rao VM, Dalinka MK, et al. Femoral head avascular necrosis: correlation of MR imaging, radiographic staging, radionuclide imaging, and clinical findings. *Radiology* 1987;162: 709–715.
98. Craig EV. The geyser sign and torn rotator cuff: clinical significance and pathomechanics. *Clin Orthop* 1984;191:213–215.
99. Craig EV. The acromioclavicular joint cyst: an unusual presentation of a rotator cuff tear. *Clin Orthop* 1986;202:189–192.
100. Cvitanic O, Schimandle J, Cruse A, Minter J. The acromioclavicular joint cyst: glenohumeral joint communication revealed by MR arthrography. *J Comput Assist Tomogr* 1999;23:141–143.
101. De la Puente, R, Boutin RD, Theodorou DJ, Hooper H, Schweitzer M, et al. Post-traumatic and stress-induced osteolysis of the distal clavicle: MR imaging findings in 17 patients. *Skel Radiol* 1999;28:202–208.

POSTOPERATIVE SHOULDER

MICHAEL B. ZLATKIN

Performing MRI in patients who have previously been operated on presents difficulties in that the normal anatomic appearances are altered by the procedures that have been carried out. For that reason, it is important to have some understanding of the more commonly performed surgical or arthroscopic procedures, or both, and how they affect the appearance of the muscles, tendons, joint capsule, labrum, and surrounding bony structures. The pathology that is discovered in these situations may be a residual or recurrent problem that remains or develops despite the surgery, a complication of the surgery itself, or a new problem unrelated to the original problem or the surgery performed for it.

This chapter will review the common surgical procedures performed for impingement and rotator cuff disease as well as those for shoulder instability and labral pathology, including SLAP lesions. The expected findings that are seen on MRI after these procedures have been done will be discussed as well as the residual and recurrent pathology that may develop and be uncovered with the use of MR imaging and MR arthrography. General complications that may occur subsequent to these procedures and their appearance in the shoulder as seen on MR imaging will also be reviewed. Similar to the nonoperated shoulder, new pathology may arise. These will not be discussed in any detail as they have been reviewed elsewhere in this book. One persistent problem in our understanding of the MRI and MR arthrographic diagnosis of the problems associated with postoperative shoulder is the lack of a large body of published data on this topic in the literature. As time passes, we are gaining more clinical experience in this area, with conventional MRI (1–10) and more recently MRI arthrography (11,12).

One of the considerable problems in imaging patients who have had prior surgery is the presence of metal artifact. This includes ferromagnetic screws or staples. Small metal shavings from the use of a burr—for example, during an acromioplast—may also yield a considerable artifact. The use of weakly ferromagnetic material such as titanium or the use of plastics may help minimize the amount of artifact generated. With respect to imaging such patients, it is useful to minimize the use of gradient echo sequences as owing to their greater sensitivity to susceptibility artifact, the imaging artifacts that may result can be considerable. This can impair visualization of important structures such as the rotator cuff, glenoid labrum, and capsule (Fig. 9.1). In this regard, turbo (TSE) or fast spin echo (FSE) imaging can be useful since the use of a longer train of 180° pulses (echo train) may help minimize the degree of magnetic susceptibility artifact (Fig. 9.2). This may yield more diagnostic images than conventional spin echo or gradient echo sequences. Additionally, fat saturation may be incomplete when imaging the postoperative shoulder, again due to the presence of magnetic susceptibility effects and ferromagnetic artifact related to the prior surgery. Fast spin echo inversion recovery sequences may prove useful in this situation. Postoperative scar formation may also help limit evaluation by distorting the anatomy and by making tissue planes difficult to differentiate. As will be discussed further in this chapter, MR arthrography can be a useful tool to help image postoperative patients more successfully (Fig. 9.2) (11–13).

IMPINGEMENT AND ROTATOR CUFF DISEASE

As is alluded to elsewhere in this text, traditional impingement involving the rotator cuff occurs when the latter is impacted against the undersurface of the anterior edge of the acromion, the coracoacromial ligament, or the acromioclavicular joint (primary impingement) (14–18). There are many different causes of this condition, including overuse syndromes as in sports activities or work-related problems, and altered acromion morphology such as the type 3 anterior acromion described by Bigliani and colleagues (19). Inferiorly projecting subacromial spurs also have a high association with the clinical syndrome of impingement. Shoulder instability may also be a factor in the development of secondary impingement, especially with respect to the throwing athlete (20,21). A spectrum of changes may occur in the cuff progressing from edema, to tendinosis, to cuff tears, partial and complete. Conservative treatment for the symptoms

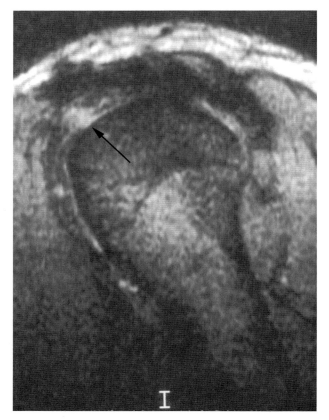

FIGURE 9.1. Sagittal oblique T2* gradient echo image. Although a small recurrent anterior supraspinatus tendon defect is identified (*arrow*), the image is significantly degraded by artifact from the prior repair.

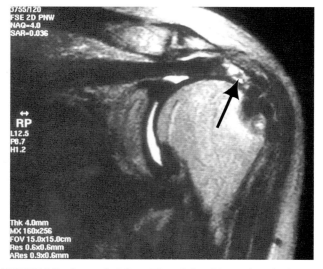

FIGURE 9.2. Coronal oblique T2-weighted fast spin echo image. The patient is status following supraspinatus tendon repair and anterior acromioplasty. A recurrent defect in the supraspinatus tendon is visualized in this patient (*arrow*). The postrepair artifact is minimized by the multiple 180° echoes.

associated with this disorder includes modification of activities, physical therapy, and anti-inflammatory medication (16,22). Various nonoperative rotator cuff programs have been described for the general population and for athletes, including throwers. Nonoperative management may be successful, especially in the patient without a significant tendon abnormality; hence, the importance of appropriately timed imaging studies. Most studies report a satisfactory result in 50% of patients treated in this manner (23). Steroid injections may be used, but repeated injections may cause tendon atrophy and inhibit repair. When patients fail conservative therapy, they usually undergo surgery. This will involve some type of decompression of the region of the coracoacromial arch, often with debridement of tendinosis or partial tear, or repair of a torn rotator cuff (14–16,22,24–26).

MRI and MR arthrographic evaluation of the rotator cuff disease and impingement in the postoperative patient may often prove much more difficult than evaluation in those patients not previously operated upon. A baseline postoperative study would be helpful. If patients do not experience pain or dysfunction after treatment, however, there is no need for posttreatment imaging; therefore, in the majority of cases after surgery no additional imaging is necessary. Recent studies however have described the MRI imaging findings in asymptomatic patients after rotator cuff surgery (8,10). If patients experience persistent or recurrent symptoms, then MRI may be of value.

The most common causes of failure after shoulder surgery for rotator cuff disease are residual bony changes of impingement after subacromial decompression, advancing rotator cuff tendinosis, residual and recurrent rotator cuff tears both partial and complete, postoperative adhesions, and weakening of the deltoid muscle from detachment or denervation (27–29).

Assessment of the symptomatic postoperative rotator cuff can be divided into two categories. The first category of postoperative patients are those who have had a prior acromioplasty for impingement, with an intact rotator cuff and no rotator cuff repair. This procedure may be done as an open procedure, via an anterolateral deltoid-splitting incision (14–17,22) or via arthroscopy (30–35) (Fig. 9.3). The anteroinferior acromion is removed, from the AC joint to the deltoid insertion, removing that portion anterior to the clavicle. Most often the subdeltoid bursa is inflamed as well and is resected at the time of the acromioplasty. There may often be removal of the insertion as well as a variable part of the coracoacromial ligament. Some surgeons may prefer to preserve, rather than excise, the coracoacromial ligament, in order to prevent superior migration of the humeral head (16). In particular, this may be true in young athletic patients, in which the CA ligament may just be thickened. In these patients, soft-tissue decompression with debridement, without release of the ligament, may be performed (22). The AC joint and the distal 2.5 cm of the clavicle may be re-

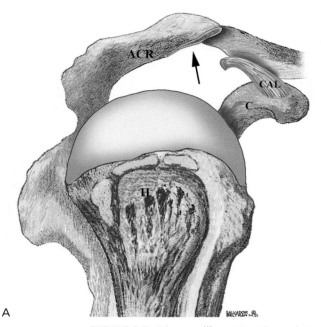
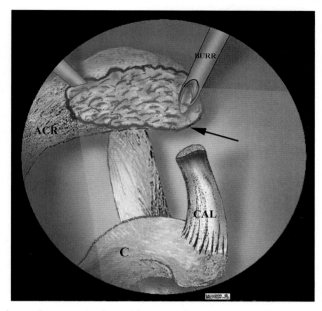

A   B

FIGURE 9.3. Diagram illustrating the technique of anterior acromioplasty. Also note the accompanying resection of coracoacromial ligament. A portion of anterior acromion has been removed (*arrow*). **A:** Open acromioplasty; **B:** arthroscopic technique. ACR, acromion; C, coracoid; CAL, coracoacromial ligament; H, humerus.

moved as well, if the patient is symptomatic or if there are large osteophytes arising from here (36,37).

Arthroscopic subacromial decompressions requires various arthroscopic shavers and burrs to remove the subacromial bursa, subdeltoid fat pad, and anterior edge and inferior surface of the acromion (30–35). A cautery is used to release the coracoacromial ligament. The distal clavicle can be resected using a burr. The advantages of the arthroscopic technique are a shorter recovery time, less pain, performance in an outpatient setting, and no need to release the anterior deltoid muscle (22). One additional advantage of the arthroscopic technique over the open technique is that the cuff can be inspected at the time of surgery for any associated disease that may not have been suspected or diagnosed prior to surgery, including rotator cuff tears, or labral pathology. Some surgeons use the arthroscopic technique mainly in younger patients, especially athletes; others may use it in all patients. Others may use a combined open and arthroscopic approach (31,32,34,38), especially if a full-thickness tear is found. MRI may help in this decision by determining the status of the cuff prior to surgery.

The incidence of failure (i.e., persistence or recurrence of pain) after subacromial decompression is reported to be between 3% and 11% (14,18,27,34,39). The interpretation of these results is difficult because of the admixture of patients with intact cuffs and those with cuff tears, partial and complete (16), in reported studies. Arthroscopic decompressions may carry a higher incidence of recurrence (31,32,34), be-

cause there is a learning curve associated with this procedure, and the view in the subacromial space is somewhat limited. One of the consequences of this is there may be insufficient excision of the acromion, which may be a cause of recurrent or residual symptoms. Arthroscopic acromioplasty has the advantage of not needing a deltoid-splitting incision to perform the procedure, therefore not putting the deltoid at risk. However, since much of the deltoid arises from the anterior acromion, neither an open nor arthroscopic acromioplasty can be performed without some compromise of the anterior deltoid (16).

MRI findings typically associated with acromioplasty (Fig. 9.4) include a flattened acromial undersurface, nonvisualization of the anterior one-third of the acromion, and decreased marrow signal in the remaining distal acromion, owing to cancellous marrow fibrosis (1). Low signal due to artifacts from small metal fragments are often present, in random fashion. These particles are typically too small to be seen on plain radiographs or computed tomographic images (2). This is usually related to burring of the acromion. The nature of the morphological changes of the acromion may vary, however, with how much of the acromion is in fact removed at the time of decompression, and this may also vary whether the decompression is open or arthroscopic. As noted, the latter procedure often shows less dramatic alterations of the appearance of the acromion, than the former. Removal of the subacromial bursa and subdeltoid fat pad results in the absence of these structures on postoperative studies.

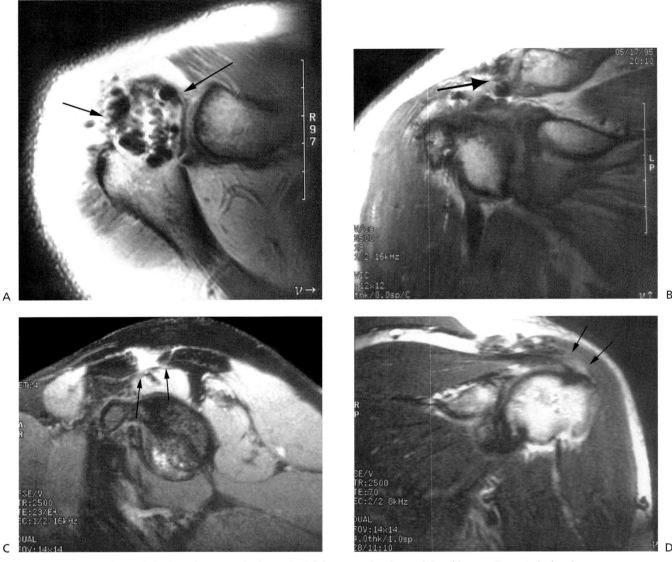

FIGURE 9.4. Anterior acromioplasty. **A:** Axial proton density–weighted image. Postsurgical artifact is seen along the anterior aspect of the acromion, following acromioplasty (*arrows*). **B:** Coronal oblique proton density–weighted image. The anterior portion of the acromion has been removed (*arrow*). **C:** Sagittal oblique proton density–weighted image. The extent of the decompression is often best seen in this position. The anterior acromion and AC joint have been excised (*arrows*). **D:** Coronal T2-weighted image. Increased signal is often identified in the subdeltoid bursal region after decompression, due to accompanying resection or debridement of the bursa (*arrows*).

These structures are often replaced by abundant scar tissue of intermediate signal intensity (6). After resection of the bursa, there is often a small amount of fluid signal identified in this region on T2-weighted images (8,10) (Fig. 9.4) or imaging sequences with similar contrast characteristics such as STIR or T2* gradient echo sequences. This renders fluid in the subdeltoid bursa not useful as a secondary sign of cuff injury or of bursal inflammation.

Assessment of the anatomy of the coracoacromial arch after decompression may be best accomplished by obtaining and reviewing sagittal oblique images (Figs. 9.4, 9.5). These are best obtained with a proton density– and T2-weighted FSE sequence. The appearance and shape of the anterior acromion and the amount of acromion that has been removed is often best seen on these images. Alterations of the coracoacromial ligament, if it has been removed, can also be identified. Preservation or excision of the acromioclavicular joint may also be readily apparent. If the AC joint has also been excised (Fig. 9.4), scar tissue may be the most prominent finding. In the more recent postoperative period, in-

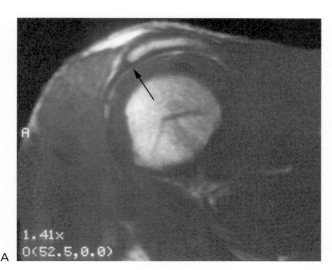 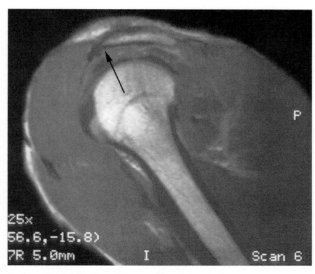

FIGURE 9.5. Sagittal oblique T1-weighted images before **(A)** and after **(B)** acromioplasty. Note the conversion from a type 2-3 acromion in A (*arrow*) to a type 1 acromion after surgery in B (*arrow*).

creased signal intensity about the margins of the excised joint may persist for a number of months (6).

With respect to the appearance of the rotator cuff after subacromial decompression, some improvement of the altered signal in the rotator cuff and in the peritendinous tissues that may be the result of inflammation may be seen over time, but resolution of any signal or morphological alterations that are related to rotator cuff tendinosis are less likely to be identified (1,4,5,6).

Most of the more common causes of failure after anterior acromioplasty have already been listed. One additional and common cause of failed subacromial decompression is the failure to recognize cases in which impingement beneath the structures of the coracoacromial arch is secondary to, or mediated by, underlying anterior shoulder instability, whereby performance of an acromioplasty without addressing the instability may in fact worsen the situation (20). Another not uncommon situation is when patients undergo acromioplasty, but the pain is related to osteoarthrosis of the acromioclavicular joint (Fig. 9.6), and this is left untreated (27). After acromioplasty, as noted earlier, patients may go on to have progression of their rotator cuff disease (Figs. 9.6, 9.7), such as the interval development of a rotator cuff tear, either partial or complete. Additionally, an unrecognized partial tear or small complete tear may extend. Progression may occur if the acromioplasty and decompression are inadequate, with persistent subacromial roughening (16,27).

The ability of MRI to detect residual bony impingement has been evaluated. One study showed a relative insensitivity to the determination of persistent bony changes of impingement (1). The sensitivity was 64%, the specificity 82%, and the accuracy 74%. In another study by Magee et al. (4), the performance of MRI was better, with a sensitivity of 84%

and a specificity of 87%. Current MR imaging criteria for persistent impingement are to some extent extrapolations of those that have been used with plain radiographic exam. Therefore, correlative plain radiographs may also be of value in the assessment of the efficacy of the decompression. As noted, however, sagittal oblique MR images to evaluate the region of the subacromial space should nonetheless best evaluate the adequacy of the decompression and any persistent impingement manifested by an insufficient acromion

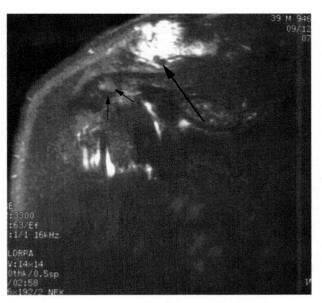

FIGURE 9.6. Postacromioplasty pain. Coronal oblique T2-weighted fast spin echo sequence with fat saturation. There is persistent AC joint arthritis, with marginal edema (*large arrow*). A small undersurface partial tear is also seen (*small arrows*).

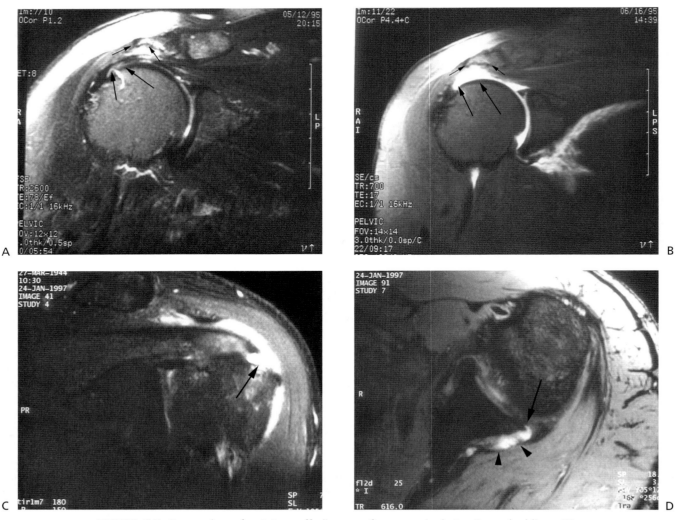

FIGURE 9.7. Progression of rotator cuff disease, after acromioplasty. Coronal oblique T2-weighted image **(A)** and MRI arthrogram **(B)**. The patient has had an acromioplasty, but the undersurface remains irregular, with a prominent lateral tip (*small arrows in A*). There is a high-grade partial-thickness undersurface tear, more evident on the MR arthrogram in B (*arrows*). **C:** Coronal oblique, turbo inversion recovery sequence, in another patient. The patient has had an anterior acromioplasty. There has been interval development of a full-thickness tear of the supraspinatus tendon, anterodistally (*arrow*). **D:** Axial T2* gradient echo image, in the same patient. There is also a posterior labral tear (*arrow*) noted with a paralabral cyst (*arrowheads*).

resection or the persistence of a large subacromial spur. Additionally, large osteophytes projecting from the acromioclavicular joint will also be best identified in the sagittal oblique plane. MR imaging may also be valuable in the determination of deltoid detachment, if the decompressive procedure was done in an open fashion; excessive acromial resection; and dense postoperative scarring between the cuff and the acromion, which may also lead to persistent or recurrent symptoms (16).

In the setting of interval development of a cuff tear or extension and/or progression of existing cuff pathology such as tendinosis or partial-thickness tears, clinical findings such as pain, including night pain, loss of motion, and weakness are

not considered to be specific (18). Reflective of this, further evaluation with an MRI is indicated, in the setting of persistent postoperative symptoms. The integrity of the cuff may typically be more difficult to determine in the postoperative setting. This is because of the distortion of the adjacent soft tissues resulting from the prior surgery, including the overlying subdeltoid fat and bursal tissues, especially if a bursectomy has been performed, as well as the metal artifact from the burring at the time of the acromioplasty. In addition, determining the normal cuff signal may be more difficult as persistent intermediate signal within the rotator cuff tendons has been described on T2-weighted images after acromioplasty (1). The precise reason for this is not clear, in the absence of any debridement or other manipulation of the cuff tissues. Studies show that in this setting MRI remains a sensitive test, but it is less specific than MRI in the patient who has not had prior surgery. Therefore, in these patients the guidelines (40–42) for a rotator cuff tear may still be applied; however, according to most studies, a tear can only be diagnosed confidently when a definite region of discontinuity in the cuff can be identified. This area of discontinuity should be accompanied by fluid signal within the defect on images with a long TR/TE acquisition (1), on STIR or T2*-weighted gradient echo sequences, or when contrast extravasation is seen through the cuff defect at MR arthrography (11–13).

The second category involves patients who have had a prior rotator cuff repair. In patients with partial-thickness tears, treatment depends on the area, depth, and severity of tendon involvement. The most common partial tears occur along the cuff undersurface and extend into the tendon substance. They occur most commonly in the anterior aspect of the supraspinatus tendon, near its insertion into the greater tuberosity. Treatment may vary from debridement of frayed tissue, in more superficial partial tears, to completely excising the area of the partial defect and repairing the remaining healthy cuff tissue (16,22,25,30,38), as if it was a small full-thickness defect. Repairs are usually done in tears involving greater than 50% of the tendon thickness, with either a side-to-side or tendon-to-bone repair being done (16,22,25,30,38). Either of these treatments may be accompanied by decompression (16,22,25,30,38). Both of these methods are often done arthroscopically (30,35,43), although the repairs and acromioplasty may be done open or with a combined approach.

Simple debridement may be used in some select groups of patients, particularly younger patients who may not have prominent bony changes about the coracoacromial arch or who may have cuff injuries related to instability or internal impingement (22,24,25,44–46). Simple debridement may be less satisfactory in older patients and in patients with deeper partial tears. These patients will usually have a decompression, along with their debridement, or repair.

Repair of full-thickness rotator cuff tears varies from surgeon to surgeon. Knowing the type of surgery performed and its extent is important when interpreting MR images of these patients. As such, it is important to obtain the details of these surgeries, if possible, from the surgical reports or other patient records, so as to best understand the postoperative anatomy.

The general principle of cuff repairs is subacromial decompression, rotator cuff mobilization, and repair of the tendon, if possible back to the tuberosity (22) (Fig. 9.8). Most open repairs are done through an anterosuperior approach through a split or takedown of the proximal deltoid. Mini-open repairs are those that employ only a split of the deltoid, without any takedown of the origin (38). Arthroscopic approaches generally involve three bursal portals: anterior, lateral, and posterior (32,47,48,49). Repair of small full-thickness tears can usually be carried out with a side-to-side suturing technique or, if distal small tears, with a tendon-to-bone repair. Larger tears with retraction require reattaching the tendon to bone. Traditionally this was done into a trough in bone at the greater tuberosity (50). Currently, this is less commonly done, with most surgeons now freshening the bone at the articular–tuberosity junction (22). The repairs are done with nonabsorbable suture material, tied to each other or with suture anchors. Suture anchors are more commonly used with arthroscopic repairs. Suture anchors can be composed of various materials, including ferromagnetic metal, nonferromagnetic metal (titanium), plastic, and bioabsorbable polymers. Larger or massive defects require mobilization of the remaining portions of the cuff (51) or

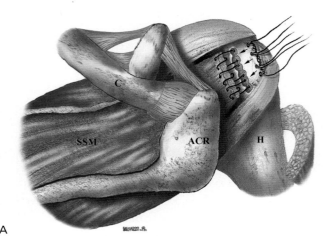
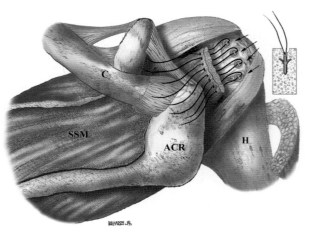

A B

FIGURE 9.8. Tendon-to-bone rotator cuff repair. **A:** A trough is formed in the humeral head (*arrows*). The edge of the torn tendon is sutured deep into this trough, via a combination of drill holes and nonabsorbable sutures. **B:** Another alternative is the use of suture anchors (*arrows*) to reattach the torn rotator cuff tendon to the humeral head. ACR, acromion; C, clavicle; H, humerus; SSM, supraspinatus muscle.

incorporation of the long head of biceps or subscapularis, to achieve an effective repair. Other authors advocate the use of allograft material or synthetic material (52,53) to reconstruct the cuff. In massive tears, some have advocated debridement alone (54).

In the majority of rotator cuff repairs, an acromioplasty is also performed; however, recently some surgeons have reserved acromioplasty for patients with definite subacromial spurs, roughening, or "abnormal acromial shapes" such as a type 3 anterior acromion (44). Again in the setting of advanced AC joint disease, removal of the osteophytes and resection of the distal one-third of the clavicle may be carried out. These procedures may be done arthroscopically or via an open approach, either a miniopen or standard superior approach. Some advocate a combination of both arthroscopic and open techniques, with the acromioplasty done arthroscopically and the tendon repair done open or miniopen (16,22). With respect to the AC joint (22), if it is tender prior to surgery, the distal clavicle may be resected. If the AC joint is nontender but the inferiorly projecting spurs are felt to contribute to impingement, then the undersurface of the AC joint is smoothed. A bursal release is generally performed for exposure and to relieve the cuff of any bursal adhesions. If the biceps is torn or subluxed, it is tenodesed or incorporated into the repair. In general, the results of rotator cuff repair are good.

Cofield (55) reviewed many different series of rotator cuff repairs and found that pain relief occurred in 87% of patients. Early results of miniopen and arthroscopic repairs (49,56) have shown similar good results. In those patients who do fail treatment, causes of recurrent pain or dimin-ished function following rotator cuff repair include failure of the repair. This can be due to fixation failure (suture anchor pullout, suture pullout, or suture failure) or tendon tissue failure. Inadequate subacromial decompression can lead to continued impingement, resulting in recurrent tendon failure. In addition, if the tendinous tissue is of poor quality due to atrophy or degenerated tissue, a new tear may develop, perhaps due to continued impingement or excessive tension at the repair site, particularly in larger tears. Another cause may be the creation of iatrogenic cuff tears due to portal placement, which may result in tears of the infraspinatus, subscapularis, or, least commonly, the supraspinatus tendons (57). Aggressive debridement of the subacromial bursa can also lead to delamination and penetration of an intact region of the rotator cuff.

Limited experience with MRI in patients after rotator cuff repairs (1–5) shows that its accuracy is decreased although the determination of an intact tendon or a recurrent complete tear remains good. MRI findings following cuff repair (Fig. 9.9) include distortion of the soft tissues adjacent to the cuff and nonvisualization of the subdeltoid fat pad and bursa, as well as fluid in the region of the subdeltoid bursa (8,10). The latter findings occur, since as mentioned earlier, most often these regions are removed at the time of surgery. Soft-tissue metal artifacts occur due to nonabsorbable sutures and suture anchors. These can be particularly problematic if ferromagnetic suture anchors are used. These can create a large balloon artifact, which can obscure anatomic details (1–3,6). Granulation tissue surrounding sutures may also result in intermediate or high signal intensity on imaging sequences with T2-weighted contrast, in the

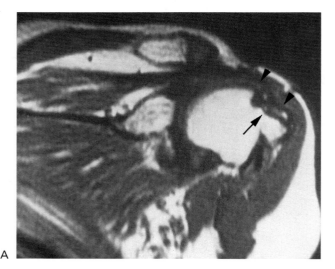
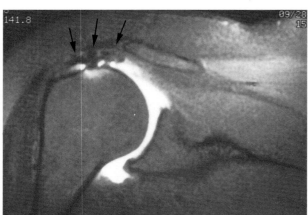

FIGURE 9.9. Intact rotator cuff, after repair. **A:** Coronal oblique proton density–weighted image. The patient has had an anterior acromioplasty and tendon-to-bone rotator cuff repair. Note the distorted soft tissues overlying the cuff, the defect from the trough in bone (*small arrow*), and the intact low-signal tendon (*arrowheads*). **B:** MRI arthrogram. Coronal oblique T1 image with fat suppression. Note the metal artifact from the suture in this tendon to tendon repair (*arrows*). The contrast remains in the joint in this intact repair.

peritendinous tissues (1,3). There is a surgical trough in the humeral head present when tendon-to-bone repairs have been performed. Intermediate signal within the rotator cuff substance may be present, on T1- and proton density–weighted images presumably due to granulation tissue (1). As such, this makes the diagnosis of tendinosis or intrasubstance degeneration not practical in the repaired tendon. Further distortion of the anatomy may occur with repair of large or massive tears if some type of allograft is utilized or if there is transfer of other tendons, including the subscapularis and biceps tendon. Mild superior subluxation of the cuff may occur, due to capsular tightening, scarring, cuff atrophy, or bursectomy (9). Decreased acromiohumeral distance does not necessarily predict a retear of the rotator cuff but may cause increased stress on the cuff by the humerus (9).

Several findings associated with full-thickness tears in the preoperative shoulder may be seen in an intact repaired shoulder. These include small to moderate joint effusions, fluid in the region of the subdeltoid bursa, and increased signal in the cuff on images with T2-weighted contrast. The increased signal in the tendon should not, however, be equivalent to fluid. Mild bone marrow edema in the humeral head may also be seen (43% of subjects) (10), even up to 5 years after surgery. Fluid in the subdeltoid bursa, although nonspecific, can be a sensitive secondary finding of a rotator cuff tear in the nonoperated tendon (40,41,58–60). As noted, alterations in signal and morphology in the region of the subdeltoid bursa may be due to a bursal resection at the time of surgery. It should not be forgotten that even functional cuff

repairs may not be watertight, and there may be some leakage of fluid from the joint, into the subdeltoid bursal region (61,62) in the absence of functional breakdown of the cuff. In the postoperative setting, this finding of fluid in the subdeltoid bursa is therefore rendered unreliable as a secondary finding of a cuff defect and thus cannot be reliably utilized in making a diagnosis (1,6,8,10). With respect to the leakage of fluid, however, it should be noted that while a nonwatertight repair can be associated with patient satisfaction and pain relief, the presence of a cuff defect does affect shoulder strength (62). Therefore, if a leak is present, it is important to quantify the presence and size of the defect that can be done with conventional MRI, but it is best done with MR arthrography.

The finding of increased signal in the tendon after rotator cuff repair can be due to postoperative hyperemic granulation tissue or disorganized granulation tissue at the repair site, which may contain or imbibe fluid. Fluid signal on T2-weighted images seen within a defect in the cuff or nonvisualization of a portion of the cuff are the more reliable indicators of full-thickness tears in the postoperative patient, according to one study (1). The authors also concluded that even fluid signal is not completely reliable, and the only specific finding of a recurrent tear is complete absence of the tendon (Figs. 9.10, 9.11). In the postoperative situation, there may be a greater incidence of obliteration of a cuff defect by scar and more chronic granulation tissue, and this may then result in a low-signal tear, which is difficult to discern with conventional imaging sequences (Fig. 9.12) (59).

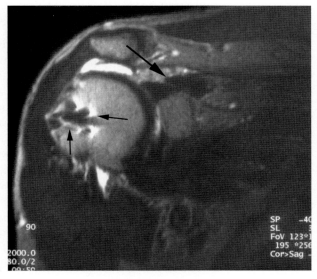 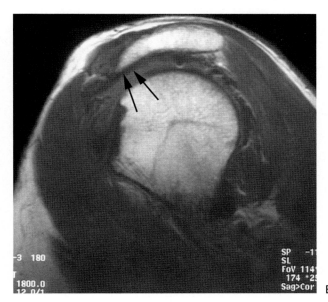

FIGURE 9.10. Recurrent rotator cuff tear. **A:** Coronal oblique T2-weighted image. The supraspinatus tendon has retracted medially from the site of repair in the humeral head, to the medial glenoid margin (*arrow*). There is severe muscle atrophy. Note the metal artifact in the humeral head from the suture anchors at the repair site (*small arrows*). **B:** Sagittal oblique turbo spin echo proton density–weighted image. Note the persistent bony impingement changes from the hook-like anterior acromion (*arrows*).

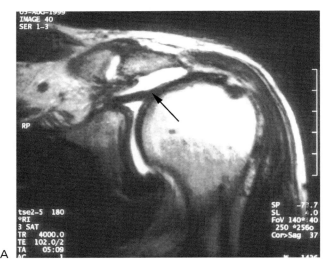

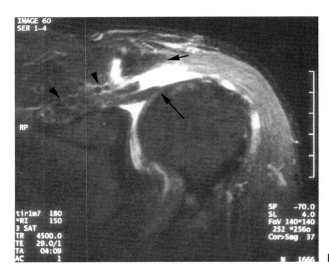

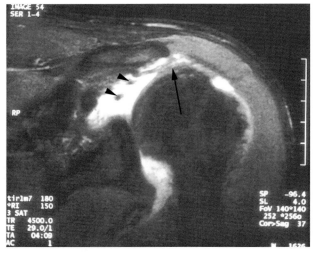

FIGURE 9.11. Recurrent rotator cuff tear. Coronal oblique turbo spin echo T2-weighted image **(A)** and turbo inversion recovery weighted images **(B, C)**. The supraspinatus tendon in A and B and the infraspinatus tendon in B are markedly thinned and retracted medially (*arrows*). The tendon is absent over the humeral head. The metal artifact in B and C (*arrowheads*) identifies the prior surgery. There is severe muscle atrophy and evidence of a prior acromioplasty (*small arrow in B*).

Secondary signs such as muscle atrophy and tendon retraction may also be of value in these cases (59). A baseline postoperative study, if it can be obtained, may be useful to separate changes from prior surgery (8,10), from those due to a recurrent tear, although this may not be possible or practical to obtain. MR arthrography, as discussed later, may therefore be particularly helpful in the evaluation of the postoperative rotator cuff (Fig. 9.12). Leakage of contrast through a cuff defect may be directly visualized, and the cuff tissues and the tendon edges better delineated.

Both conventional MRI (Fig. 9.13) and MR arthrography (Fig. 9.14) in the postoperative situation are useful in the determination of severe muscle atrophy, tendon retraction, or fragmentation of the tendon edges in patients who develop a recurrent tear (Fig. 9.13). This is of importance as it can often help the surgeon decide whether any further operative repair is feasible, and the MR and MR arthrographic images can be used to explain these findings to the patient, for prognostic purposes. Muscle retraction may be visible in larger defects, but it should also be remembered that the lo-

cation of the musculotendinous junction is not a reliable secondary finding of a cuff tear after surgery. This is because its position may change if the cuff is mobilized during surgery, particularly in trying to close large defects (6).

Recurrent partial tears may also not be easily distinguished from intact repaired tendons. The criteria for a partial tear, according to Gaenslen and coworkers (3), is fluid signal on images with T2-weighted contrast replacing a portion of the tendon. In this study, however, this fluid signal could not always be distinguished from edematous degeneration of the tendon as seen around sutures (3). In another earlier study (1), it was noted that occasionally a small recurrent full-thickness tear might be underestimated to be a partial tear. Many of these difficulties in distinguishing partial tears with conventional MRI should be resolved with the use of MR arthrography (13).

The prior discussion is based on data and experience evaluating patients who have returned for MRI due to recurrent or residual symptoms after rotator cuff repair. Spielmann and coworkers in a recent study (10) evaluated MRI imaging

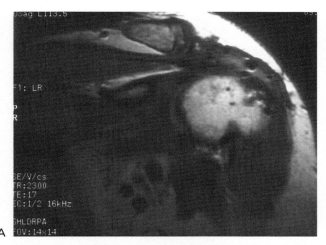

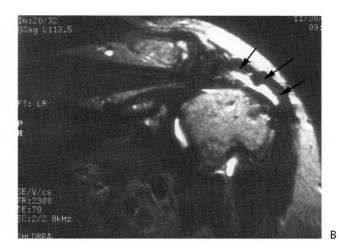

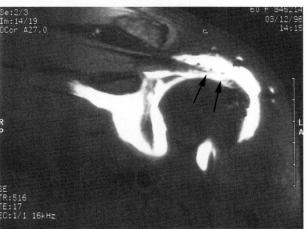

FIGURE 9.12. Recurrent rotator cuff tear, MR arthrography. **A, B:** Coronal oblique proton density–weighted image in A and T2-weighted image in B. The patient is status after acromioplasty and tendon-to-bone repair. The cuff is scarred, and the metal artifact also helps obscure the anatomy. Fluid in the subdeltoid bursa seen in B (*arrows*) is a very common finding after cuff repair, related to the bursal debridement or resection. **C:** MRI arthrogram. Coronal oblique T1-weighted image with fat suppression. The MR arthrogram reveals a defect in the tendon, not seen on the conventional sequences, with contrast extravasating through the defect (*arrows*), into the subdeltoid bursa.

in asymptomatic individuals after rotator cuff repair. They made a number of important observations in their study of 15 patients. They found that only 10% of patients after surgery had "normal" tendons. Mildly increased signal in the tendon was present in 53% of subjects, felt to be due to inflammation or scarring, but difficult to distinguish from tendinosis. Even more troublesome was that in more than one-third of the patients, MR findings similar to those seen in partial and complete tears were found, although these were not surgically confirmed. Other imaging findings in these patients included partial or complete loss of the peribursal fat in all, subacromial-subdeltoid bursal fluid in 67%, and small or moderate effusions in 93%. They also found mild bone marrow edema in 40%, subchondral cysts in 60%, and AC joint osteophytes in 70%. They concluded based on this small study that postoperative MRI findings similar to those considered pathologic may be commonly seen and therefore should be interpreted with caution and careful clinical correlation.

Zanetti and coworkers (8) also studied 15 asymptomatic volunteers after rotator cuff repair. They found recurrent tears in 33% of patients, although the retears were small, with a mean of 8 mm, whereas a similar-sized sample of pa-

tients studied with recurrent or residual pain had retears in 45%, but the mean size was 3.4 cm. Fluid in the subacromial-subdeltoid bursa was seen in nearly all patients.

The sensitivity and specificity of MRI for rotator cuff tears in the postoperative shoulder have also been evaluated. In the study by Magee et al. (4), the sensitivity and specificity for rotator cuff tears (partial and complete) were 100% and 87%, respectively. For partial-thickness tears, only the sensitivity was 83%, and the specificity was 83%. In an earlier study (1), for complete cuff tears, the sensitivity was 86%, and the specificity was 92%. Partial-thickness tears were felt to be indistinguishable from repaired tendons in this earlier study. It was felt that the lack of fat-suppressed images such as fast STIR or T2-weighted FSE with fat saturation may have contributed to this poorer sensitivity to partial tears.

As has already been alluded to, MR imaging after intraarticular contrast injection may be useful in the postoperative rotator cuff (Figs. 9.2, 9.7, 9.9, 9.12, 9.14–9.17). A 1/200 dilution of gadolinium in saline is used. T1-weighted images with fat suppression are performed in the axial, coronal, and sagittal oblique planes. In addition, postinjection T2-weighted FSE with fat saturation images are

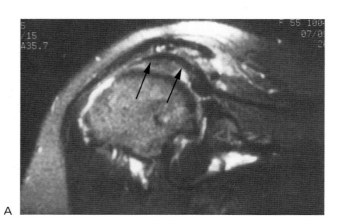

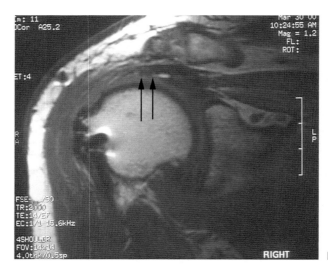

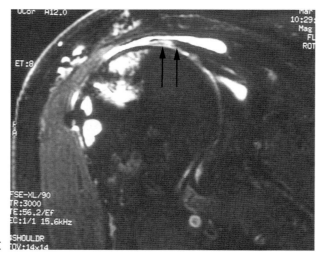

FIGURE 9.13. Recurrent rotator cuff tears, status of tendon and muscle. **A:** Coronal oblique T2-weighted spin echo image. Conventional MR images nicely illustrate the poor quality of the torn tendon after repair (*arrows*). There is moderate muscle atrophy and glenohumeral joint degenerative change. **B, C:** Coronal oblique proton density–weighted image in B and fast spin echo T2-weighted image in C with fat suppression. Again, note the attenuated, frayed tendon edges of the supraspinatus tendon in B and infraspinatus tendon in C (*arrows*). Muscle atrophy and AC joint degenerative change is also noted in B.

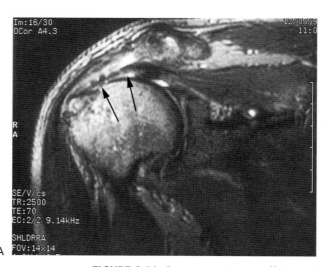

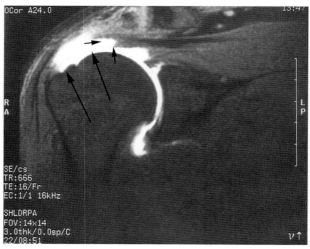

FIGURE 9.14. Recurrent rotator cuff tears, status of tendon and muscle, MR arthrography. **A, B:** Coronal oblique T2-weighted image in A and MR arthrogram in B. MR athrography reveals the moderately sized supraspinatus tendon defect (*arrows*) and contrast imbibing into the degenerated tendon edges in B (*small arrows*), more difficult to appreciate in A, owing to the artifact from prior surgery.

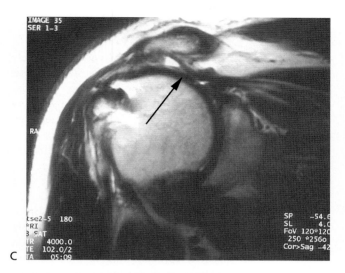

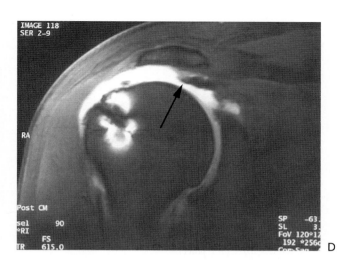

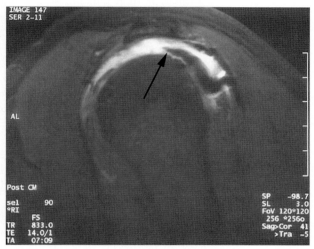

FIGURE 9.14 (continued). C, D, E: Coronal oblique T2-weighted image in C; MR arthrogram in D; sagittal oblique proton density–weighted images in E. Similar to the patient in A and B, MR arthrography better reveals the presence, size, and extent of the recurrent tendon defect in the supraspinatus tendon (*arrows*).

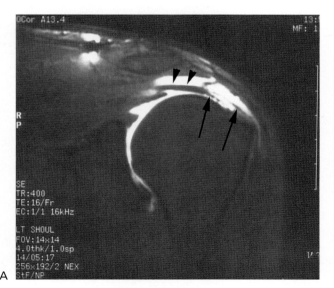

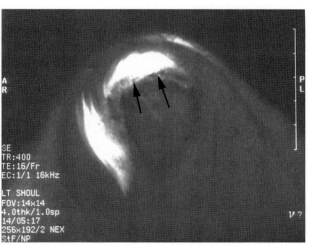

FIGURE 9.15. Small recurrent rotator cuff tear, MR arthrogram. Coronal oblique T1-weighted image in A and sagittal oblique T1-weighted image in B, with fat suppression. A small defect in the central aspect of the supraspinatus tendon is identified (*arrows*), with contrast extravasation into the subdeltoid bursa. The supraspinatus tendon appears diffusely thin as well, as best seen in A (*arrowheads*).

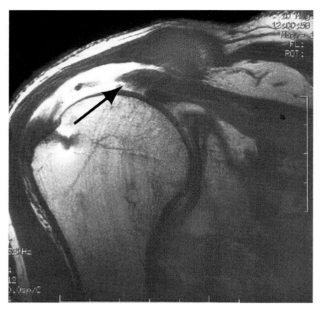

FIGURE 9.16. Coronal oblique T1-weighted high-resolution, MR arthrogram. A moderate-size recurrent tear of the supraspinatus tendon is identified (*arrow*). Images were carried out with small field of view and larger matrix (512 × 384). Fat suppression was also not applied to maintain better signal to noise. Note the excellent depiction of the tear size and status of the tendon edges with MR arthrography.

because contrast material may leak through an incompletely healed but well-repaired tendon, and, conversely, contrast material may fail to leak from the joint due to scar tissue, despite a tear. With the addition of MRI after contrast injection, the size and nature of the defect leading to the leak can be directly visualized to determine its significance. If there is scar formation, intraarticular contrast improves visualization of the cuff anatomy over conventional MRI and better outlines the morphological alterations needed to diagnose these types of tears. It may also better reveal any tendon defects that may be obscured by the low-signal scar tissue. Intraarticular contrast can help confirm the presence of an intact cuff, in a situation in which the cuff may have high signal on images with T2-weighted contrast, due to postoperative granulation tissue, edema, or fluid contained in residual nonabsorbable sutures; by the absence of contrast material extending into the cuff; or through the cuff, into the bursa. If a cuff defect is found, MR arthrography can be helpful in determining the size and location of the defect and better determine the integrity of the tendon edges for preoperative planning. MRI arthrography may also potentially increase the sensitivity for recurrent partial tears of the cuff undersurface. A recent study has described the use of MR arthrography in evaluating the postoperative rotator cuff (11,12).

Another complication of rotator cuff surgery is postoperative detachment of the deltoid from its insertion to the acromion. With open repairs through an arthrotomy, the shoulder is accessed through a deltoid-splitting incision. If the closure of the deltoid muscle is inadequate or if it dehisces, deltoid detachment may occur. Another cause can be due to aggressive resection of the anterior portion of the

often carried out, in the coronal and often the axial plane (Fig. 9.17). Conventional arthrography has been used in the past to try to diagnose recurrent rotator cuff tears (29,61). Conventional arthrography has been considered unreliable

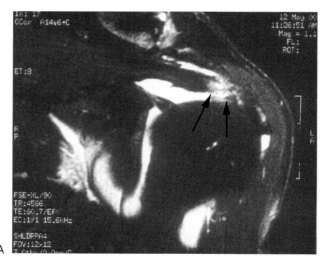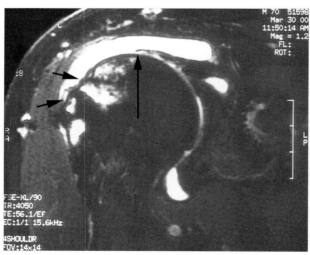

FIGURE 9.17. Coronal oblique T2-weighted fast spin echo, MR arthrogram images, with fat suppression. **A:** A small tear in the more anterior supraspinatus tendon is identified (*arrows*). **B:** A larger recurrent tear in the posterior supraspinatus tendon is observed (*larger arrow*). The tears are well delineated, with MR arthrography; the fat-suppressed T2 weighting aids in conspicuity. The multiple refocusing echoes used help to limit the metal artifacts, including those from the suture anchors in the greater tuberosity in B (*smaller arrows*), while still allowing for the use of fat suppression.

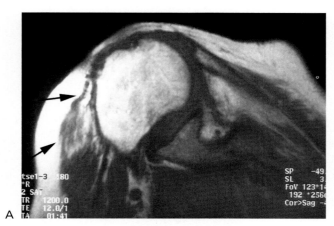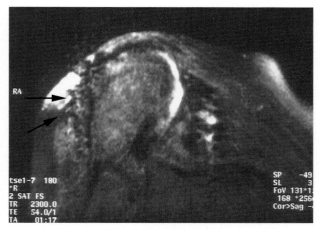

FIGURE 9.18. Deltoid detachment, coronal oblique proton density– (A) and T2-weighted (B) turbo spin echo images. The deltoid muscle is retracted distally and shows atrophy (*arrows*). The patient has a large rotator cuff tear after open rotator cuff surgery and subacromial decompression. There is no anatomic or functional depressor of the humeral head, which has migrated superiorly.

acromion at the time of decompression. Since much of the deltoid inserts here, this can result in inadvertent deltoid release from its acromial attachment. On MRI images (Fig. 9.18), the presence of deltoid detachment can be identified by observing retraction of the deltoid from the acromion, with fluid filling the defect (63). If the detachment is chronic, atrophy will be present as well. In the study by Magee et al. (4) all five cases of deltoid muscle retraction found at surgery were correctly diagnosed on preoperative MRI.

MRI was also found to be accurate in the diagnosis of biceps tendon rupture (4) in patients who had prior surgery. Biceps tendon rupture was diagnosed based on lack of visualization of the biceps tendon in the intertubercular groove. In the study by Magee et al. (4), this was correctly identified in eight of ten shoulders found to have this complication after surgery. Biceps tendon dislocations with associated tears of the subscapularis tendon were found in 8 of the 50 patients studied by these authors (4). In this situation, the diagnosis of tendon dislocation is made by visualizing the empty intertubercular groove and medial displacement of the biceps tendon. The subscapularis, if torn, will seem to be retracted from its insertion into the lesser tuberosity.

INSTABILITY

The clinical features of shoulder instability are covered in greater detail elsewhere in this text. Instability is most commonly unidirectional and may be anterior, posterior, inferior, or very rarely superior. Of these, anterior instability is by far the most common direction of instability and represents approximately 95% of cases (64). Instability can be traumatic, due to either a single episode or repetitive microtrauma, as in athletics. It may be atraumatic as well, often related to ligament and capsular laxity. Anterior instability is most commonly due to prior trauma, most commonly prior anterior dislocation, and is usually associated with avulsion of the complex of the labrum, adjacent capsule, and glenohumeral ligaments (anterior inferior labroligamentous complex) from the bony glenoid (Bankart lesion and its variants).

The other more common clinical situation encountered is multidirectional instability, which by definition is instability in more than one direction. This is often seen in patients with ligamentous laxity, in which case it may often be bilateral. It is also encountered in overhead athletes such as baseball pitchers, who perform repetitive overhead maneuvers such as throwing, which may lead to stretching of the capsule and laxity on this basis. Whereas patients with unidirectional instability most commonly are treated surgically, many patients with multidirectional instability will be treated conservatively with a vigorous rehabilitation regime, prior to any consideration of surgery.

Conservative treatment of an acute subluxation or dislocation is most commonly symptomatic. This is with pain medication, often nonsteroidal anti-inflammatory drugs, and rest. This initial treatment is then followed by a period of rehabilitation designed to restore full range of motion and to strengthen the dynamic stabilizers such as the rotator cuff and periscapular muscles. While this regime may be successful in atraumatic anterior instability, posterior instability, or patients with multidirectional instability, it usually is not as efficacious in patients with traumatic anterior instability. If these patients, after an adequate trial of conservative treatment, continue to experience instability, pain, apprehension, and loss of shoulder function, which is extremely common, especially in younger patients, they are then considered for early operative treatment.

The surgical treatment of patients with anterior instability has involved different approaches. Currently a direct repair of the labral and capsular lesions is done most

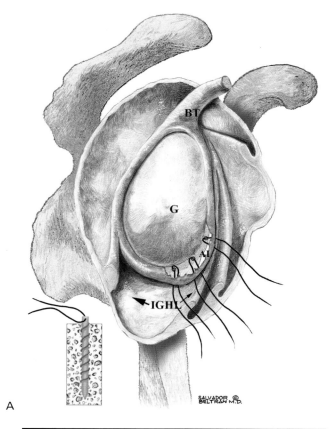

A

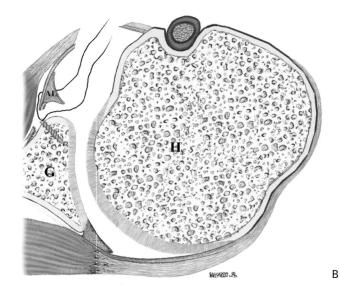

B

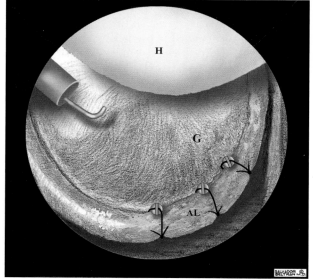

C

FIGURE 9.19. Bankart repair. Three suture anchors are placed in the anterior inferior aspect of the bony glenoid. The capsule and labrum are sutured back in an anatomic position. **A:** Artist's depiction of open repair, sagittal view; **B:** Artist's depiction of open repair, axial view; **C:** Artist's depiction of arthroscopic Bankart repair. AL, anterior inferior labrum; BT, biceps tendon; G, glenoid; H, humerus; IGHL, inferior glenohumeral ligament.

commonly, usually a Bankart-type repair (65), or less commonly the staple capsulorrhaphy described by Du Toit and Roux (66). Other types of repair are those that tighten the capsule indirectly, usually through manipulation of the subscapularis, most commonly the Putti-Platt (67) or Magnusson-Stack procedure (68), and those that involve movement of the coracoid process, most commonly the Bristow (69) procedure.

As noted earlier, the approach that is currently most commonly utilized and favored is to treat the contributing pathology specifically and to aim repairs at restoring as best as possible the normal anatomy. That is, it is aimed at repairing the essential lesion of instability, as described by Perthes (70) and Bankart (65,71). This is usually done via some modification of the repair originally described by Bankart in 1938 (65) (Fig. 9.19). This was originally described as an

Postoperative Shoulder **267**

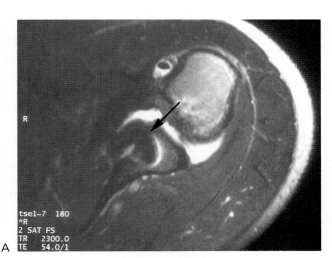 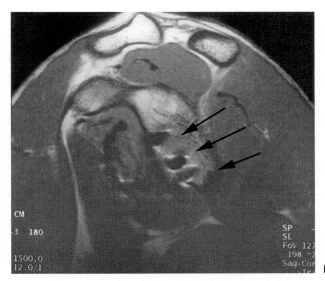

FIGURE 9.20. Post Bankart repair. **A:** Axial turbo spin echo T2-weighted image. Note the artifact from the suture anchor in the anterior inferior glenoid (*arrow*). **B:** Sagittal oblique fast spin echo proton density–weighted image in another patient. Postsurgical artifact outlines the sites of fixation in the anterior glenoid (*arrows*).

open procedure via the deltopectoral interval to accomplish a reattachment of the torn capsulolabral complex to the bony glenoid rim. Drill holes are made in the glenoid, through which sutures may be passed to secure the labrum and capsule. In place of drill holes, suture anchors may be used. These are usually placed at the 3, 4, and 5 o'clock positions. These suture anchors may have different compositions and can be ferromagnetic (Fig. 9.20), especially in older repairs, but others may be made of nonferromagnetic substances, including plastic and bioabsorbable materials.

Capsulolabral repairs may also be done arthroscopically, and this approach has become more common in recent years. Arthroscopic techniques have theoretic advantages compared with open procedures, including minimizing surgical dissection, damage to surrounding tissues, and scarring (72). Caspari (73,74) described a technique in which the torn capsulolabral tissues are repaired via the passage of sutures from the capsulolabral tissue, through the glenoid neck and scapular body, and secured over the fascia above the scapula. Newer techniques use suture anchors placed in the bony glenoid with arthroscopic graspers and knot pushers used to secure the labrum to the glenoid (75). Another type of fixation used in arthroscopic repairs is fixation with a stapling or tacking device (76). Currently bioabsorbable tacks are used (77).

In addition to repairing the torn labrum and capsule, many surgeons also perform a capsulorrhaphy of the stretched-out and redundant capsule, which may also often be present in cases of recurrent anterior instability. This can be done as part of an open procedure or arthroscopically. When performed arthroscopically, this may be done with absorbable sutures or with a holmium laser. The use of the laser has been developed since arthroscopic techniques are not that

well suited to performing capsular shifts (78). The recurrence rate after open Bankart repair is 5% or less (79), but it has been reported to be somewhat higher with arthroscopic repair (80,81,82). Caspari (73,74), using his technique, had results close to those with open techniques.

The staple capsulorapphy described by Du Toit and Roux (66) employs a staple to reattach the anterior capsulolabral complex to the glenoid margin. It has apparently fallen into disfavor among orthopedic surgeons (6), because of a high rate of failure due to loss of fixation and staple migration. This procedure has also been done arthroscopically (83) but again has had a similar high rate of failure.

In the presence of glenoid deficiency, a glenoid fracture that involves more than 25% of the glenoid fossa and is associated with shoulder instability is an indication for surgery. This is usually done as an open reduction of the fragment with screw fixation. Often this is determined with the use of a CT scan, which is generally felt to be the best method of determining fragment size and displacement (72). Obviously the presence of fixation screws, depending on their composition, can lead to significant metal artifact that will impair visualization, so that when these patients are seen in follow-up, one or the other of MR arthrography with fast spin echo imaging or CT arthrography may be attempted to best evaluate such patients.

Many surgeons also believe that pathology in the rotator interval may also contribute to shoulder instability (87), and this may be identified on MRI. Consequently, closure of this interval is often performed in conjunction with procedures for shoulder instability (85).

The Putti-Platt (67) and Magnuson-Stack (68) procedures are not anatomic reconstructions and as noted tighten

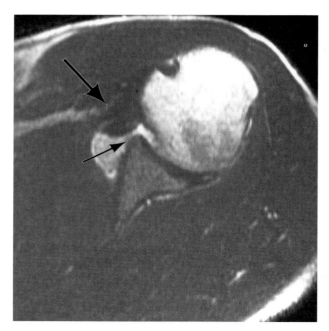

FIGURE 9.21. Post Putti-Platt repair, axial conventional spin echo T2-weighted image. Note the deformity in the subscapularis tendon after repair (*thick arrow*). Note the absent anterior labrum (*thin arrow*) in this nonanatomic repair.

the capsule indirectly, through manipulations of the subscapularis (Fig. 9.21). They prevent recurrent dislocations via restricting natural motion. They realign and tighten the subscapularis and limit external rotation. As indicated, these are less commonly done as the current trend in orthopedics is away from subscapularis-based procedures. These procedures have a higher rate of patient dissatisfaction because of the decrease in motion and have higher rates of osteoarthritis. Patients who have had these procedures may still be seen for complications and recurrences and therefore it is important to review them. The subscapularis tendon is split at its midpoint in the Putti-Platt procedure. Its lateral portion is attached to the glenoid, and its medial portion is then imbricated over it. The humerus must be rotated internally to a near neutral position (67). The recurrence rate with this procedure is reported as between 2% and 10%. In the Magnuson-Stack procedure (M-Stack) (68), the subscapularis is removed from its insertion into the lesser tuberosity and transferred distal and lateral to the greater tuberosity. The loss of external rotation is usually less than with the Putti-Platt procedure. Note that in these nonanatomic procedures, the anatomic lesion is not fixed, so that the detached labrum and/or capsule will still be present on imaging examinations, after repair.

Bony procedures have been developed to augment the bony anterior glenoid. The Bristow procedure (69) involves moving the coracoid process and using it as a bone block to prevent recurrent anterior dislocation. This procedure was utilized much more commonly in the past. There is also some static and dynamic reinforcement of the anterior cap-

sule with this method. The bony tip of the coracoid process is transferred with the conjoined tendon and attached to the anterior inferior glenoid rim through a split made in the subscapularis. The conjoined tendon can then act as a reinforcement of the capsule. The coracoid is fixed with a cancellous screw. A high rate of subluxation and hardware complications (86) has been reported with the modified Bristow procedure. Failure of this procedure may also be related to the fact that it does not address the detached labrum and capsule (72).

Imaging of patients with Bristow procedures can often be challenging, due to the significant metal artifact arising from the cancellous screw, and is again best done with one or the other of MR arthrography with fast spin echo imaging or CT arthrography. Assessing for failure of fixation or for hardware complications may be best done with CT scanning.

As with anterior instability the initial treatment for posterior instability is nonoperative, but surgical options are chosen if these fail. Initial results in treating these patients were often poor, but more recently the approach has been to correct the underlying pathology anatomically (87). Repair for posterior instability is generally modified from that done for anterior instability. Most commonly this is a repair of the reverse Bankart lesion, and if this is combined with a redundant posterior capsule, then a posterior capsular plication or shift is needed. If there is a bony deficiency, it is treated with a posterior glenoid bone graft or posterior opening wedge osteotomy (88). In these patients, the repair is approached from posterior, through the infraspinatus muscle and tendon.

The pathology in patients with multidirectional instability is generally the presence of a loose redundant joint capsule. When treated surgically, patients are usually treated with an inferior capsular shift procedure (89,90,91). This procedure was devised for multidirectional anteroinferior instability. It reduces the volume of the glenohumeral joint anteriorly, inferiorly, and posteriorly. This procedure may also be used for posteroinferior and other combinations of instability, with the region of capsular shift adjusted accordingly. The deltopectoral interval is used as the approach and the subscapularis traversed to expose the capsule. A T-shaped incision is made in the capsule to allow the inferior capsule to be advanced in a superior direction and the superior capsule to overlap it by advancing it inferiorly. On MRI exam, the findings associated with this procedure will mainly be reflected by the presence of thickening of the anteroinferior capsule due to scar formation (6). Owing to the capsular plication, on coronal views in particular, the axillary pouch will be diminished in size. Low-signal foci from suture material may be seen in the subscapularis and anterior capsule. To assess the efficacy of the repair, the degree of capsular plication may be best assessed with MRI arthrography, as it may be difficult to determine whether there is any residual redundancy without distending the joint.

Labral tears such as SLAP lesions are often treated with debridement of the torn portion of the labrum, generally via

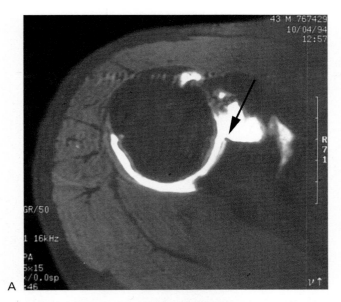

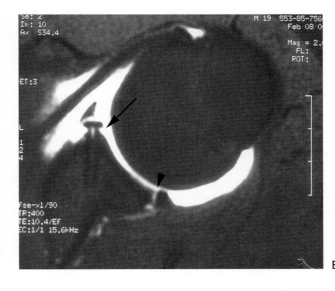

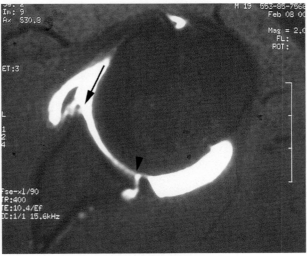

FIGURE 9.22. A: Labral debridement, MR arthrogram, axial 3D volume gradient echo image. A smooth but attenuated anterior superior labrum is seen (*arrow*). **B:** Labral repair with tack, MR arthrogram, axial T1-weighted image with fat suppression. A tack is seen in the anterior superior glenoid (*arrow*). Note contrast outlining of a detached posterior labrum (*arrowhead*). **C:** MR arthrogram, axial T1-weighted image with fat suppression, same patient as in B. The labrum below the tack is blunted and frayed (*arrow*). Contrast is again seen to outline a detachment in the posterior labrum (*arrowhead*).

an arthroscopic approach (92) (Fig. 9.22). In some situations, especially where there is an avulsion of the anterior superior labrum or avulsion of the biceps labral anchor complex, the lesions are debrided of loose tissue, and a suture or staple repair back down to the bony glenoid bone may be carried out (72). Labral fraying or tearing may be present in regions other than SLAP lesions or anteroinferiorly (Bankart lesions). For example, posterior labral fraying or detachment may occur in patients with internal impingement. In such patients, the frayed portions can be debrided under arthroscopic visualization to minimize mechanical catching (43).

As with imaging after surgery for rotator cuff disease, the artifacts that result from surgery for instability impair visualization of any residual lesions. These include metal artifacts, especially, as noted earlier, with the use of screw fixation of the coracoid in the Bristow procedure or the placement of suture anchors, staples, or tacks with some of the other techniques

described (Fig. 9.20). Scarring from the incisions as well as suture repair may impair visualization, resulting in disruption of normal tissue contrast, with areas of more prominent signal void arising. In Bankart repairs, even nonferromagnetic suture anchors or other materials may be apparent within the glenoid neck (6). If transglenoid sutures are placed, there will be channels seen traversing the glenoid neck and scapula. In addition, the suture knot placed posteriorly—that is, tied over fascia—may show some surrounding intermediate or high signal on images with T2-type contrast, due to the formation of hyperemic granulation tissue. In patients with anatomic repairs such as the Bankart repair, there should be an anatomic position and morphology of the labrum and capsule after repair (79). In certain procedures, especially those that do not directly repair the labral and capsular lesions, as noted earlier, the abnormality from these lesions remains on subsequent imaging. This makes assessment of the cause of persistent or recurrent instability difficult.

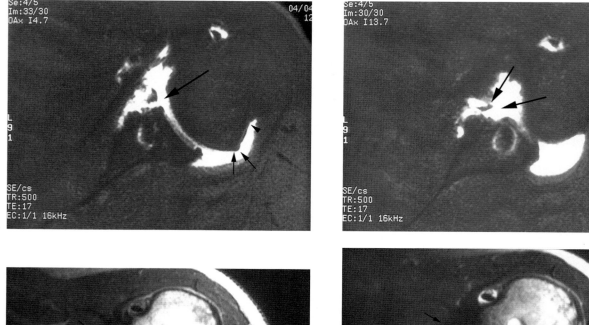

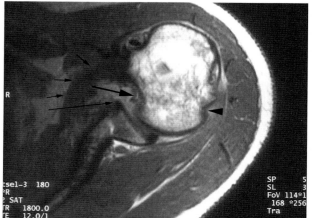

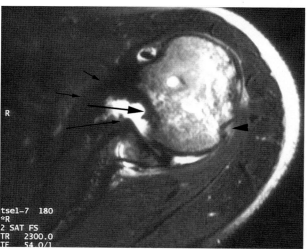

FIGURE 9.23. Post Bankart repair, recurrent lesions, degenerative joint disease. **A, B**: MR arthrogram, axial T1-weighted images with fat suppression. The anterior inferior labrum is detached and blunted (*arrows*) in this patient after open Bankart repair. Note the early glenohumeral joint degenerative change. Note also the small osteophyte projecting from the humeral head in A (*small arrows*) and the early articular cartilage loss. A Hill-Sachs lesion is present (*arrowhead*). Axial proton density– **(C)** and T2-weighted **(D)** turbo spin echo images; same patient as in Figure 9.20. The anterior labrum is blunted (*long thin arrow*). The humeral head is displaced posteriorly, with a wedgelike defect in the anteromedial humeral head (*thicker arrow*), with subjacent marrow edema. These latter two findings were felt to reflect an overtight anterior repair, thought to have resulted in posterior laxity/instability. There is joint space narrowing, reflective of glenohumeral joint degenerative change. Also note the small Hill-Sachs lesion of the posterolateral humeral head (*arrowhead*).

There is little known on the utility of MRI in patients who have been operated upon for instability. The success rates for surgery for typical patterns of anterior glenohumeral instability are usually good. The recurrence rate for most instability procedures done in an open manner is 1% to 10% (72,79,93–95). Procedures done arthroscopically may have a higher rate of recurrence, in the range of 15%–20% (73,74,80–82,96–98). If there are recurrent problems after surgery, patients may be treated based on clinical grounds or assessed via arthroscopy. The volume of cases referred for MRI for recurrent instability after surgical treatment has

therefore been limited, and there is little in the literature on this topic. MRI may be helpful in diagnosing some of the abnormalities that may be present, although discerning true recurrent pathology from artifacts, scarring, and residual untreated lesions is often quite difficult. In our experience, MRI arthrography is often helpful, particularly to improve visualization, by improving tissue contrast (13).

Causes of recurrent instability include inadequate or incorrect procedures and the uncovering of missed anterior or posterior instability with isolated treatment of one. An overtight repair either may lead to degenerative change (95) or may precipitate instability in the other direction (Fig. 9.23). This may be particularly the case in such procedures as the Putti-Platt (67) or Magnuson-Stack (68), which may also result in loss of external rotation. In these latter procedures, an internal rotation contracture may be present but may only be apparent if axial images are performed in internal and external rotation. Inferior capsular shifts or other types of capsular plications can also be overtightened. Signs of an overtightened inferior capsular shift may include prominent loss of the axillary pouch, which is often the first sign. Subtle posterior subluxation of the humeral head relative to the glenoid is another finding of overtightening in an inferior capsular shift or other shoulder plication. Degenerative arthritis may also occur, if there is persistent instability from inadequate repair (Fig. 9.23). The articular cartilage will appear thin, and osteophytes will most commonly be seen at the humeral head neck junction. Marginal glenoid cysts may also be present. Misplaced or detached staples or tacks from labral and capsular repairs (Fig. 9.24) or misplaced screws or coracoid nonunion in a Bristow procedure may also cause joint derangement. If left unrecognized, it may lead to degenerative changes as well. These can be identified with MRI but are better seen with MR arthrography and, if needed, CT scanning. It should be noted, however, that the presence of coracoid nonunion in the Bristow procedure does not by itself indicate instability, as there is a 5% to 10% nonunion rate even in patients who are clinically stable with this procedure (69,86,99).

In patients after repair of the labrum and capsule, the postoperative labrum may be thickened and irregular, due to scar tissue or suture material; however, it should not be de-

tached. Signal alterations may be present within the labrum as well as postoperatively, and high signal on images with T2 contrast may be present in the earlier postoperative periods due to hyperemic granulation tissue (9). As such, outlining the labrum and capsule with intraarticular contrast is the best means of discerning recurrent tears and detachments, by outlining any surface irregularities and revealing any contrast extension into or beneath the labrum (11,12). Failed Bankart repairs may show persistence or recurrence of the detachment of the labrum and capsule (Fig. 9.23). This is often due to breakdown of the fixation, suture breakage, anchor device pullout, or failure of the reapproximated labral and capsular tissues. The repaired labrum may also become blunted, attenuated, or fragmented.

With respect to the joint capsule, postoperatively it may appear thickened and nodular as a response to the surgery. Measurements of capsular thickening have been described for adhesive capsulitis (100) and can be measured best in the axillary recess on MR arthrography, as a band of low signal adjacent to the hyperintense signal of contrast medially and the hyperintense signal of the fat stripe laterally, on T1-weighted images. Whereas a measurement of 4 mm has been believed to be indicative of adhesive capsulitis, a measurement of 2 to 4 mm is thought to be consistent with the thickening expected in the postoperative state in patients after Bankart repair. The glenohumeral ligaments may also appear thickened and nodular following repair. In patients with recurrent instability, the repaired capsule may become stretched out and redundant. These changes are best identified by MR arthrography.

One criterion suggested for the diagnosis of residual or recurrent capsular stripping may be the presence of a capsular attachment that is more medial than would be expected for a type 3 insertion (9,101). Tirman and associates (102) recommended measuring the anterior and posterior capsular widths in nonoperated patients using MR arthrography. Rand and coworkers (9) indicated that an anterior capsular width/posterior capsular width ratio of <1 on MR arthrography may predict a good outcome after surgery particularly if a capsulorapphy, open, or arthroscopic has been done. Imaging patients in abduction and external rotation may be useful to demonstrate any subtle persistent laxity. The glenohumeral ligaments, if abnormal, may appear thin, elongated, irregular, and discontinuous.

One potential pitfall even with MR arthrography is the Bankart repair that is partly adherent related to fibrous tissue and granulation tissue, even when the joint is distended with contrast. This may be missed on MR arthrography but evident at arthroscopy when this area is probed. Intravenous gadolinium enhancement with T1 weighting and fat suppression may potentially be helpful in such cases by outlining these areas of granulation tissue, which should enhance (9).

It is well known now that secondary occult impingement and rotator cuff injury can also be an outcome of or a cause of continual problems in patients with persistent or recurrent

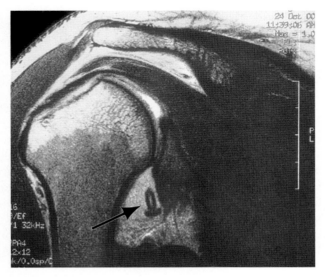

FIGURE 9.24. Displaced, tack, coronal oblique image, fast spin echo T1-weighted MR arthrogram, without fat suppression. Note the displaced tack from a prior Bankart repair axillary, in the axillary recess (*arrow*). Note the Hill-Sachs lesion in the superior humeral head.

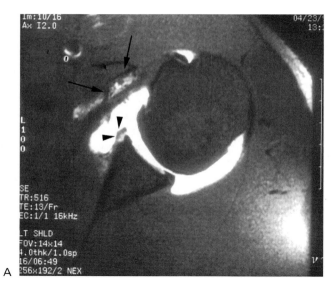

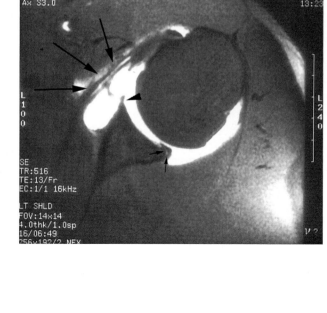

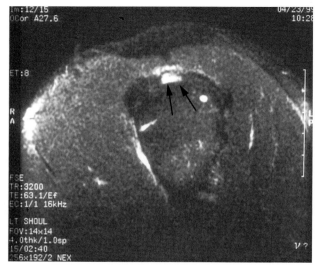

FIGURE 9.25. Persistent anterior instability, partial rotator cuff tear. **A, B:** MR arthrogram, axial T1-weighted images with fat suppression. The patient is status post subscapularis plication. Note the attenuated subscapularis tendon after surgery (*arrows*). The anterior labrum is blunted and attenuated in A and B and is also separated in A (*arrowheads*). Also note the posterior labral tear (*small arrow*). There is mild glenohumeral joint degenerative arthritis. **C:** Sagittal oblique T2-weighted fast spin echo image with fat suppression, same patient as in A and B. A high-grade partial tear of the supraspinatus tendon undersurface is seen (*arrows*).

instability, and these should be searched for as well, on MRI or MR arthrography (Fig. 9.25). Other postoperative findings that can be visualized on MRI that may be a cause of persistent or recurrent symptoms include avascular necrosis and paralabral or ganglion cysts (4) (Fig. 9.7).

Paralabral cysts may occur and arise from the glenoid labrum. They may extend into the spinoglenoid notch (103,104). Patients with ganglion cysts in the spinoglenoid notch may present with clinical findings similar to impingement. MRI will reveal a fluid-filled sac in the region of the notch. The intraarticular portion may be visualized and excised arthroscopically. If it is too large, the visible portion can be unroofed and decompressed (35, 43), or it may need to be removed in an open fashion. Failure of this procedure can be due to incomplete removal of the cyst, intraoperative injury to the suprascapular nerve or artery, and continued compression due to hematoma. In patients with incomplete

cyst removal or with recurrence, MRI may reveal cyst remnants or a recurrent cyst on images with T2-type contrast or with MRI arthrography.

Other complications of surgery (Fig. 9.26) include hematoma formation, wound infection, osteomyelitis, septic arthritis, and synovitis. MRI can be useful to diagnose these abnormalities as well. The appearance of a hematoma will depend on its age. Blood products at the appropriate stage may be bright on T1- and T2-weighted images. Fluid-fluid levels may also be present. Postoperative wound abscess formation may present as a localized cavity with signal characteristics similar to fluid. There may be a rim of inflamed tissue surrounding the abscess cavity, which may be bright on images with T2-type contrast and STIR imaging and enhance with intravenous administration of gadolinium.

Osteomyelitis may be best detected with the use of fat-suppressed imaging, such as T2-weighted fast spin echo im-

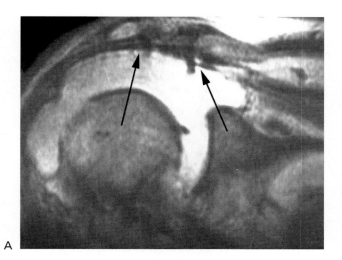

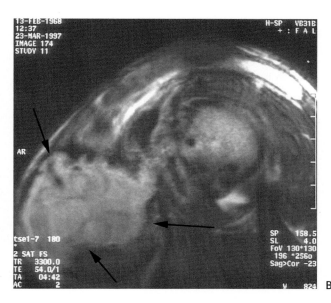

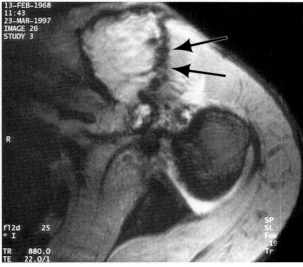

FIGURE 9.26. Postoperative complications. **A:** Coronal oblique T2-weighted image. A large to massive effusion is present in this patient who developed septic arthritis after a rotator cuff repair (*arrows*). **B, C:** Sagittal oblique T2-weighted turbo spin echo image in B and axial 2D T2* gradient echo image in C. A large anterior hematoma is seen in the deltoid muscle (*arrows*). The patient had an open Bankart repair 2 days prior to this scan.

ages with fat saturation or with fast STIR images. These sequences will increase the conspicuity of the lesions. Synovitis may also follow surgery. It may be infectious or reactive (2). A joint effusion may then be present. Synovial thickening may be present, and synovial proliferation may give rise to a bumpy contour of the inner surface of the joint capsule. The intermediate signal synovial nodules present may stand out against the joint fluid. Intravenous gadolinium may reveal enhancement of the inflamed synovium. If the synovitis is infectious, joint destruction, including cartilage loss, cysts, and erosions, may be identified. Unfortunately, it may at times be difficult to differentiate signal alterations seen in infection and inflammation from those that are due to the postoperative status of the patient, particularly in patients who have more recently had surgery. Interval follow-up is therefore very useful in these circumstances, to differentiate normal postoperative changes from those due to inflammation or infection (9).

Damage to nerve and vessels such as in the axilla may also occur, but this is not common. In the rare situation of pseudoaneurysm formation, this condition may be evaluated with MR angiographic techniques, including those with intravenous contrast injection. Damage to nerves may be manifest by secondary evidence of muscle atrophy and in the acute phase by diffusely increased signal on imaging sequences with T2-type contrast or on fast STIR images.

REFERENCES

1. Owen RS, Iannotti JP, Kneeland JB, Dalinka MKD, Deren JA, Oleaga L. Shoulder after surgery: MR imaging with surgical validation. *Radiology* 1993;186:443–447.
2. Haygood TM, Oxner KG, Kneeland JB, Dalinka MK. Magnetic resonance imaging of the postoperative shoulder. *MRI Clin North Am* 1993;1:143–155.
3. Gaenslen ES, Stterlee CC, Hinson GW. Magnetic resonance

imaging for evaluation of failed repairs of the rotator cuff: relationship to operative findings. *J Bone Joint Surg* 1996;78A:1391–1396.

4. Magee TH, Gaenslen ES, Seitz R, Hinson GA, Wetzel LH. MR imaging of the shoulder after surgery. *AJR* 1997;168:925–928.

5. Gusmer PB, Potter HG, Donovan WD, O'Brien SJ. MR imaging of the shoulder after rotator cuff repair. *AJR* 1997;168:559–563.

6. Longobardi RSF. Rafii M, Minkoff JM. MR imaging of the postoperative shoulder. *MRI Clin North Am* 1997;5:841–859.

7. Feller JF, Howey TD, Plaga BR. MR imaging of the postoperative shoulder. In: Steinbach LS, Tirman PFJ. Peterfy CG, Feller JF, eds. *Shoulder magnetic resonance imaging*. Philadelphia: Lippincott-Raven, 1998:187–221.

8. Zanetti MD, Jost B, Hodler J. MR findings in asymptomatic patients after supraspinatus reconstruction. *Radiology* 1999;213(P):157.

9. Rand T, Trattnig S, Breitenseher M, Wurnig C, Marchner B, Imhof H. The postoperative shoulder. *Top Magn Reson Imaging* 1999;10:203–213.

10. Speilman AL, Forster BB, Kokan P, Hawkins RH, Janzen DL. Shoulder after rotator cuff repair: MR imaging findings in asymptomatic individuals—initial experience. *Radiology* 1999; 213:705–708.

11. Rand T, Trattnig S, Breitenseher M, Feilinger W. Postoperative MR arthrography of the shoulder joint. *Radiologe* 1996:36: 966–970.

12. Rand T, Feilinger W, Breitenseher M, et al. Magnetic resonance arthrography in the postoperative shoulder. *Magn Resn Imaging* 1999;10.

13. Zlatkin MB. Arthro-IRM de l'épaule. In: Laredo JD, ed. Arthrographie, arthroscanner, arthro-IRM. Paris: Masson, 2000:93–117.

14. Neer CS II. Anterior acromioplasty for the chronic impingement syndrome of the shoulder: a preliminary report. *J Bone Joint Surg Am* 1972;54A:41–50.

15. Neer CS II. Impingement lesions. *Clin Orthop* 1983;173:70–77.

16. Matsen FA, Artnz CT, Lippitt SB. Rotator cuff. In: Rockwood CE, Matsen FA, eds. *The shoulder*. Philadelphia: WB Saunders, 1998:755–795.

17. Rockwood CA, Lyons FR. Shoulder impingement syndrome: diagnosis, radiographic evaluation, and treatment with a modified Neer acromioplasty. *J Bone Joint Surg Am* 1993;75:409–424.

18. Fu FH, Harner CD, Klein AH. Shoulder impingement syndrome: a critical review. *Clin Orthop* 1991;269:162–173.

19. Bigliani LU, Morrison DS, April EW. The morphology of the acromion and its relationship to rotator cuff tears. *Orthop Trans* 1986;10:228.

20. Kvitne RS, Jobe FW. Diagnosis and treatment of anterior instability in the throwing athlete. *Clin Orthop* 1993;291:107–123.

21. Arroyo JS, Hershorn SJ, Bigliani LU. Special considerations in the athletic throwing shoulder. *Orthop Clin North Am* 1997:28: 69–78.

22. Arroyo JS, Flatow EL. Management of rotator cuff disease: intact and repairable cuff. In: Iannotti JP, Williams GR Jr., eds. *Disorders of the shoulder: diagnosis and management*. Philephia: Lippincott, Williams and Wilkins, 1999:31–56.

23. Bokor DJ, Hawkins RJ, Huckell GH, Angelo RL, Schikendantz MS. Results of nonoperative management of full thickness tears of the rotator cuff. *Clin Orthop* 1993;294:103–110.

24. Burkhead WZ, Burkhart SS, Gerber C, Harryman DT, Morrison DS, Uhthoff HK, Williams GR, Jr. Symposium on the rotator cuff: debridement vs. repair—Part II. *Contemp Orthop* 1995;31: 313–326.

25. Burkhart SS. Reconciling the paradox of rotator cuff repair versus debridement: a unified biomechanical rationale for the treatment of rotator cuff tears: current concepts. *Arthroscopy* 1994;10:4–19.

26. Burkhart SS. Shoulder arthroscopy: new concepts. *Clin Sports Med* 1996;15:635.

27. Ogilvie-Harris D, Wiley A, Sattarian J. Failed acromioplasty for impingement syndrome. *J Bone Joint Surg Br* 1990;72:1070–1072.

28. Bigliani LU, Cordasco FA, McIlveen SJ, Musso ES. Operative treatment of failed repairs of the rotator cuff. *J Bone Joint Surg Am* 1992;74:1505–1515.

29. DeOrio JK, Cofield RH. Results of a second attempt at surgical repair of a failed initial rotator-cuff repair. *J Bone Joint Surg* 1984; 66A:563–567.

30. Esch J. Rotator cuff disease and impingement. In: Esch JC, Baker CL, eds. *Arthroscopic surgery: the shoulder and elbow*. Philadelphia: JB Lippincott, 1993:151–175.

31. Gartsman GM. Arthroscopic acromioplasty for lesions of the rotator cuff. *J Bone Joint Surg* 1990;72A:169–180.

32. Beach WR, Caspari RB. Arthroscopic management of rotator cuff disease. *Orthopedics* 1993;16:1007–1015.

33. Hurley JA, Anderson TE, Dear W, Andrish JT, Bergfeld JA, Weiker GG. Posterior shoulder instability: surgical versus conservative results with evaluation of glenoid version. *Am J Sports Med* 1992;20:396–400.

34. Paulos LE, Franklin JL. Arthroscopic shoulder decompression development and application: a five year experience. *Am J Sports Med* 1990;18:235–244.

35. Peterson II CA, Altchek DW. Arthroscopic treatment of rotator cuff disorders. *Clin Sports Med* 1996;15:715–736.

36. Mumford EB. Acromioclavicular dislocation: a new operative treatment. *J Bone Joint Surg* 1941;23:799–802.

37. Flatow EL, Duralde XA, Nicholson GP, Pollock RG, Bigliani LU. Arthroscopic resection of the distal clavicle from a superior approach. *J Shoulder Elbow Surg* 1995;4:41–50.

38. Blevins FT, Warren RF, Cavo C, Altchek DW, Dines D, Palletta G, Wickiewicz TL. Arthroscopic assisted rotator cuff repair: results using a mini-open deltoid splitting approach. *Arthroscopy* 1996; 12:50–59.

39. Hurley JA, Anderson TE. Shoulder arthroscopy: its role in evaluating the shoulder disorders in the athlete. *Am J Sports Med* 1990: 18:480–483.

40. Zlatkin MB, Iannotti JP, Roberts MC, et al. Rotator cuff disease: diagnostic performance of MR imaging: comparison with arthrography and correlation with surgery. *Radiology* 1989;172: 223–229.

41. Iannotti JP, Zlatkin MB, Esterhai JL, Kressel HY, Dalinka MK, Spindler KP. Magnetic resonance imaging of the shoulder. *J Bone Joint Surg Am* 1991;73:17–29.

42. Needel SD, Zlatkin MB. Comparison of fat-saturation fast spin echo versus conventional spin-echo MR in the detection of rotator cuff pathology. *JMRI* 1997;7:674.

43. Peterson CA, Altcheck DW, Warren RF. Shoulder arthroscopy. In: Rockwood CE, Matsen FA, eds. *The shoulder*. Philadelphia: WB Saunders, 1998.

44. Budoff JE, Nirschl RP, Guidi EJ. Debridement of partial thickness tears of the rotator cuff without acromiplasty. *J Bone Joint Surg Am* 1988;80:733–748.

45. Andrews JR, Broussard TS, Carson WG. Arthroscopy of the shoulder in the management of partial tears of the rotator cuff: a preliminary report. *Arthroscopy* 1985;1(2):117–122.

46. Snyder SJ, Pachelli AF, Del Pizzo W, Friedman MJ, Ferkel RD, Patten G. Partial thickness rotator cuff tears: results of arthroscopic treatment. *Arthroscopy* 1991;7:1–7.

47. Ellman H, Kay SP, Wirth M. Arthroscopic treatment of full-thickness rotator cuff tears: 2- to 7-year follow-up study. *Arthroscopy* 1993;9:195–200.

48. Baker CL, Liu SH. Comparison of open and arthroscopically assisted rotator cuff repairs. *Am J Sports Med* 1995;23:99.

49. Gartsman GM, Hammerman SM. Full thickness tears: arthroscopic repair. *Orthop Clin North Am* 1997;28:83–98.

50. McLaughlin HL. Repair of major cuff ruptures. *Surg Clin North Am* 1963;43:1535–1540.
51. Hawkins RJ, Misamore GW, Hobeika PE. Surgery for full thickness rotator cuff tears. *J Bone Joint Surg Am* 1985;67:1349–1355.
52. Neviaser JS, Neviaser RJ, Neviaser TJ. The repair of chronic massive ruptures of the rotator cuff. *J Bone Joint Surg Am* 1978:60:681–684.
53. Ozaki J, Fujimoto S, Masuhara K, et al. Reconstruction of chronic massive rotator cuff tears with synthetic materials. *Clin Orthop* 1986;202:173–183.
54. Melilo AS, Savoie FH III. Field LD. Massive rotator cuff tears: debridement versus repair. *Orthop Clin North Am* 1997:28:117–124.
55. Cofield RH. Rotator cuff disease of the shoulder. *J Bone Joint Surg Am* 1985;67:974–979.
56. Weber SC. All arthroscopic versus mini open repair in the management of complete tears of the rotator cuff. *Arthroscopy* 1997;13:368–372.
57. Norwood L, Fowler FH. Rotator cuff tears: a shoulder arthroscopy complication. *Am J Sports Med* 1989;17:837–841.
58. Mitchell MJ, Causey G, Berthoty DP, et al. Peribursal fat plane of the shoulder: anatomic study and clinical experience. *Radiology* 1988:168;699–704.
59. Rafii M, Firooznia H, Golimbu C, Weinreb J. Magnetic resonance imaging of glenohumeral instability. *MRI Clin North Am* 1993;1:87–104.
60. Farley TE, Neumann CH, Steinbach LS, Jahnke AJ, Peterson SS. Full-thickness tears of the rotator cuff: diagnosis with MR imaging. *AJR* 1992;158:347–351.
61. Calvert PT, Packer NP, Stoker DJ, Bayley JIL. Kessel L. Arthrography of the shoulder after operative repair of the torn rotator cuff. *J Bone Joint Surg Br* 1986;68:147–150.
62. Harryman DT II, Mack LA, Wang KY, Jackins SE, Richardson ML, Matsen FA III. Repairs of the rotator cuff: correlation of functional results with integrity of the cuff. *J Bone Joint Surg Am* 1991;73:982–989.
63. Oxner KG. Magnetic resonance imaging of the musculoskeletal system. *Clin Orthop* 1997;334:354–373.
64. Cain PR, Mutschler TA, Fu FH. Anterior stability of the glenohumeral joint: a dynamic model. *Am J Sports Med* 1987;15:144–148.
65. Bankart ASB. The pathology and treatment of recurrent dislocation of the shoulder. *Br J Surg* 1938;26:23–39.
66. Du Toit GT, Roux D. Recurrent dislocation of the shoulder. *J Bone Joint Surg Am* 1956;38:1–12.
67. Osmond-Clarke H. Habitual dislocation of the shoulder: the Putti-Platt operation. *J Bone Joint Surg Br* 1948;30:19–25.
68. Magnuson PB, Stack JK. Recurrent dislocation of the shoulder. *JAMA* 1943;123:889–892.
69. Helfet A. Coracoid transplantation for recurring dislocation of the shoulder. *J Bone Joint Surg Br* 1958;40:198–202.
70. Perthes G. Uber Operationen der habituellen Schulterluxation. *Dtsche Z Chir* 1906:85:199.
71. Bankart ASB. Recurrent or habitual dislocation of the shoulder joint. *Br Med J* 1923;2:1132–1133.
72. Matthews LS, Pavlovich LJ Jr. Anterior and anteroinferior instability: diagnosis and management. In: Iannotti JP, Williams GR Jr. *Disorders of the shoulder: diagnosis and management.* Philadelphia: Lippincott, Williams and Wilkins, 1999:251–294.
73. Caspari R, Savoir B. Arthroscopic reconstruction of the shoulder: the Bankart repair. In: Pariesen JS, ed. *Operative arthroscopy.* New York: Raven Press, 1990:65–74.
74. Caspari RB. Arthroscopic reconstruction for anterior shoulder instability. In: Paulos LE, Tibone JD, eds. *Operative techniques in shoulder surgery.* Gaithersburg, MD: Aspen, 1991:57–63.
75. Wolf E, Walk R, Richmond J. Arthroscopic Bankart repair using suture anchors. *Oper Technique Orthop* 1992;1:184–191.
76. Lane JG, Sachs RA, Riehl B. Arthroscopic staple capsulorrhaphy: a long term follow up. *Arthroscopy* 1993;9:190–194.
77. Speer KP, Warren RF, Pagnani M, Warner JJ. An arthroscopic technique for anterior stabilization of the shoulder with a bioabsorbable tack. *J Bone Joint Surg Am* 1996;78:1801–1807.
78. Hayashi K, Thabit G III. Bogdanske JJ, Mascio LN, Markel MD. The effect of nonlaser ablative energy on the ultrastructure of joint capsular collagen. *Arthroscopy* 1996;12:474–481.
79. Rowe, CR, Patel D, Southmayd WW. The Bankart procedure: a long-term end-result study. *J Bone Joint Surg Am* 1978;60:1–16.
80. Morgan CD, Bodenstab AB. Arthroscopic Bankart suture repair: technique and early results. *Arthroscopy* 1987;3:111–122.
81. Morgan C. Arthroscopic transglenoid Bankart suture repair. *Oper Tech Orthop* 1991;1:171–179.
82. Hawkins, RB. Arthroscopic stapling repair for shoulder instability: a retrospective study of 50 cases. *Arthroscopy* 1989;5:122–128.
83. O'Driscoll S, Evans D. Long term results of staple capsulorrhaphy for anterior instability of the shoulder. *J Bone Joint Surg Am* 1993;75:249–258.
84. Nobuhara K, Ikeda H. Rotator interval lesion. *Clin Orthop* 1987;223:44–50.
85. Field LD, Warren RF, Obrien SJ, et al. Isolated closure of rotator interval defects for shoulder instability. *Am J Sports Med* 1995;23:557–563.
86. Young DC, Rockwood CA Jr. Complications of failed Bristow procedure and their management. *J Bone Joint Surg Am* 1991;73:969–981.
87. Fronek J, Warren RF, Bowen M. Posterior subluxation of the glenohumeral joint. *J Bone Joint Surg Am* 1989;71:205–216.
88. Ramsey ML, Klimkiewica JJ. Posterior instability: diagnosis and management. In: Iannotti JP, Williams GR Jr. *Disorders of the shoulder: diagnosis and management.* Philadelphia: Lippincott, Williams and Wilkins, 1999:295–319.
89. Neer CS II, Foster CR. Inferior capsular shift for involuntary inferior and multidirectional instability of the shoulder: a preliminary report. *J Bone Joint Surg Am* 1980;62:897–908.
90. Altcheck DW, Warren RF, Skyhar MJ, Ortiz G. T plasty modification of the Bankart procedure for multidirectional instability of the anterior and inferior types. *J Bone Joint Surg Am* 1991;73:105–112.
91. Bigliani LU, Kurzwell PR, Schwartzbach CC, et al. Inferior capsular shift procedure for anterior inferior shoulder instability in athletes. *Am J Sports Med* 1994;22:578–584.
92. Altchek DW, Russell WF, Wickiewicz TL, Ortiz G. Arthroscopic labral debridement: a three-year follow-up study. *Am J Sports Med* 1992;20:702–706.
93. Matsen FA III. Thomas SC, Rockwood CA, Wirth MA. Glenohumeral instability. In: Rockwood CA, Matsen FA III. eds. *The shoulder,* 2nd ed. Philadelphia: WB Saunders, 1998:611–754.
94. Rowe, CR, Zarins B, Ciullo JV. Recurrent anterior dislocation of the shoulder after surgical repair: apparent cause of failure and treatment. *J Bone Joint Surg Am* 1984;66:159–168.
95. Rosenberg BN, Richmond JC, Levine WN. Long term follow up of Bankart reconstruction: incidence of late glenohumeral arthrosis. *Am J Sports Med* 1995;23:538–544.
96. Guanche CA, Quick DC, Sodergren K, et al. Arthroscopy vs. open reconstruction of the shoulder in patients with isolated Bankart lesions. *Am J Sports Med* 1996;24:144–148.
97. Pagnani MJ, Warren RF, Altcheck DW, et al. Athroscopic shoulder stabilization using transglenoid sutures: a four year minimum follow up. *Am J Sports Med* 1996;24:459–567.
98. Snyder SJ, Stafford BB. Arthroscopic management of instability of the shoulder. *Orthopedics* 1993;16:993–1002.
99. May VR Jr. A modified Bristow operation for recurrent anterior dislocation of the shoulder. *J Bone Joint Surg Am* 1970;52:1010–1016.

100. Emig EW, Schweitzer ME, Karasick D, Lubowitz J. Adhesive capsulitis of the shoulder: MR diagnosis. *AJR* 1994;164: 1457–1459.
101. Neumann CH, Peterson SA, Jahnke AH, et al. MR. in the evaluation of patients with suspected instability of the shoulder joint including CT arthrography. *Fortschr Roentgenstr* 1991:154: 593–600.
102. Tirman PFJ, Stauffer AE, Crues JV, et al. Saline magnetic resonance arthrography in the evaluation of glenohumeral instability. *Arthroscopy* 1993; 9:550–559.
103. Daumas JL, Padovani B, Rafelli C, et al. Compression du nerf sus-scapulaire dans le défile spinoglenoidien par un kyste synovial. *J Radiol* 1995;76:25–28.
104. Tirman PF, Feller JF, Janzen DL, et al. Association of glenoid labral cysts and tears and glenohumeral instability: radiological findings and clinical significance. *Radiology* 1994;190:653–658.

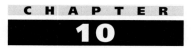

MAGNETIC RESONANCE ARTHROGRAPHY OF THE SHOULDER

WILLIAM E. PALMER

In magnetic resonance (MR) imaging of the shoulder, diagnostic success requires the delineation of complex anatomic structures and the demonstration of subtle abnormalities. MR arthrography extends the capabilities of conventional MR imaging because contrast solution separates intraarticular structures and outlines abnormalities.

There are several major contributions of MR arthrography. In assessment of the rotator cuff, for example, arthrographic MR images enable the accurate differentiation between full- and partial-thickness tears, as well as the ability to determine tendon quality. In shoulders with suspected glenohumeral instability, arthrographic MR images demonstrate nondisplaced labral tears and their locations relative to the origins of glenohumeral ligaments.

MR arthrography exploits the natural advantages gained from joint effusion. In conventional MR imaging, it is known that intraarticular structures and abnormalities are better delineated in shoulders with effusions (1–4). Joint fluid distends the capsule, separates glenohumeral ligaments from the labrum, outlines the cuff tendon, and fills tears. Without a joint effusion, signal differences between intraarticular structures may be insufficient to allow the differentiation of normal and abnormal findings.

Either saline or gadolinium can be injected as the arthrographic MR contrast material, but the majority of authors have chosen to investigate the role of gadolinium (5–12). Saline has diagnostic disadvantages compared to gadolinium and does not overcome several major shortcomings encountered in conventional MR imaging. Injected saline has the identical signal characteristics as a subacromial-subdeltoid bursal effusion. Thus, despite the leak of saline across the cuff tendon, it still may not be possible to differentiate a partial- from a full-thickness tear.

Intravenous administration of gadolinium also has been investigated as an alternative to direct intraarticular injection (13). Intravascular contrast material leaks from the capillary bed into the interstitial space and diffuses from the synovium into the glenohumeral joint. The rate of diffusion is increased in joints that are inflamed (e.g., rheumatoid arthritis) or exercised vigorously following injection. Thus, intravenous technique can produce an arthrographic effect, depending on the degree of joint enhancement. Unfortunately, indirect MR arthrography does not achieve the most important benefits of intraarticular injection, because the capsule does not become distended. The enhancement of vascularized structures may create other diagnostic problems. Enhancing synovium in the subacromial-subdeltoid bursa, for example, may simulate the extraarticular leak of contrast solution and lead to the false-positive diagnosis of rotator cuff tear.

Several factors have slowed the widespread utilization of MR arthrography in radiological practices. The procedure converts MR imaging from a noninvasive examination into a mildly invasive one, exposing patients to ionizing radiation as well as the risk of intraarticular needle placement. The study requires the coordination of scheduling in two procedure rooms and becomes impractical if the fluoroscopy suite is too distant from the MR scanner. Many radiologists have felt obliged to obtain approval from an institutional review board because gadolinium contrast agents have not been approved by the Food and Drug Administration for intraarticular injection. Finally, the test is more expensive than either arthrography or MR imaging by itself. As economic forces increasingly dominate patient care and dictate choices in diagnostic testing, MR arthrography must be proven to be cost-effective in the clinical management of patients and in the outcome of treatments.

MR ARTHROGRAPHIC TECHNIQUE
Gadolinium Arthrography

The T1 relaxation time of contrast solution is dependent on the concentration of gadolinium (14). To optimize the paramagnetic effect on T1-weighted images, gadolinium formulations currently marketed by pharmaceutical companies must be diluted to a concentration of 2 mmol/L (15). To obtain this concentration, 0.8 ml of gadopentetate dimeglumine (Magnevist; Berlex Laboratories, Wayne, NJ) is added to 100 ml of normal saline. Ten milliliters of this solution is mixed with 5 ml of 60% iodinated contrast material, 5 ml of lidocaine 1%, and a drop of epinephrine 1:1,000 (final dilution ratio equals 1:250). Following aspiration of joint effusion (to avoid excessive dilution of gadolinium), contrast solution is injected until the joint capsule becomes distended (approximately 12 cc in the shoulder). Single contrast technique is necessary to avoid magnetic susceptibility artifact from intraarticular gas. Iodinated contrast material enables the fluoroscopic confirmation of intraarticular needle placement and the acquisition of standard pre- and post-exercise arthrographic spot films.

MR Imaging

MR imaging is initiated within 30 minutes following arthrography to minimize the absorption of contrast solution and the loss of capsular distension. The same dedicated coils and imaging planes are used in both arthrographic and conventional MR imaging. The arm is positioned in mild external rotation by elevating the patient's elbow close to the torso. In MR arthrography, the field of view often can be decreased since the examination is not directed at the visualization of extraarticular abnormalities.

T1-weighted spin echo pulse sequences, with or without fat suppression, maximize the signal intensity from contrast solution. They generate high signal-to-noise ratio, excellent spatial resolution, and contiguous slices (interleaved acquisition) within relatively short examination times. A T2-weighted sequence is helpful in the identification of extraarticular fluid collections, such as glenoid labral cysts, and the characterization of incidental bone marrow lesions or periarticular masses. Using fast spin echo technique, T2-weighted images can be obtained in a short time.

Fat suppression is critical in MR arthrography. Diagnostic difficulty may arise because fat and gadolinium have similar signal intensities on T1-weighted images. In high field systems, frequency-selective fat suppression utilizes the difference (chemical shift) in the precessional frequencies of fat and water by applying a presaturation pulse that is identical to the precessional frequency of fat. Mid- and low-field systems can achieve fat suppression by using phase shift techniques that create separate sets of water and fat images. Because the signal from fat is decreased and the signal from contrast solution is preserved, fat-suppressed images delineate the boundary between contrast solution and fat and accurately demonstrate extraarticular contrast material. However, fat-suppressed images cannot completely replace standard T1-weighted images because they obscure juxtaarticular structures and marrow abnormalities. As in conventional MR imaging, the final pulse sequence choices depend on radiologist preference and MR system capabilities.

Arthrographic MR Pitfalls

Diagnostic difficulty can result from extraarticular injection or leak of contrast material. If contrast solution passes out of the joint through a needle track, for example, it can spread along fascial planes into the subacromial-subdeltoid space, creating a bursogram that can be mistaken for a full-thickness rotator cuff tear. The likelihood of extraarticular leak is decreased by injecting less than 15 ml into the joint. Extraarticular injection of contrast can mimic partial tears of the subscapularis tendon or the inferior glenohumeral ligament.

Inadvertent injection of gas into the joint may lead to the false-positive diagnosis of intraarticular loose bodies. Gas bubbles, however, will elevate to nondependent regions of the joint, whereas loose bodies will gravitate to dependent locations.

Image degradation occurs if the injected gadolinium is too concentrated or diluted. The use of full-strength gadolinium results in marked T1 and T2 shortening, and nearly absent signal intensity from the intraarticular fluid. If the contrast solution is injected into a large effusion, the gadolinium becomes diluted, decreasing its signal intensity. The signal from a gadolinium solution also depends on the magnet's field strength. On low-field systems, the optimal concentration of gadolinium is greater than on high-field systems.

MR ARTHROGRAPHY OF THE ROTATOR CUFF

In the patient with suspected rotator cuff disorder, the decision to perform MR arthrography depends on the clinical need to identify and distinguish partial cuff tears from small complete tears. It also depends on the importance of preoperative assessment of the size and location of a cuff tear or the quality of the retracted tendon margin. In older patients in whom surgery would only be performed to repair a complete cuff tear, conventional MR images are sufficient to differentiate torn, retracted tendons from normal tendons. Single- or double-contrast arthrography is accurate, safe, and cost-effective. In athletes and younger patients in whom surgery would be performed to repair partial cuff tears and remove bony abnormalities of the coracoacromial arch, MR arthrography can maximize anatomic resolution and diagnostic confidence.

On conventional MR images, nonspecific diagnostic criteria permit subjectivity in the interpretation of images. Partial- and full-thickness cuff tears may demonstrate identical appearances. Partial-thickness tear may be confused with tendinopathy (inflammation or degeneration), normal anatomic variation (interposed muscle slips), or MR imaging artifact (magic angle phenomenon, volume averaging). The majority of these diagnostic problems can be resolved using MR arthrography.

Both conventional and arthrographic MR images can demonstrate the uniform thickness and hypointensity of a

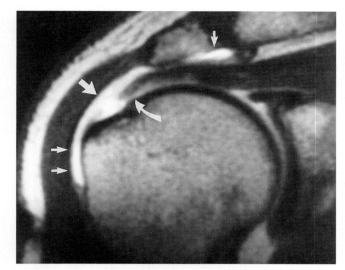

FIGURE 10.1. Small full-thickness rotator cuff tear proved surgically in a 48-year-old patient. On a T1-weighted (450/18) coronal oblique arthrographic MR image, contrast solution extends through a full-thickness cuff tear (*thick straight arrow*) and fills the subacromial-subdeltoid bursa (*thin straight arrows*). The distal supraspinatus tendon (*curved arrow*) is retracted from its attachment site on the greater tuberosity.

the inferior cuff surface, fills partial cuff tears, and, in complete tears, leaks from the glenohumeral joint into the subacromial-subdeltoid space (5–7). If contrast solution leaks into the subacromial-subdeltoid space, the diagnosis of full-thickness cuff tear is confirmed (figs. 10.1–10.4). Thus, the presence or absence of extraarticular contrast solution distinguishes partial and complete cuff tears. The sensitivity and specificity of arthrographic MR images in the diagnosis of full-thickness tear are comparable to those of conventional arthrography (i.e., approach 100%).

Both the anteroposterior dimension of tears and their degree of retraction can be accurately measured on arthrographic MR images. Full-thickness cuff tears usually begin anteriorly at the critical zone of the supraspinatus tendon and propagate posteriorly into the infraspinatus tendon (Figs. 10.2, 10.3). This predictable pattern of propagation explains why larger tears always show a greater degree of tendon retraction anteriorly than posteriorly. To identify the location of the smallest cuff tears, it is necessary to visualize the most anterior attachment site of the supraspinatus tendon on the greater tuberosity. This region should be inspected on axial and sagittal oblique images, since it can be difficult to assess on coronal oblique images when the shoulder is positioned in excessive internal rotation. Vertical cuff tears are relatively uncommon and difficult to diagnose on conventional MR images because they represent a longitudinal split in the tendon. Since vertical tears parallel the cuff fibers, there is no tendon retraction. Arthrographic MR images can

normal cuff tendon or the retracted margin of a large cuff tear. In both examinations, subacromial-subdeltoid fat or fluid delineates the bursal surface of the tendon. On arthrographic MR images, intraarticular contrast solution outlines

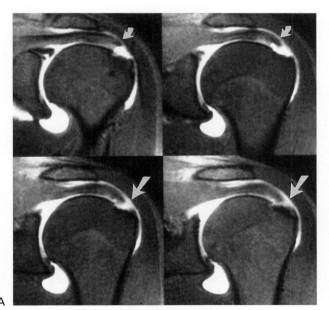

A

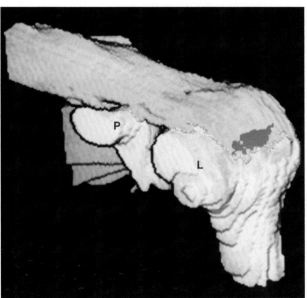

B

FIGURE 10.2. Full-thickness rotator cuff tear, with posterior propagation and tapering, repaired surgically in a 52-year-old patient. **A:** Following arthrography, sequential T1-weighted (450/18) coronal oblique arthrographic MR images with fat suppression show retraction of the anterior supraspinatus tendon (*curved arrows*). More posteriorly, the tear (*slanted arrows*) tapers in width. **B:** The 3D image in the same patient simulates the expected appearance of the cuff tear (*blue*) at surgery. Typical for most tendon tears, anteroposterior propagation results in retraction anteriorly and tapering posteriorly. P, coracoid process; L, lesser tuberosity.

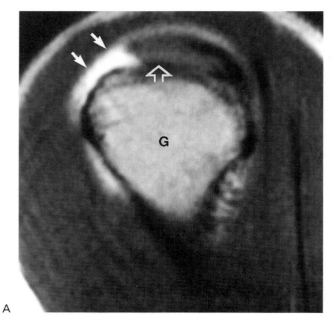

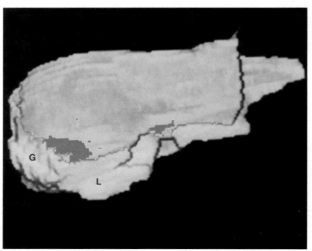

A   B

FIGURE 10.3. Small rotator cuff tear repaired arthroscopically. **A:** A T1-weighted (450/18) sagittal oblique arthrographic MR image through the greater tuberosity (*G*) shows contrast solution defining the exact location and size of the cuff tear (*closed arrows*). Tendon thickening and increased signal intensity (*open arrow*) indicate tendinosis and contrast imbibition in the adjacent cuff, where tear propagation would be expected. **B:** The 3D image in the same patient depicts the usual anterior location of a rotator cuff tear (*blue*). G, greater tuberosity; L, lesser tuberosity.

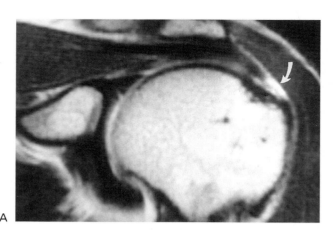

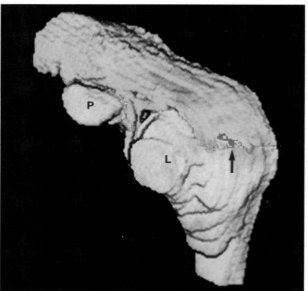

A   B

FIGURE 10.4. Small, vertical rotator cuff tear repaired at arthroscopy. **A:** A T1-weighted (450/18) coronal oblique arthrographic MR image through the midsupraspinatus tendon demonstrates contrast solution (*arrow*) crossing a full-thickness defect in the cuff tendon. Adjacent coronal oblique images showed normal tendon, suggesting vertical orientation of the tear. **B:** The 3D image in the same patient depicts the vertical tear location (*arrow*) posterior to the anterior attachment site of the cuff on the greater tuberosity. P, coracoid process; L, lesser tuberosity.

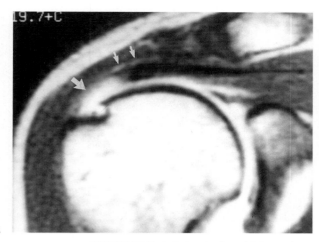 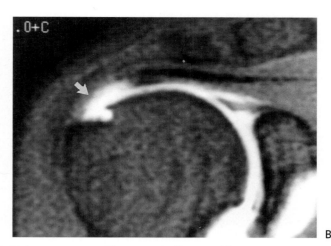

FIGURE 10.5. Inferior surface, high-grade partial-thickness rotator cuff tear surgically proved in 64-year-old patient. **A:** On a T1-weighted (450/18) coronal oblique arthrographic MR image without fat suppression, contrast solution (*large arrow*) appears to cross the entire cuff tendon. Linear high signal intensity in the subacromial-subdeltoid space (*small arrows*) could represent fat or contrast solution. **B:** On a corresponding fat-suppressed image, contrast (*arrow*) remains contained within the supraspinatus tendon, confirming the diagnosis of a high-grade partial-thickness cuff tear.

demonstrate their locations (Fig. 10.4), which are more variable compared with the anterior positions of classical horizontal tears.

Arthrographic MR images are particularly well suited to the diagnosis of partial-thickness tears, since they usually begin at the articular (inferior) surface of the supraspinatus tendon (Figs. 10.5, 10.6). In this location, high-signal contrast solution can fill focal cuff defects. Whenever partial-thickness tears involve the superior (bursal) surface or the interstitium of the tendon, they do not fill with contrast material and, therefore, may be overlooked on T1-weighted arthrographic images. For this reason, the arthrographic MR protocol should include T2-weighted images, which can reveal extraarticular bursal collections or fluid disrupting cuff fibers (Fig. 10.7).

Diagnostic accuracy is increased when fat-suppressed images are acquired (7). Partial- and full-thickness cuff tears may not be distinguishable on standard T1-weighted images

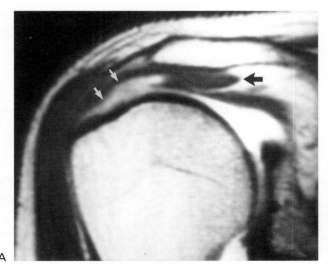 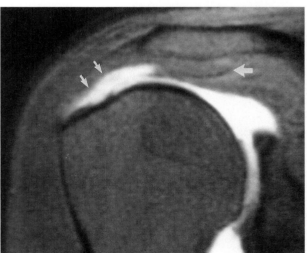

FIGURE 10.6. Large partial-thickness rotator cuff tear proved surgically in a 50-year-old patient. **A:** At the junction of supra- and infraspinatus tendons, a T1-weighted (450/18) coronal oblique arthrographic MR image shows contrast solution filling a large tendon defect (*white arrows*). Low-signal material is present in the subacromial space (*black arrow*). **B:** On corresponding fat-suppressed image, contrast solution (*thin arrows*) is confined to the cuff tendon. The bursal region remains low in signal intensity (*thick arrow*).

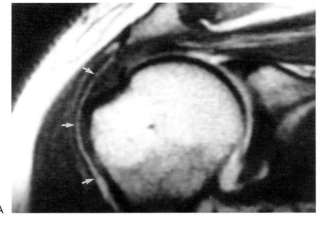

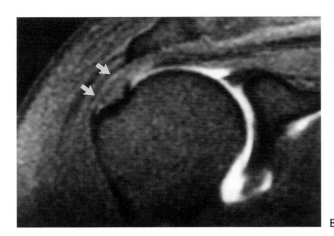

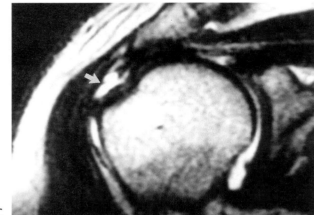

FIGURE 10.7. Large superior surface partial-thickness rotator cuff tear in a 48-year-old patient. **A:** A T1-weighted (450/18) coronal oblique arthrographic MR image without fat suppression demonstrates minimal thickening of distal supraspinatus tendon. The subdeltoid fat plane (*arrows*) appears intact. **B:** The corresponding fat-suppressed image shows normal contour of the inferior tendon surface. No contrast is present in the subdeltoid bursa (*arrows*). **C:** At the same slice location, a T2-weighted image shows focal fluid at the superior tendon surface (*arrow*). A large bursal sided partial-thickness cuff tear was surgically repaired.

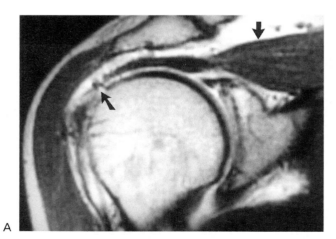

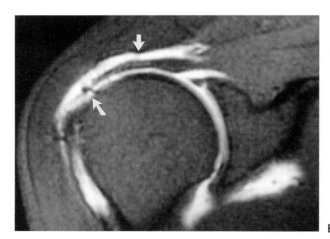

FIGURE 10.8. Recurrent supraspinatus tear following rotator cuff repair in a 56-year-old patient with pain and decreased strength. **A:** On a T1-weighted (450/18) coronal oblique arthrographic MR image without fat suppression, susceptibility artifact (*slanted arrow*) is present in the region of the tendon repair. The distal cuff tendon is attenuated, but the supraspinatus muscle remains normal in size without fatty replacement (*straight arrow*). **B:** On the corresponding fat-suppressed image, contrast leaks into the subacromial-subdeltoid space (*straight arrow*) and appears to cross the tendon in the region of susceptibility artifact (*slanted arrow*).

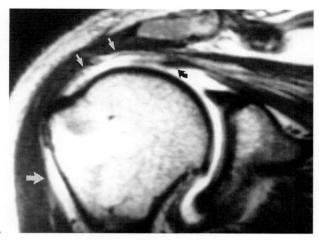
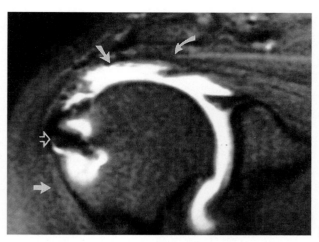

A

B

FIGURE 10.9. MR arthrogram in 45-year-old patient with recurrent full-thickness rotator cuff tear following surgical repair. **A:** On a T1-weighted (450/18) coronal oblique arthrographic MR image without fat suppression, contrast solution fills a large defect (*small white arrows*) in the supraspinatus tendon (*black arrow*), which appears retracted to the level of the acromion. The subdeltoid high signal (*large white arrow*) could represent fat or contrast solution. **B:** On the corresponding fat-suppressed image, contrast solution remains contained (*slanted arrow*). Lack of contrast leak into the subacromial-subdeltoid bursa (*straight arrow*) may lead to an underestimation of the extent of a rotator cuff defect. At surgery, the retracted tendon (*curved arrow*) was difficult to mobilize due to severe scarring in the subacromial-subdeltoid bursa. Scar tissue prevented the free flow of contrast into the subacromial-subdeltoid bursa and therefore resulted in underestimating the extent of the cuff tear at arthrographic MR diagnosis. Susceptibility artifact (*open arrow*) from prior surgery is seen at the greater tuberosity.

because fat and gadolinium have similar signal intensities (6,7). The greatest diagnostic difficulty occurs whenever cuff tendons show contrast solution that extends to the bursal surface, but not definitely through it (Figs. 10.5, 10.6). On fat-suppressed T1-weighted images, the signal from contrast solution is unchanged, whereas the signal from normal fat is selectively decreased. Thus, persistent high signal intensity in the subacromial-subdeltoid space indicates a full-thickness cuff tear, whereas low signal intensity indicates a partial-thickness tear. This benefit is valuable in the assessment of the postoperative cuff, although severe scarring in the subacromial-subdeltoid space can prevent the free flow of contrast solution despite the presence of recurrent tear (Figs. 10.8, 10.9). Fat suppression also improves diagnostic accuracy in the detection of small partial-thickness tears whenever they are located at the inferior cuff surface (7). Whereas focal collections of contrast solution indicate actual disruptions of tendon fibers, mild irregularities in tendon contour and signal intensity indicate fraying of inferior surface fibers.

Arthrographic MR images show anatomic features that are useful in the prediction of cuff repairability and postoperative prognosis. They depict the location and size of the cuff tear, the degree of tendon retraction, and the contour of the torn tendon margin (Figs. 10.10, 10.11). This information adds value to the diagnostic report and may influence preoperative planning. For example, the surgeon may elect to perform an open procedure rather than an arthroscopic repair, depending on the size of the cuff tear.

Decreased quality of tendon tissue has been correlated with the presence of imbibition (7). Tendons that imbibe contrast solution have increased signal intensity on fat-suppressed T1-weighted images, indicating the diffusion of gadolinium into the substance of tendon (Figs. 10.12–10.14). At surgery, these tendons are swollen and friable

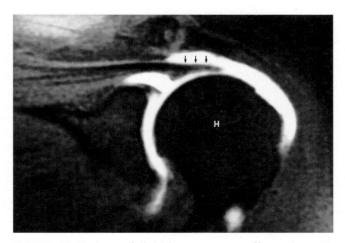

FIGURE 10.10. Large full-thickness rotator cuff tear in a 63-year-old patient. The fat-suppressed T1-weighted (450/18) coronal oblique arthrographic MR image shows contrast solution crossing a large retracted tear of supraspinatus tendon. The tendon margin (*arrows*) is low in signal intensity and sharp in contour, corresponding with adequate tendon substance for surgical repair. H, humeral head.

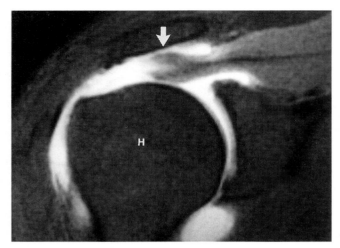

FIGURE 10.11. Large full-thickness rotator cuff tear in a 57-year-old patient. On a fat-suppressed T1-weighted (450/18) coronal oblique arthrographic MR image, the retracted supraspinatus tendon (*arrow*) shows thickening and an irregular contour. At surgery, the tendon was soft and frayed, requiring debridement. H, humeral head.

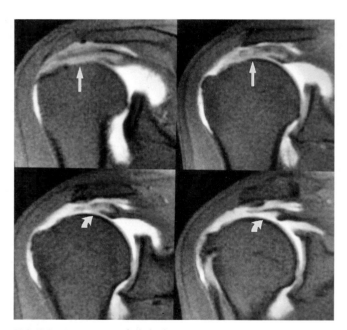

FIGURE 10.12. Large full-thickness rotator cuff tear and imbibition in a 56-year-old patient. Contiguous fat-suppressed T1-weighted (450/18) coronal oblique arthrographic MR images demonstrate large full-thickness cuff tear. The anterior cuff tendon (*curved arrows*) is retracted to the level of the acromion. The posterior cuff tendon (*straight arrows*) is thickened and increased in signal intensity, indicating imbibition of contrast into its substance. At open cuff repair, the infraspinatus tendon required extensive surgical debridement

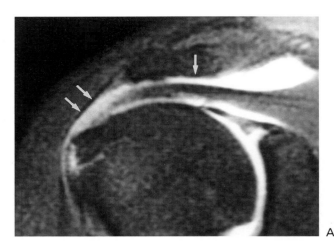

A

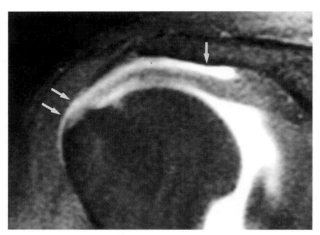

B

FIGURE 10.13. Severe tendinosis resulting in full-thickness diffusion of contrast solution in a 52-year-old patient. **A:** On a T1-weighted (450/18) coronal oblique arthrographic MR image with fat suppression, the anterior cuff tendon shows attenuation and increased signal intensity (imbibition). Contrast solution has diffused across the tendon into the subacromial-subdeltoid space (*arrows*). **B:** More posteriorly, the infraspinatus tendon also shows thinning and contrast imbibition, with contrast solution extending through it, into the subacromial-subdeltoid space (*arrows*). During open surgical repair, the entire cuff tendon was boggy and friable but remained attached to the greater tuberosity.

due to severe inflammation or degeneration. They require debridement to expose adequate tissue for suturing, increasing the technical difficulty of cuff repair and decreasing the likelihood for operative success. Imbibition usually involves the torn tendon along its retracted margin, which can be thickened or attenuated. Imbibition may also extend posterior to the cuff tear, involving a tendon that remains intact on the greater tuberosity. In this case, imbibition is located between the completely torn and completely normal segment of rotator cuff, and it represents the transition zone of an abnormal tendon that is at imminent risk for posterior tear propagation.

In severe tendinosis, imbibition may occur without a focal cuff defect (Figs. 10.13, 10.14). In rare cases, contrast may diffuse across the full tendon thickness, leaking into the subacromial-subdeltoid space and simulating a complete cuff tear. At surgery, these tendons are diffusely boggy but attached to the greater tuberosity. The cuff surfaces are frayed but intact.

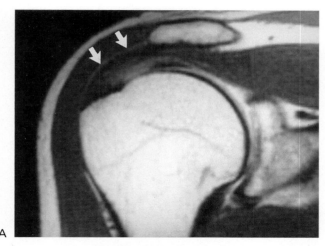
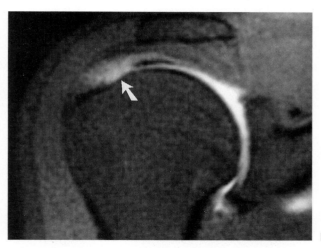

A   B

FIGURE 10.14. Rotator cuff imbibition identified on fat-suppressed images in a 53-year-old patient. **A:** On a T1-weighted (450/18) coronal oblique arthrographic MR image without fat suppression, the distal supraspinatus tendon (*arrows*) appears thickened. Mildly increased signal intensity could represent tendinosis or magic angle artifact. **B:** On a corresponding fat-suppressed image, an amorphous region of increased signal indicates diffusion of contrast solution into the tendon from the inferior cuff surface (*arrow*). At arthroscopy, undersurface fraying was present without an arthroscopically evident partial-thickness cuff tear.

MR ARTHROGRAPHY OF THE GLENOID LABRUM

Conventional MR imaging has been used with mixed results to evaluate the glenoid labrum. Anterior labral lesions have been diagnosed with sensitivities ranging from 44% to 95% and specificities ranging from 67% to 86% (1–4,16). Diagnostic confidence is limited by the normal variability in labral size and shape, and by the difficulty in distinguishing tears of the labrum from pseudotears caused by either articular cartilage that undercuts the labral fibrocartilage or glenohumeral ligaments that pass close to the glenoid rim (17). Unless a joint effusion is present, the inferior glenohumeral ligament and its origin from the glenoid labrum are collapsed against the glenoid rim and cannot be followed into the axillary pouch.

On arthrographic MR images, the majority of anatomic variations are easily differentiated from labral abnormalities. Investigators have reported diagnostic sensitivities and specificities ranging from 90% to 95% (8–11). Articular cartilage that undercuts the labral fibrocartilage is rarely a source of diagnostic difficulty because the cartilage is lower in signal intensity than the contrast solution. Whereas cartilage shows uniform thickness, sublabral contrast in a tear shows variable width. Normal glenohumeral ligaments are distinguished from torn labra because the ligaments can be followed away from the glenoid rim until they merge with the distended capsule. In contrast, torn labral fragments can be followed back to the glenoid rim on sequential arthrographic MR images.

Some anatomic variations continue to create diagnostic problems on arthrographic MR images. Morphological criteria may not be sufficient to distinguish a small, normal labrum from a blunted, deficient labrum. Normal sublabral sulci can mimic tears because they occur at the interface of the labrum with the articular cartilage and become filled with contrast solution (9,18). Occasionally, the labrum can be completely detached (sublabral hole or foramen). As normal sulci increase in size with aging, the labrum becomes progressively separated from the glenoid rim, mimicking a displaced labral fragment. These variations in the appearances of sulci lead to both false-negative and false-positive diagnoses. The most common locations of sulci include the superior labrum at its junction with the bicipital tendon, and the anterosuperior labrum between the origins of middle and inferior glenohumeral ligaments (Fig. 10.15). Since sublabral sulci are not present in all shoulders, they further cause diagnostic confusion.

Labral-Ligamentous Complex

One of the major advantages of MR arthrography is visualization of the labral-ligamentous complex, which consists of the glenoid labrum in combination with the superior, middle, and inferior glenohumeral ligaments. The glenohumeral ligaments reinforce the joint capsule and function as a unit with the glenoid labrum, which anchors the ligaments to the glenoid rim (9,10,19,20).

On arthrographic MR images, the glenohumeral ligaments can be identified in three imaging planes (21). The superior and middle glenohumeral ligaments have conjoined origins from the labrum immediately anterior to the labral-bicipital junction. The superior glenohumeral ligament courses anteriorly (parallel to the coracoid process) and merges with the coracohumeral ligament in the rotator interval. The middle

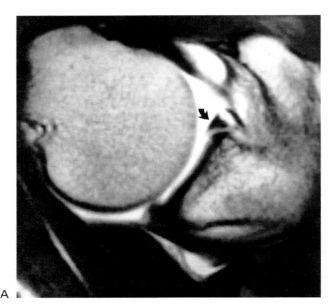

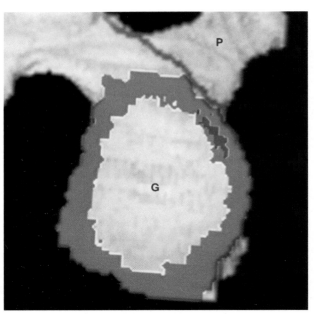

FIGURE 10.15. Normal anterosuperior sublabral sulcus in a 26-year-old patient. **A:** Following arthrography, a T1-weighted (TR:450, TE:18) axial image shows linear contrast underlying the anterior glenoid labrum (*arrow*). Normal anterosuperior sulci usually occur between the origins of the middle and inferior glenohumeral ligaments. **B:** On a 3D image in the same patient, sublabral contrast (*red*) shows the typical location of a normal sublabral sulcus. During arthroscopic repair of rotator cuff tear, the labrum (*blue*) was proven to be normal. G, glenoid fossa; P, coracoid process.

glenohumeral ligament passes caudally, adjacent to the glenoid rim, and merges with the subscapularis tendon before inserting onto the lesser tuberosity. The middle glenohumeral ligament shows normal variations in size from threadlike to cordlike. There tends to be an inverse relationship between the sizes of the middle glenohumeral ligament and the adjacent anterior labrum: the larger the ligament, the smaller the labrum. When the ligament is cordlike, for example, the labrum can be completely absent (Buford complex) (22). The location of the middle glenohumeral ligament depends on shoulder positioning (11). The ligament lies medial to the anterior glenoid rim when the shoulder is internally rotated, and it moves lateral to the glenoid rim when the shoulder is externally rotated.

The inferior glenohumeral ligament has three components (anterior band, posterior band, and intervening axillary pouch), but the anterior band has greatest functional significance because of its role in maintaining passive anterior stability of the shoulder (19,20). In shoulder adduction (the usual scanning position), the anterior band is lax as it courses caudally from the anteroinferior labrum to its insertion on the anatomic neck of the humerus. The inferior glenohumeral ligament is usually thicker than either the superior or middle glenohumeral ligaments and has a broader-based glenolabral origin. It arises from a 1- to 2-cm segment of labrum at approximately 4 to 6 o'clock on the anteroinferior glenoid rim (9,11).

Glenohumeral Instability

Anterior glenohumeral instability causes significant morbidity in young patients, particularly athletes, and often requires surgical reconstruction to restore shoulder function. The clinical spectrum of instability ranges from obvious recurrent dislocations to equivocal symptoms that may mimic other shoulder disorders, such as rotator cuff tear and biceps tendon dislocation. In patients with inconclusive clinical evaluations, imaging studies are commonly used to guide preoperative planning and to select appropriate therapy.

By demonstrating the inferior labral-ligamentous complex, MR arthrography makes a major contribution to the evaluation of patients with suspected glenohumeral instability. The anterior band of the inferior glenohumeral ligament is critical in maintaining passive anterior stability of the shoulder and functions as a unit with the glenoid labrum, which anchors the ligament to the glenoid rim (19,20). The origin of the inferior glenohumeral ligament creates a stress point on the labrum. During shoulder dislocation or abduction-external rotation, tension is transmitted through the inferior glenohumeral ligament to the labral attachment site. Excessive tension can avulse the labrum from the glenoid rim, rendering the ligament incompetent. Thus, the inferior glenohumeral ligament can appear normal but lose its stabilizing function if its labral anchor is partially or completely detached. Rupture of the inferior GHL is a much less com-

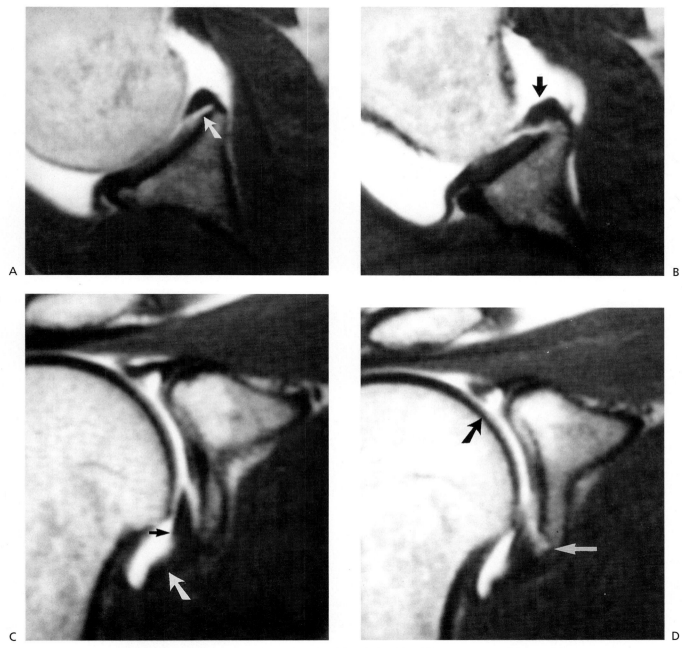

FIGURE 10.16. Twenty-eight-year-old male with inferior labral-ligamentous avulsion and anterior instability proved at arthroscopy. **A:** A T1-weighted (450/18) axial arthrographic MR image through inferior glenoid fossa shows contrast solution filling anterior labral tear (*arrow*). **B:** On a more caudal image, the torn labral fragment (*arrow*) is displaced from the glenoid rim. **C:** On a T1-weighted (450/18) coronal oblique arthrographic MR image, the inferior glenohumeral ligament (*white arrow*) attaches to the labrum (*black arrow*), which is separated from the glenoid rim. **D:** On a more posterior coronal oblique image, the inferior labral tear extends under the capsule (*white arrow*), which is stripped medially on the glenoid neck. The tear extended into the superior labrum (*black arrow*).

mon cause of anterior instability than avulsion of the glenolabral attachment site (11).

This functional anatomy of the inferior labral-ligamentous complex enables a biomechanical approach to the diagnosis of anterior shoulder instability. Specific arthrographic MR criteria can be used in the differentiation of stable and unstable shoulders because these images can show the location and length of labral abnormalities relative to the origin of the inferior glenohumeral ligament (Figs. 10.16, 10.17). If the torn labral segment extends into the attachment site of

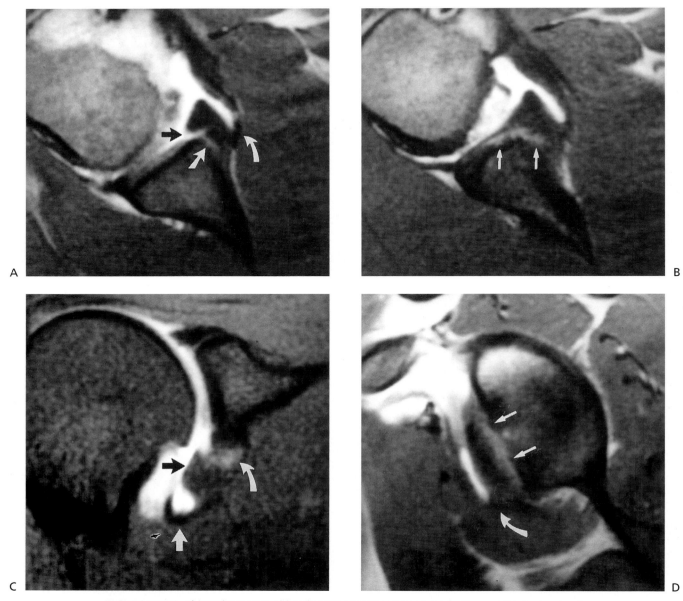

FIGURE 10.17. Thirty-three-year-old male with anterior glenoid rim fracture and anterior shoulder instability proved at arthroscopy. **A:** Following arthrography, a T1-weighted (450/18) axial image through the inferior glenoid fossa shows contrast solution (*black arrow*) filling a labral tear. Contrast also passes into a fracture (*slanted white arrow*) of the anterior glenoid rim. The anterior capsule inserts normally at the base of the osseous fragment (*curved white arrow*). **B:** On a more caudal axial image, contrast solution (*arrows*) fills both the inferior labral tear and anteroinferior glenoid rim fracture. **C:** On a fat-suppressed T1-weighted (450/18) coronal oblique image, the inferior glenohumeral ligament (*straight white arrow*) attaches to the displaced osteochondral fragment (*black arrow*). Contrast solution fills the fracture plane (*curved white arrow*). **D:** A T1-weighted (450/18) sagittal oblique image shows the fracture (*straight arrows*) filled with contrast solution and the attachment site of the inferior glenohumeral ligament (*curved arrow*) on the displaced glenoid rim fragment.

the inferior glenohumeral ligament, there is a high likelihood of anterior instability (9,11). This information may guide the orthopedic surgeon in preoperative planning and in the selection of appropriate surgical or conservative treatments. Rarely, patients develop trauma-related instability due to ligamentous stretching and laxity without an associated labral tear. MR arthrography is less valuable in these cases because the entire inferior labral-ligamentous complex appears intact. Currently, no accurate MR imaging criteria are recognized in the diagnosis of capsular laxity.

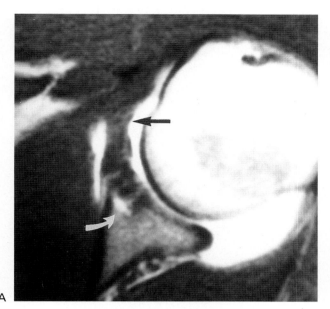 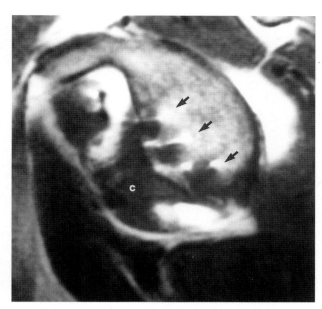

A

B

FIGURE 10.18. Normal arthrographic MR appearance of anterior capsular repair in a 23-year-old patient with persistent shoulder pain. **A:** A T1-weighted (450/18) axial arthrographic MR image shows thickening of the anterior capsule (*black arrow*). The capsule is attached to the glenoid rim adjacent to artifact from a metallic anchor (*white arrow*). **B:** On a T1-weighted (450/18) sagittal oblique arthrographic MR image, the thickened capsule (*c*) shows continuity between glenoid rim and subscapularis tendon. Three metallic anchors (*arrows*) create artifact along the antero-inferior glenoid rim.

Capsular insertion sites have been used to evaluate joint stability (1,2). Type I capsule arises from the glenoid labrum, Type II arises from the scapular neck within 1 cm of the labral base, and Type III arises from the scapular neck more than 1 cm medial to the labral base. MR arthrography of the shoulder has helped to shift diagnostic emphasis onto the labral-ligamentous complex and away from the capsular insertion site. Appearances of the capsular insertion site are markedly variable in individuals and are heavily dependent on both the position of the shoulder (e.g., internal vs. external rotation) as well as the degree of capsular distension due to effusion or injected contrast solution. The three types of capsular insertions represent normal variations in the size, morphology, and location of the subscapularis recess. Since the incidences of capsular insertion types are statistically similar in stable and unstable shoulders, Type III capsular insertion cannot be used to predict anterior glenohumeral instability (9). Following anterior stabilization procedure, however, it is most important to assess the integrity of the capsular reconstruction site, since the inferior labral-ligamentous complex has been surgically distorted. (Figs. 10.18, 10.19)

The lexicon of glenohumeral instability has evolved into a complex collection of eponyms that refer to closely related abnormalities of the inferior labral-ligamentous complex (Figs. 10.20–10.22) (23). *Bankart lesion* generally refers to a complete labral tear at the origin of the inferior glenohumeral ligament, resulting in disruption of the scapular periosteum and detachment of the labrum from the glenoid rim. *Partial Bankart lesion* is sometimes used to describe an incomplete labral tear in the same location. *Osseous Bankart lesion* indicates an osteochondral fracture of the glenoid rim at the inferior labral-ligamentous attachment site (Fig. 10.17).

Perthes lesion also refers to labral detachment from the glenoid rim, but the inferior labral-ligamentous complex remains attached to the scapular periosteum, which is stripped medially on the glenoid neck. If the Perthes lesion is nondisplaced, the tear may become synovialized or filled with granulation tissue, preventing the sublabral leak of contrast solution and leading to the false-negative diagnosis of labral tear. Although the Perthes lesion can appear deceptively normal on arthrographic MR images, the shoulder remains susceptible to anterior subluxation and recurrent instability.

Anterior labral-ligamentous periosteal sleeve avulsion (ALPSA) is similar to the Perthes lesion, except the inferior labral-ligamentous complex becomes bunched and retracted medially, similar to a rolled-up sleeve. Thus, the labrum is permanently displaced from the glenoid rim in the ALPSA lesion, but it may reapproximate its normal position in the Perthes lesion. *Glenolabral articular disruption* (GLAD) refers to a partial anteroinferior labral tear that is associated with an adjacent articular cartilage defect involving the glenoid fossa. The GLAD lesion may not always be associated with anterior instability but may progress to rapid joint degenerative with intraarticular loose bodies. Loose bodies may also result from cartilage defects involving the humeral head (Fig. 10.23). *Humeral avulsion of the glenohumeral*

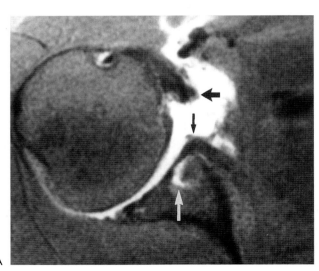

A

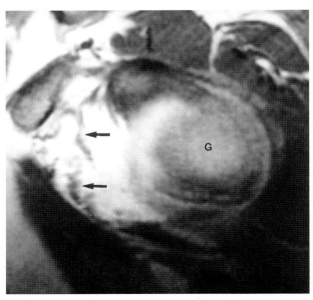

B

FIGURE 10.19. Recurrent anterior instability and capsular rupture following Bankart repair in a 32-year-old patient. **A:** On a fat-suppressed T1-weighted (450/18) axial arthrographic MR image, there is discontinuity of the subscapularis tendon (*thick black arrow*). Contrast solution leaks into the anterior soft tissues. At the site of artifact due to metallic anchor (*white arrow*), the anterior glenoid rim demonstrates labral deficiency (*thin black arrow*). **B:** At level of the glenohumeral joint (*G*), a T1-weighted (450/18) sagittal oblique arthrographic MR image shows discontinuity and marked attenuation of anterior capsular ligaments (*arrows*). The subscapularis tendon is not visualized due to rupture with retraction.

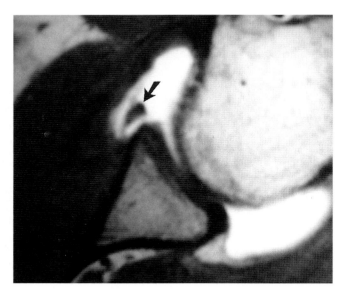

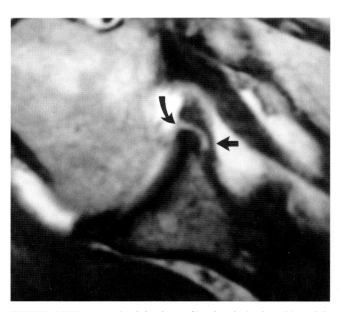

FIGURE 10.20. Bankart lesion proved at arthroscopy in a 38-year-old patient. At the level of lower glenoid fossa, a T1-weighted (450/18) axial arthrographic MR image shows displacement of the anterior labrum (*arrow*) from the glenoid rim. Contrast solution distends the joint capsule, creates tension on the glenohumeral ligaments, and displaces torn labral fragments from the glenoid rim. Bankart repair was performed arthroscopically.

FIGURE 10.21. Anterior labral tear (Perthes lesion) and instability proved at arthroscopy in a 34-year-old patient. At the level of lower glenoid fossa, a T1-weighted (450/18) axial arthrographic MR image demonstrates sublabral contrast solution (*curved arrow*). The torn, displaced labral fragment is attached to the scapular periosteum (*straight arrow*), which has stripped medially along the glenoid neck. Bankart repair was performed arthroscopically.

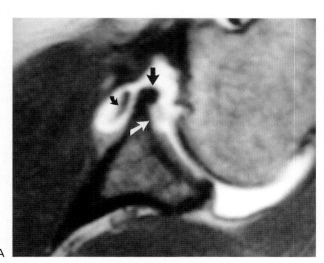
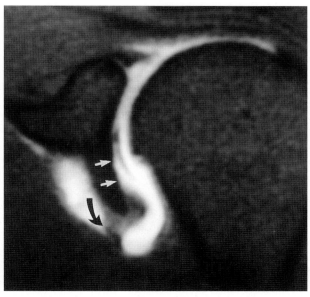

A

B

FIGURE 10.22. Surgically proven cartilage flap and an intraarticular loose body in a 32-year-old patient. **A:** A T1-weighted (450/18) axial arthrographic MR image through the inferior glenoid fossa demonstrates a full-thickness defect involving articular cartilage. Contrast solution undermines an adjacent cartilage flap (*white arrow*) and surrounds a detached cartilage fragment (*curved black arrow*). The anterior labrum (*straight black arrow*) remains attached to the glenoid rim, consistent with glenolabral articular disruption (GLAD). **B:** On a T1-weighted (450/18) coronal oblique arthrographic MR image, the chondral flap (*white arrows*) is mildly displaced from the glenoid rim. The inferior glenohumeral ligament (*black arrow*) and inferior labrum are unremarkable. The shoulder was stable during examination under general anesthesia.

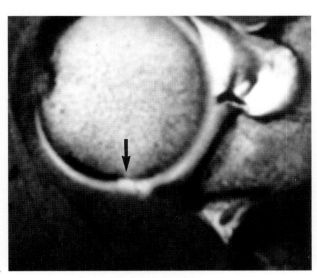
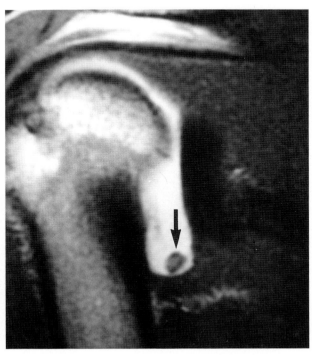

A

B

FIGURE 10.23. Focal cartilage defect and an intraarticular loose body proved at arthroscopy in a 40-year-old patient. **A:** A T1-weighted (450/18) axial arthrographic MR image shows focal full-thickness cartilage defect (*arrow*) involving the posterior humeral head. **B:** On a T1-weighted (450/18) coronal oblique arthrographic MR image through posterior glenoid rim, a loose body (*arrow*) is surrounded by contrast in the axillary pouch. A single intraarticular loose body was removed at arthroscopy.

ligament (HAGL) is a rare cause of debilitating anterior instability. The HAGL lesion results from anterior dislocation and may be associated with subscapularis tendon avulsions from the lesser tuberosity.

Although arthrographic MR images have demonstrated greater than 90% accuracy in the detection of anteroinferior glenoid labral tears, diagnostic confidence may be further increased when the shoulder is imaged in abduction and external rotation (ABER) (24,25). The ABER position is achieved by flexing the elbow and placing the patient's hand posterior to the contralateral aspect of the head or neck (24). In the ABER position, MR images of the shoulder are prescribed in an axial oblique plane from a coronal localizer image, parallel to the long axis of the humerus.

In unstable shoulders, the most important abnormality is a tear of the inferior labral-ligamentous complex at the glenoid attachment site. When shoulders are imaged in the ABER position, diagnostic confidence is increased because the anterior band of the inferior glenohumeral ligament is stretched, transmitting tension to the labrum (Fig. 10.24). Thus, an anteroinferior glenoid labral tear that is nondisplaced when the shoulder is neutral in position has a greater likelihood of being displaced from the glenoid rim and becoming more conspicuous when the shoulder is in ABER (Fig. 10.25). For the same reason, ABER images

may demonstrate the degree of medial stripping of the scapular periosteum following anterior labral-ligamentous detachment from the glenoid rim. Preliminary reports also suggest that the ABER position is valuable in the detection of partially healed labral tears (e.g., Perthes lesion), in which the surface of the tear becomes resynovialized, although the labral-ligamentous anchor remains incompetent. These tears may not fill with contrast on arthrographic MR images obtained in the usual adducted position, but they may become visible on ABER images because the labrum is more likely to become displaced from the glenoid rim (24).

There are potential limitations in ABER imaging. Approximately 20% of patients may be unwilling or unable to assume the ABER position due to shoulder pain or apprehension (24). Even motivated, experienced technologists require substantial extra time for repeat patient positioning, coil placement, and ABER image acquisition. Therefore, the ABER technique can be time-consuming, adding at least 10 minutes to the routine MR protocol.

Superior Labral Disorders

MR arthrography shows labral tears in any location on the glenoid rim, but it is particularly helpful in the evaluation of the complex anatomic features that characterize the superior

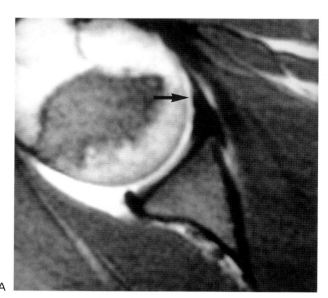

A

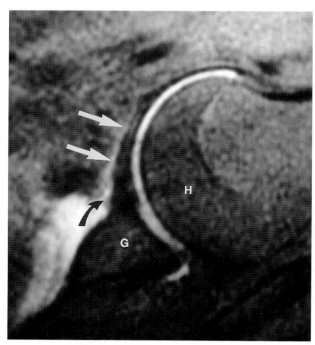

B

FIGURE 10.24. Sixteen-year-old patient with normal inferior labral ligamentous complex in abduction-external rotation (ABER) position. **A:** A T1-weighted (450/18) axial arthrographic MR image through the inferior glenoid fossa demonstrates apparent thickening of the labrum at the attachment site of the inferior glenohumeral ligament (*arrow*). **B:** A T1-weighted ABER image with fat suppression shows the inferior glenohumeral ligament (*white arrows*) along its entire course from the labral origin (*black arrow*) to the humeral attachment site. G, glenoid; H, humerus.

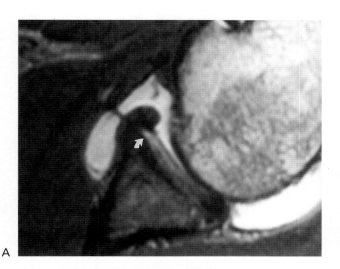

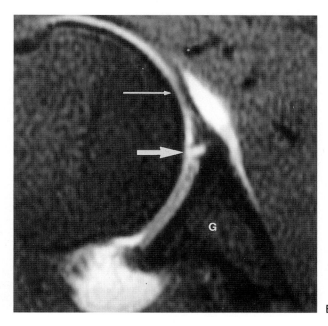

A

B

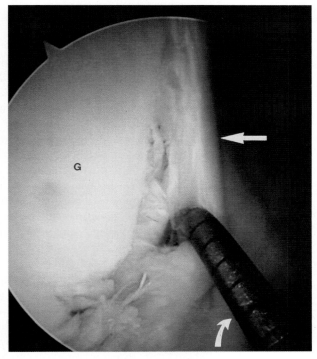

C

FIGURE 10.25. Twenty-eight-year-old patient with a surgically proved anteroinferior labral tear, identified on abduction-external rotation (ABER) images. **A:** A T1-weighted (450/18) axial arthrographic MR image shows a nonspecific focus of increased signal intensity (*arrow*) that partially undercuts the base of labrum. Since the labral position is normal on the glenoid rim, this finding is equivocal for tear. **B:** On a fat-suppressed ABER image, a partial-thickness anterior labral tear (*thick arrow*) is filled with contrast solution. Diagnostic confidence is increased because the labrum is displaced from the glenoid rim by the inferior glenohumeral ligament (*thin arrow*). G, glenoid. **C:** At arthroscopy, the anteroinferior labrum (*straight arrow*) was displaced from the glenoid rim using a probe (*slanted arrow*). Bankart procedure was performed for shoulder stabilization. G, glenoid fossa.

labrum (18). Superior labral tears have gained recognition as common and clinically important abnormalities that may cause persistent pain and limit the competitive performance of athletes that use repetitive overhead motions (e.g., baseball pitchers, tennis players, and swimmers). The most likely biomechanical explanation for superior labral tear involves the labral-bicipital anchor. The bicipital tendon (long head) originates from the supraglenoid tubercle and unites histologically with the superior labrum through a network of in-

termingled collagen fibers. Excessive tension on the bicipital tendon stresses the labral-bicipital junction, places traction on the superior labrum, and avulses it from the glenoid rim.

Superior labral tears must be differentiated from normal sublabral sulci that commonly occur at the labral-bicipital anchor. Two criteria enable this differentiation with greatest diagnostic confidence: (a) extension of sublabral contrast solution posterior to the bicipital anchor and (b) displacement of the labrum from the glenoid rim (Figs. 10.26, 10.27).

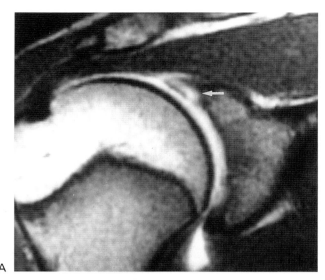

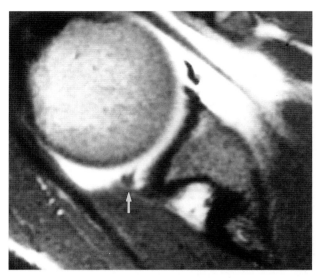

FIGURE 10.26. Arthroscopically proved superior bucket handle tear in a 16-year-old baseball player with posterosuperior glenoid impingement. **A:** Following arthrography, a T1-weighted (450/18) coronal oblique MR image shows sublabral contrast solution (*arrow*) with linear extension into the labral substance. **B:** On a T1-weighted (450/18) axial arthrographic MR image, the tear passes posteriorly, typical for a SLAP (superior labrum, from anterior to posterior) lesion. The labral fragment (*arrow*) was reattached at arthroscopy.

Thus, sublabral contrast confined to the bicipital anchor can be assumed to represent normal anatomic variation. True tears propagate posterior to the labral-bicipital junction (so-called SLAP lesion: superior labrum, anterior to posterior).

FIGURE 10.27. Arthroscopically proved superior labral tear in a 35-year-old patient. A fat-suppressed T1-weighted (450/18) coronal oblique arthrographic MR image shows displacement of the superior labrum (*arrow*) from the glenoid rim and extension of sublabral contrast solution posterior to the bicipital anchor. A superior labral tear was debrided at arthroscopy.

Larger superior labral tears become displaced from the glenoid rim and may develop a bucket handle configuration (18).

Superior labral tears are often associated with bicipital tendinopathy, partial tearing, or complete rupture. A tear involving the superior labrum may dissect into the tendon at the labral-bicipital junction. The orthopedic surgeon is more likely to repair a superior labral tear if it involves the bicipital tendon and therefore places the tendon at increased risk of rupture. Arthrographic MR images can be helpful in the differentiation of a bicipital tear from tendinopathy because contrast solution leaks into the substance of a tendon that is torn but outlines the thickened peripheral contour of a tendon that is simply inflamed or degenerated.

Arthrographic MR images may be helpful in delineating the location and length of posterior tears and in assessing the presence of posterior instability (Figs. 10.28–10.30). Glenoid labral cysts may occur whenever a labral tear extends peripherally across the joint capsule, analogous to the mechanism that is believed to explain the development of meniscal cysts in the knee. A labral cyst, therefore, represents an extraarticular collection of joint fluid that has leaked through a labral tear. Labral cysts most commonly arise at the posterosuperior glenoid rim in conjunction with a superior labral tear (Fig. 10.31) (27). These cysts may enlarge in the spinoglenoid notch and compress the suprascapular nerve, occasionally causing denervation atrophy in the supraspinatus and infraspinatus muscles. Because the usual cyst contains thick, gelatinous material, contrast solution can only diffuse slowly into the lesion. Thus, arthrographic MR images may show minimal enhancement or partial enhancement of the labral cyst.

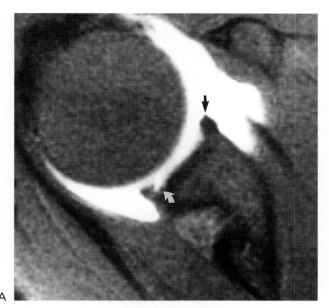

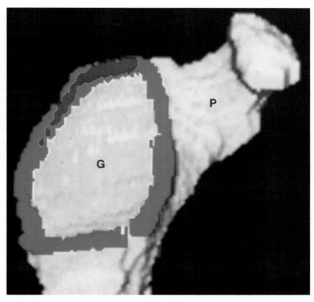

FIGURE 10.28. Posterosuperior labral tear in a 31-year-old patient with grand mal seizures. **A:** Following arthrography, a T1-weighted (TR:450, TE:18) fat-suppressed axial image through the upper glenoid shows extension of contrast solution (*white arrow*) under the posterior labrum. The anterior labrum (*black arrow*) is normal. **B:** The 3D image in the same patient depicts the glenoid fossa (*G*), coracoid process (*P*), and labrum (*blue*). The location and length of the labral tear (*red*) were confirmed at arthroscopy.

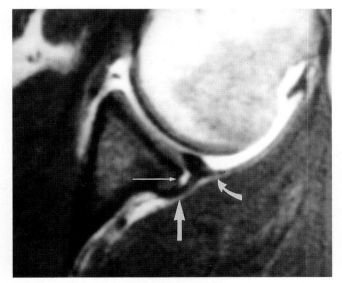

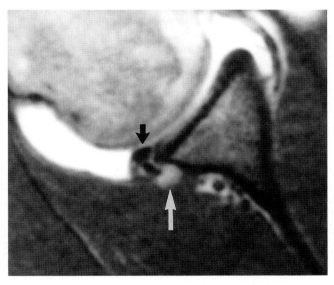

FIGURE 10.29. Posterior labral tear and posterior instability surgically proved in a 30-year-old patient. At midglenoid level, a T1-weighted (450/18) axial arthrographic MR image shows normal location of the posterior labrum on the glenoid rim. Although the joint capsule inserts normally on the posterior labrum (*curved arrow*), the periosteum (*thick straight arrow*) is stripped medially on the glenoid neck. On MR arthrographic images, the presence of contrast solution (*thin straight arrow*) under the stripped periosteum correlates closely with posterior instability.

FIGURE 10.30. Posterior labral tear and posterior instability surgically proved in a 42-year-old patient. At midglenoid level, a T1-weighted (450/18) axial arthrographic MR image shows mild displacement of the posterior labrum (*black arrow*) and associated extraarticular contrast collection (*white arrow*). Both of these findings strongly suggest posterior instability.

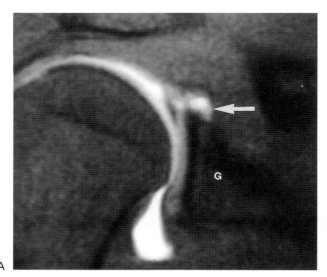
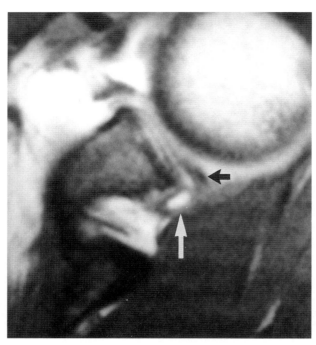

A

B

FIGURE 10.31. Posterosuperior labral tear with a small labral cyst in a 44-year-old patient. **A:** On a fat-suppressed T1-weighted (450/18) coronal oblique arthrographic MR image, extraarticular contrast solution (*arrow*) collects at the posterosuperior glenoid rim. The labrum is minimally displaced. G, glenoid. **B:** On a T1-weighted (450/18) axial arthrographic MR image, the collection (*white arrow*) is located adjacent to the posterosuperior glenoid labrum (*black arrow*), which shows sublabral contrast and mild displacement from the glenoid rim. In shoulders with nondisplaced posterosuperior labra, the leak of contrast into a cyst confirms the presence of a labral tear.

REFERENCES

1. Seeger LL, Gold RH, Bassett LW. Shoulder instability: evaluation with MR imaging. *Radiology* 1988;168:695–697.
2. Kieft GJ, Bloem JL, Rozing PM, Obermann WR. MR imaging of recurrent anterior dislocation of the shoulder: comparison with CT arthrography. *AJR* 1988;150:1083–1087.
3. Garneau RA, Renfrew DL, Moore TE, El-Khoury GY, Nepola JV, Lemke JH. Glenoid labrum: evaluation with MR imaging. *Radiology* 1991;179:519–522.
4. Legan JM, Burkhard TK, Goff WB, Balsara ZN, et al. Tears of the glenoid labrum: MR imaging of 88 arthroscopically confirmed cases. *Radiology* 1991;179:241–246.
5. Flannigan B, Kursunoglu-Brahme S, Snyder S, Karzel R, Del Pizzo W, Resnick D. MR arthrography of the shoulder: comparison with conventional MR imaging. *AJR* 1990;155:829–832.
6. Hodler J, Kursunglu-Brahme S, Snyder SJ, et al. Rotator cuff disease: assessment with MR arthrography versus standard MR imaging in 36 patients with arthroscopic correlation. *Radiology* 1992;192:431–436.
7. Palmer WE, Brown JH, Rosenthal DI. Fat-suppressed MR arthrography of the shoulder: evaluation of the rotator cuff. *Radiology* 1993;188:683–687.
8. Chandnani VP, Yeager TD, DeBerardino T, et al. Glenoid labral tears: prospective evaluation with MR imaging, MR arthrography, and CT arthrography. *AJR* 1993;161:1229–1235.
9. Palmer WE, Brown JH, Rosenthal DJ. Labral-ligamentous complex of the shoulder: evaluation with MR arthrography. *Radiology* 1994;190:645–651.
10. Chandnani, VP, Gagliardi JA, Murnane TG, Bradley YC, De-

Berardino TA, Spaeth J, Hansen MF. Glenohumeral ligaments and shoulder capsular mechanism: evaluation with MR arthrography. *Radiology* 1995;196:27–32.
11. Palmer WE, Caslowitz PL. Anterior shoulder instability: diagnostic criteria determined from prospective analysis of 121 MR arthrograms. *Radiology* 1995;197:819–825.
12. Willemsen UF, Wiedemann E, Brunner U, Scheck R, Pfluger T, Kueffer G, Hahn K. Prospective evaluation of MR arthrography performed with high-volume intraarticular saline enhancement in patients with recurrent anterior dislocations of the shoulder. *AJR* 1998;170:79–84.
13. Vahlensieck M, Peterfy CG, Wischer T, et al. Indirect MR-arthrography: optimization and clinical applications. *Radiology* 1996;200:249–254.
14. Weinman HJ, Brasch RC, Press WR, Wesbey GE. Characteristics of gadolinium DTP complex: a potential NM contrast agent. *AJR* 1984;142:619–624.
15. Hajek PC, Sartoris DJ, Neumann CH, Resnick D. Potential contrast agents for MR arthrography: in vitro evaluation and practical observations. *AJR* 1987;149:97–104.
16. Iannotti JP, Zlatkin MB, Esterhai JL, Kressel HY, Dalinka MK, Spindler KP. Magnetic resonance imaging of the shoulder. *J Bone Joint Surg Am* 1991;73(1):17–29.
17. Liou JTS, Wilson AJ, Totty WG, Brown JJ. The normal shoulder: common variations that simulate pathologic conditions at MR imaging. *Radiology* 1993;186:435–441.
18. Kreitner KF, Botchen K, Rude J, Bittinger F, Krummenauer F, Thelen M. Superior labrum and labral-bicipital complex: MR imaging with pathologic-anatomic and histologic correlation. *AJR* 1998;170:599–605.
19. Bowen MK, Warren RF. Ligamentous control of shoulder stabil-

ity based on selective cutting and static translation experiments. *Clin Sports Med* 1991;10(4):757–782.

20. O'Connell PW, Nuber GW, Mileski RA, Lautenschlager E. The contribution of the glenohumeral ligaments to anterior stability of the shoulder joint. *Am J Sports Med* 1990;18(6):579–584.
21. Palmer WE, Caslowitz PL, Chew FS. MR Arthrography of the shoulder: normal intraarticular structures and common abnormalities. *AJR* 1995;164:141–146.
22. Tirman PFJ, Feller JF, Palmer WE, Carroll KW, Steinbach LS, Cox I. Buford complex—variation of normal shoulder anatomy: MR arthrographic imaging features. *AJR* 1996;166:869–873.
23. Tirman PFJ, Palmer WE, Feller JF. MR arthrography of the shoulder. *Magn Reson Imaging Clin N Am* 1997;5(4):811–839.
24. Cvitanic O, Tirman PFJ, Feller JF, Bost FW, Minter J, Carroll KW. Using abduction and external rotation of the shoulder to increase the sensitivity of MR arthrography in revealing tears of the anterior glenoid labrum. *AJR* 1997;169:837–844.
25. Kwak SM, Brown RR, Trudell D, Resnick D. Glenohumeral joint: comparison of shoulder positions at MR arthrography. *Radiology* 1998;208:375–380.
26. Tirman PFJ, Bost FW, Garvin GJ, et al. Posterosuperior glenoid impingement of the shoulder: findings at MR imaging and MR arthrography with arthroscopic correlation. *Radiology* 1994;193:431–436.
27. Tirman PFJ, Feller JF, Janzen DL, Peterfy CG, Bergman AG. Association of glenoid labral cysts with labral tears and glenohumeral instability: radiologic findings and clinical significance. *Radiology* 1994;190:653–658.

Fractures of greater tuberosity of humerus
    affecting rotator cuff, 124, 126
    occult, 242, 242f
Fraying
    bursal, with tendinosis, 141f, 143
    labral, debridement in, 269, 269f
Free induction decay signal, 7, 7f
Frequency encoding, 6

G

Gadolinium
    affecting signal enhancement, 3t, 11, 12f
    in MR arthrography, 105, 131, 279–280
Ganglion cysts
    paralabral, 217f–219f, 218
    with SLAP lesions of superior labrum, 80, 80f
Garth view in glenohumeral instability studies, 72,
        73f
Geyser sign in rotator cuff tears, 244
Giant cell tumor of tendon sheaths, 236
Glenohumeral joint
    anatomic variants in joint space, 38, 40, 113
    capsular hyperlaxity in, 68, 69f, 69–70
    causes of pain in, 50t
    dislocation of, 65
    fluid in, 155
    instability of, 65–76. *See also* Instability
    laxity, 179
    neuroarthropathy, 238, 239f
    stability of
        dynamic factors in, 66, 119, 179
        static factors in, 65–66, 179
    stabilizers of, 88, 89f, 91, 93, 119
    subluxation of, 65, 179
Glenohumeral ligaments, 66, 66f, 89f, 91–93, 92f,
        93f
    anatomic variants in, 42, 110
    Buford complex in, 41–42, 42f, 66, 67f,
        111–112, 112f, 288
    humeral avulsion of, 196, 196f, 197f, 291, 294
    inferior, 91, 93, 95f, 106
        anterior band of, 89f, 91, 92f, 93f, 106
        axillary pouch of, 89, 91, 93f, 106
        posterior band of, 89f, 91, 106
        superior band of, 93
    labral-ligamentous complex. *See* Glenoid
        labrum, labral-ligamentous complex
    middle, 91, 95f
    superior, 91, 94, 95f, 227
Glenoid fossa, 88, 89f, 90
    articular rim divot or disruption, 243
    fracture reduction and fixation, 267
    osteochondral lesions, 242f, 242–243
Glenoid labrum, 88–91, 89f
    anatomic variants in, 41f, 41–42, 42f, 108–112,
        287
    articular disruption of, 218–220, 219f–220f,
        291
    biceps-labral complex, 91, 92f, 105–106, 113,
        114f
    cysts of, 296, 298f
        paralabral, 217f–219f, 218, 256f, 272
    debridement of, 268–269, 269f
    instability repair affecting, 271
    labral-ligamentous complex
        abnormalities of, 291–294, 292f–293f
        anatomic variants in, 111, 111f
        anterior inferior, injury or avulsion of, 185
        MR arthrography of, 287–288
    labrocapsular ligamentous complex, 188
    labrocapsular periosteal sleeve avulsion,
        posterior, 199
    labroligamentous periosteal sleeve avulsion,
        anterior, 193, 194f–195f, 291

lesions in anterior instability, 185–190
    classification of, 185–186
    MR arthrography of, 187–188, 188f
MR arthrography of, 187–188, 188f, 190,
        287–298
ovoid mass sign, 41, 187
quadrants of, 188, 189f
SLAP lesions, 78–81, 79f, 208–218, 296. *See
    also* SLAP lesions of superior labrum
tears of
    anterior inferior, 188–190, 189f
    articular disruption with, 218–220,
        219f–220f
    differential diagnosis of, 216
    isolated, 206–207
        anterior, 188
        posterior, 200
    paralabral cysts with, 217f–219f, 218
    posterior superior, 200, 200f, 201f
    with rotator cuff lesions, 206–207, 207f
    superior labral, 294–296, 296f–298f
    undercutting by articular cartilage, 41, 42, 103f,
        108, 110, 110f, 186f
Glenoid rim
    bony lesions of. *See* Bankart lesions
    in internal glenoid impingement, 76–77, 77f
Gradient coils, 17
Gradient echo, 7, 8, 9f
    in shoulder imaging, 32, 32f
    spin echo hybrid, 9
Granulation tissue after rotator cuff repair, 258,
        259

H

Half acquisition single shot turbo spin echo
        imaging, 8
Hardware considerations, 17
Hawkins reinforcement test in rotator cuff
        pathology, 56, 57f
Helmholtz coils, 22–23, 23f, 29
Hematoma, postoperative, in instability repair,
        272, 273f, 276f
Hemophilic arthropathy, 237, 238f
High-field magnets, 17
Hill-Sachs lesions, 72, 73f, 180, 181, 181f–183f
    differential diagnosis of, 37, 113
    reverse, 197, 198f, 199
    simulation of, 181, 183f, 207
Hornblower's sign in rotator cuff pathology, 56,
        57f
Humeral head, 87, 88f, 89f
    avascular necrosis of, 243, 243f
    cysts of, 136, 137f
        differential diagnosis of, 37
Humeral ligament, transverse, 87, 88f, 94, 227
Humeral notch, normal, 181, 183f
Humerus
    anatomy of, 87
    bone marrow in epiphyses, 37–38, 39f,
        112–113
    greater tuberosity
        contusions, 168f, 169
        fractures affecting rotator cuff, 124, 126
        occult fractures of, 242, 242f
    surgical neck of, 87
Hyaline articular cartilage. *See* Cartilage, hyaline
Hydroxyapatite crystal deposition disease, 167f,
        167–169, 168f, 237–238, 239f

I

Iatrogenic conditions affecting signal intensity, 42,
        43f
Imaging principles and concepts
    acquisition time, 7–8

artifacts. *See* Artifacts
coil types. *See* Coils
contrast-to-noise ratio, 13
flow affecting signal intensity, 14
Fourier transformation, 6, 33
frequency encoding, 6
hardware considerations, 17
magnetic susceptibility, 14–15
    artifacts from, 15, 16f
    suppression of, 33
overview of, 3
phase encoding, 6
pulse sequences, 7–13, 31–32
reconstruction of images, 6–7
signal production, 3–5, 4f, 5f
signal-to-noise ratio, 13
slice selection, 6
spatial resolution, 13
spin density, 13
T1 relaxation time, 5, 14, 14f
T2 relaxation time, 5, 14, 14f, 15f
T2* weighting, 5, 13
techniques in shoulder imaging, 29–34,
        130–133
    options in, 32–34
three-dimensional methods, 6
Imbibition of contrast agents, 285–286, 286f,
        287f
Impingement
    biceps tendon, 77–78, 166, 166t, 229–230
    coracoid, 52
        surgical management of, 64
    internal, 207
        glenoid, 76–77, 77f
    rotator cuff, 51–53, 120–124. *See also* Rotator
        cuff, impingement syndrome
    signs in rotator cuff pathology, 56–58, 57f, 58f
    subacromial, 138
    subglenoid
        with partial tears of rotator cuff, 145, 145f
        posterior superior, 181, 183f, 200, 200f, 207
Infraglenoid tubercle, 87
Infraspinatus bursa, 96
Infraspinatus muscle, 88f, 93
    denervation syndrome, 234
    partial volume averaging with, 35
Infraspinatus tendon, 87, 88f, 93, 95f
    tears of, 129, 163, 163f
Instability, 65–76, 179–220
    anterior, 180–197, 265
        bone abnormalities in, 181f–183f, 181–185
        in capsular and intraligamentous tears, 196
        capsular lesions in, 190–191
        clinical features of, 180
        in humeral avulsion of glenohumeral
            ligament, 196, 196f, 197f
            with capsular disruption from humeral
                neck, 187f, 196–197
        labral lesions in, 185–190
        MR arthrography in, 288–294
        pathologic lesions in, 180–181
        posterior lesions with, 187f, 188f, 199–200
        surgery in, 265–268
    anterior apprehension test in, 70, 71f
    atraumatic, 179, 265
    Bankart lesions in. *See* Bankart lesions
    biceps tendon, 78
    bidirectional, 199–200
    in chronic dislocations, 203–206
    classification of, 68t, 68–69, 179
    clinical features of, 69–72
    functional, 179
    imaging studies, 72–73, 73f
    in labral tears. *See* Glenoid labrum, tears of